Hospitals and Healing from Antiquity to the Later Middle Ages

Peregrine Horden

Hospitals and Healing from Antiquity to the Later Middle Ages

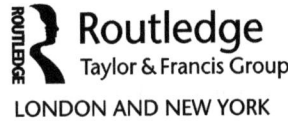
Routledge
Taylor & Francis Group

LONDON AND NEW YORK

First published 2008 by Ashgate Publishing

2 Park Square, Milton Park, Abingdon, Oxfordshire OX14 4RN
52 Vanderbilt Avenue, New York, NY 10017

Routledge is an imprint of the Taylor & Francis Group, an informa business

First issued in paperback 2018

British Library Cataloguing in Publication Data
Horden, Peregrine
  Hospitals and healing from antiquity to the later Middle Ages.
  - (Variorum collected studies series; no. 881)
  1. Medicine, Medieval 2. Hospitals, Medieval 3. Medicine,
  Greek and Roman
  I. Title
  610.9'02

  ISBN 978-0-7546-6181-8 (hbk)
  ISBN 978-0-367-18701-9 (pbk)

Library of Congress Control Number 2007943061

VARIORUM COLLECTED STUDIES SERIES CS881

CONTENTS

This volume contains xii + 338 pages

PUBLISHER'S NOTE

The articles in this volume, as in all others in the Variorum Collected Studies Series, have not been given a new, continuous pagination. In order to avoid confusion, and to facilitate their use where these same studies have been referred to elsewhere, the original pagination has been maintained wherever possible.

Each article has been given a Roman number in order of appearance, as listed in the Contents. This number is repeated on each page and is quoted in the index entries.

PREFACE

Asked what he did, W.H. Auden was tempted to forestall the obvious enquiries that would follow if he confessed to being a poet by answering 'medieval historian'. Never having had the effrontery to try the converse, I admit when pressed that I am a medievalist and that I study the large and loosely defined historical domain where disease, poverty, poor relief, family history, medicine and healing all intersect. This volume reprints a selection of my published papers reflecting that interest, a selection loosely grouped under two headings.[1] First come those that concentrate on institutions of mutual support, charity, and health care, predominantly hospitals but also confraternities and those collective rituals that can be seen as a form of public health. The second part attempts to relate the usual subject matter of medical history – doctors and their writings – to a much wider spectrum of sources of therapy, domestic, saintly, even musical.

When prefacing collected writings of this kind, it is customary to justify the reprint by recalling that the contents were published over a long period in diverse and now often inaccessible periodicals and proceedings, and by expressing the confidence that, for all the original diversity, the papers exhibit, in retrospect, a consistent, even unitary, point of view. I find the bibliographical argument easier to invoke than the intellectual one. As far as an explicit theoretical stance is concerned I have been, and remain, a sceptical *bricoleur*, finding any single approach to social history uncomfortably reductive, but willing to try out different ones according to the task in hand. It will be evident, however, that I am no partisan of social construction or of the language of site, contestation, and discourse. Within the pertinent historiography, I admire comparativists who apply a historical intelligence – as distinct from a method or a theory – to more than one period and who move between countries and cultures.[2] Outside

---

[1] I have excluded a number of papers that feed directly into a forthcoming monograph on 'The First Hospitals'; my several contributions to Horden (ed.), *Music as Medicine: The History of Music Therapy since Antiquity* (Aldershot: Ashgate, 2000); papers connected to another research project on the environmental history of the Mediterranean world; and a foray into the history of psychoanalysis in Horden (ed.), *Freud and the Humanities* (London: Duckworths, 1985).

[2] Like so many I have been inspired by the writings of Peter Brown and Arnaldo Momigliano, but also, in different ways, by the publications of that Hume and Hegel of early medieval historical scholarship, Michael Wallace-Hadrill and Walter Ullmann.

historiography, my limited interdisciplinarity has normally resolved itself into reading the work of social anthropologists, not only of medicine but of a range of other topics: anthropologists of an older generation, both familiar names and neglected masters.[3] It is as a historical anthropology of hospitals, healing and poor relief that I hope what follows may be read.

PEREGRINE HORDEN

Oxford,
September 2007

---

[3] Among the many anthropologists who have helped me, either in person or in print, I single out the late Rodney Needham.

ACKNOWLEDGEMENTS

Grateful acknowledgement is made to the following institutions and publishers for their kind permission to reproduce the essays included in this volume: Centro di Documentazione per la Storia dell'Assistenza e della Sanità Fiorentina, Florence (I); The Ecclesiastical History Society, Manchester (II, X, XI); Ashgate Publishing, Aldershot (III, V); Boydell and Brewer, Woodbridge and Rochester, NY (IV); Casa Editrice Università La Sapienza, Rome (VI); Oxford University Press, Oxford (VII, IX, XII, XV); Kegan Paul International, London and New York (VIII); Cambridge University Press, Cambridge (XIII, XIV); Besa Editrice (XVI). I am also most grateful to Ms Noha Mohamed for her help with the required correspondence.

The research for these articles was variously but generously supported by All Souls College, Oxford; Royal Holloway University of London; and, above all, the Wellcome Trust, to which the author is enormously beholden.

ABBREVIATIONS

An Bol	*Analecta Bollandiana*
BMGS	*Byzantine and Modern Greek Studies*
BZ	*Byzantinische Zeitschrift*
CC	Corpus christianorum
CMG	Corpus medicorum graecorum
CS	P. Horden and N. Purcell, *The Corrupting Sea: A Study of Mediterranean History* (Oxford: Blackwell, 2000)
CSCO	Corpus scriptorum christianorum orientalium
DACL	*Dictionnaire d'archéologie chrétienne et de liturgie*
DOP	*Dumbarton Oaks Papers*
GCS	Die griechischen christlichen Schriftsteller
HE	*Historia ecclesiastica*
JÖB	*Jahrbuch der Österreichischen Byzantinistik*
MGH	Monumenta germaniae historica
PG	Patrologia graeca
PO	Patrologia orientalis
PP	*Past and Present*
REB	*Revue des études byzantines*
SCH	*Studies in Church History*
SRM	Scriptores rerum merovingicarum
TU	Texte und Untersuchungen

I

How Medicalised
Were Byzantine Hospitals?

Philanthropic social welfare and medical assistance institutions [in Byzantium]
[...] were in every respect perfect and nearly similar to present day institutions
of this kind. In any case, they were the first fully equipped European hospitals.

So wrote the physician and medical historian G. C. Pournaropoulos[1].
Even the most ardent of Byzantine hospitals' more recent admirers might
find his verdict somewhat hyperbolic. Yet many scholars would pardon the
hyperbole and acknowledge an element of truth within it. Only two
monographs have been devoted to Byzantine philanthropic institutions, and
neither is wholly opposed to Pournaropoulos in outlook. The first monograph
surveys the whole range of hospitals, hospices, orphanages, old-age homes
and the like that were founded during the Byzantine millennium. Its author,
Demetrios J. Constantelos, takes the space to quote Pournaropoulos's
judgement - as an exaggeration, but not, it is implied, as a complete distortion

---

[1] Pournaropoulos, 1960, p. 378.

I

- and he lauds one Byzantine hospital as 'a medical center in the modern sense of the term'[2]. The second book, by Timothy S. Miller, announces its narrower scope, and its conviction of the subject's significance, in the title, 'The Birth of the Hospital in the Byzantine Empire': the birth, that is, of the modern hospital[3]. 'Byzantine xenones [hospitals]', he writes, 'resemble more closely modern hospitals than they do any of the institutions of pagan antiquity or any of the houses of charity in the Latin West during the Middle Ages'[4]. Miller takes the huge medical personnel of one exceptionally documented establishment as broadly indicative of the whole trajectory of Byzantine hospitals, and argues that east Roman hospitals were, quite generally, highly medicalised. They were staffed by doctors whose purpose was cure rather than care. More than that, after the mid-sixth century they were the focus of the entire medical profession: leading physicians concentrated their activities within them. Those activities were regularly supported by facilities for the copying and conservation of medical manuscripts (i.e. scriptoria and libraries) and the education of doctors. In Miller's pages, hospitals become decisive for the character and evolution of the entire medical profession in the Byzantine Empire.

My aim in this paper is not to review or question this bold interpretation in its every aspect. Rather, I want to concentrate on medicalisation, straightforwardly defined as the regular presence of doctors in hospitals in order to tend the sick. I shall ask how frequent their presence was and what it signified. I am thus joining a debate among students of Byzantine hospitals in which the chief division is between the optimists (as I shall call them) such as Timothy Miller and pessimists such as Vivian Nutton, perhaps the most trenchant critic of Miller's work[5].

For the optimists, Byzantine hospitals were clearly ancestors of modern hospitals in focusing on cure by doctors, and they characteristically functioned at a high level of medical sophistication – approximately the level of the best known and most striking examples. In this they distinguished themselves from contemporary medical hospitals in western Europe, where (with the exception of Italian institutions) doctors were hardly in evidence until the end of the

---

[2] Constantelos, 1991, pp. 118, 128.

[3] Miller, 1997. What follows is written in friendly debate with Professor Miller. I hope that our disagreement obscures neither my debt to his bold and pioneering work nor my admiration for the stimulus that he has given to the whole subject.

[4] Miller, 1997, p. 207.

[5] Nutton, 1986. For the further bibliography of the debate see Miller, 1997, p. xxix.

Middle Ages and the distinctions between curative hospital and caring hospice can scarcely be drawn[6].

The pessimists, in contrast, discern many fewer signs of precocious modernity in the hospitals of the Middle Ages. They think that the majority of Byzantine establishments were more like a hospice than a hospital, and that the well-documented medicalised ones cannot be taken as any guide to the capabilities of the rest. Byzantine hospitals were thus for the most part not so different from contemporary western ones. *A fortiori* they could not have assumed the role in the development of the medical profession and in the transmission of medical learning that the optimists (chiefly Miller) attribute to them. Not surprisingly there is – so the pessimists contend – very little substantial evidence that that role was ever played[7].

The easiest way to contribute to any debate in which there are two strongly polarised positions is to suggest that the truth lies in between them. To some extent that is what I shall be proposing below. To leave the matter there, however, would be to accept the terms in which the debate has been conducted. I shall suggest that to do so would be a mistake, and at the end of the paper I want to consider whether the question of the presence or absence of medical personnel in a hospital is an appropriate and worthwhile one to ask.

II

For the moment, though, let us think straightforwardly in terms of personnel and institutions. First, what is uncontroversial in this debate? What would both sides accept? Looking at the common ground may provide a way of gaining a fresh perspective on the whole topic and thereby starting to dissolve some of the implacable confrontations that beset it. Three general statements are, I think, beyond reasonable challenge.

The first is this: from at least the mid-fourth century up to the late twelfth (and to a much lesser extent from the end of the Latin conquest until the fall of Constantinople) a very wide variety of philanthropic institutions were founded in the Byzantine empire by emperors, churchmen, monks, and lay individuals; and many of those institutions must be regarded as basically therapeutic in character. We encounter the *xenodocheion* (house for strangers), the *xenon* (literally meaning much the same), the *nosokomeion* (house for the

---

[6] Horden, 1988; Horden, forthcoming; Park and Henderson, 1991.
[7] Some preliminary remarks along these lines, comparing East and West, Byzantium and Islam, may be found in Horden, 2000, pp. 214-215.

sick), the *ptochotropheion* (poor house), the *orphanotropheion* (orphanage), *gerokomeion* (home for the elderly), and others. This array has especially impressed those optimists who see Byzantium as, by medieval standards, a uniquely charitable society. But the specialised designations may reflect changing fashion, or perhaps the desire of donors to individuate their achievements, rather than the functions actually performed by the institutions in question, either at their inception or as they evolved. A lesson to be learned from the study of western European foundations is that hospitals may have many more functions than their various labels suggest, and that the principal function can change quite rapidly over time. In the case of Byzantium, it is clear that the sick, whether transient or not, might be received in a *xenon* or *xenodocheion*, that the poor in a *ptocheion* or *ptochotropheion* might be impoverished because chronically ill, and so on. *Xenodocheion, nosokomeion*, and *xenon* have all, moreover, sensibly been translated as 'hospital'. In short, it is clear that the particular designation in the written evidence is no guide to type of clientèle. We may find the sick in a variety of (superficially) different institutions[8].

The second point to be made about Byzantine charitable institutions is that no scholar, however optimistic, supposes that doctors were available in all of them, or even in all those in which the sick predominated among inmates. The pessimist views this lack as a matter of economics: doctors were too expensive for the smaller or poorer establishments. It is not a question of which foundations were hospitals and which were not. On a minimal definition of the hospital as a more or less independent institution for the overnight relief of the poor and/or sick, of course, most of the philanthropic establishments we know about would qualify. It would follow that – out of poverty or some other reason – there were numerous hospitals without doctors. The optimists naturally view the availability of doctors in a different light. They adopt a more stringent definition of the 'true hospital' as one that focuses exclusively on medical treatment of the sick (whether it is called *nosokomeion* or *xenon* or *ptochotropheion*) rather than just nursing. On this argument, the statement 'all Byzantine hospitals were medicalised' becomes, optimistically speaking, true by definition rather than through historical enquiry. Yet even the optimists are then, like the pessimists, left with other types of foundation, not (on their definition) true hospitals, in which the attendance of doctors

---

[8] Constantelos, 1991, part III; Miller, 1997. The latter is now supplemented by Miller, 2003; see also Brown, 2002, p. 33. For the later Middle Ages see for example Orme and Webster, 1995, ch. 3; Rawcliffe, 1999.

was at least unusual. On either account we have to deal only with a portion of the whole range of Byzantine philanthropic foundations for the sick[9].

The third general statement is that, even on the minimal definition of the hospital (that is, the most inclusive definition), doctors were indeed on a number of occasions explicitly associated with hospitals in Byzantium. This is true of the very beginnings of Christian hospital history in the later-fourth century, as exemplified in the Basileias, the medical-philanthropic complex established outside Caesarea (modern Kayseri, Turkey) by St Basil the Great[10]. (The hospital really was, to that extent, 'born' in the Byzantine Empire, as Miller advocates.) It is even true of the later phase of the empire's history – after the end of Latin occupation in 1261 – at least in Constantinople[11]. We can find traces of doctors (*iatroi*) active in hospitals in late Egyptian papyri, in inscriptions, correspondence and encomia, and, perhaps most vividly, in hagiography[12]. As we shall see below, we can also reasonably infer the presence of doctors from the titles and, occasionally, the contents of Byzantine medical manuscripts.

III

The problem is one of how to estimate proportions. Here we are leaving common ground behind and begin to re-enter the arena of controversy. Let us confine discussion to the pre-1204 period because it is the better documented. My very rough count of the number of specific hospitals in which doctors are attested is at the most 23–25. This figure is based on evidence collected by Miller so to an extent reflects the optimistic view[13]. I shall not take the space here to go through the texts one by one, because all I am seeking to establish is an order of magnitude. A precise figure is impossible, given the ambiguous nature of some of the evidence. It is also meaningless, because the absence of evidence of doctors in a given hospital is not, of course, evidence of their absence. (Nor, incidentally, can we be confident about what is meant in all the attestations of doctors by the term *iatros*, a problem to which I return at the end of this paper).

Against what aggregate figure should we set these, at most, 25 'doctored'

[9] I am indebted here to Nutton, unpublished.

[10] Basil's philanthropic foundations are discussed in Brown, 2002, pp. 38-42; Holman, 2001, pp. 74-75; Miller, 1997, pp. 85-88. For context see also, among recent works, Van Dam, 2002, ch. 2.

[11] Miller, 1997, ch. 10, with new evidence presented on pp. xvi-xvii. See also Constantelos, 1992, chs 8-9.

[12] Miller, 1997, pp. 21-23, 81-84, 90-96; Constantelos, 1991, ch. 9; Nutton, 2004, p. 30.

[13] Miller, 1997.

hospitals? Counting Byzantine hospitals and their like began over three centuries ago when du Cange published his *Constantinopolis Christiana*, listing some 35 charitable institutions[14]. Janin's more recent tabulation for the capital – not wholly reliable – finds 28 *xenones*, some 6 hospitals, and 27 old people's homes[15]. The most recent general survey for the provinces of the Byzantine empire (excluding the capital), up to the mid-ninth century, gives a total of over 160 charitable facilities of various kinds, of which the most numerous are those called *xenodocheia (59)*, *nosokomeia (49)*, and *ptocheia* (poor-houses; 22)[16]. How many of these actually admitted the sick and included medical facilities is, naturally, unknowable. But on any estimation it is clear that explicitly 'doctored' hospitals were a minority. If we inflate the number of the latter by making allowance for those of which we have only an imprecise record, we must also inflate the total number of institutions. True, medieval hospitals were always going 'out of business'; they were, often, by modern standards, ephemeral creations. So we cannot tell how many known foundations were actually functioning at any given date.

On the other hand there are always likely to have been more hospitals than we know about because of the great scarcity of archaeological evidence and the disappearance of texts. The Egyptian papyri have, of late, markedly increased the number of identifiable hospitals from just one corner of the early Byzantine Empire[17]. Yet there is no reason to suppose that Egypt was atypical in its philanthropic provision, which extended to small towns, and even to villages. Close regional studies of charitable activity in later periods nearly always substantially increase the numbers of foundations. One such study, of East Anglia (England) in the fifteenth and sixteenth centuries, expanded the dossier by almost thirty per cent[18]. So the hidden foundations probably more than compensate for those known to us that quickly ceased to function.

Of all these institutions, to repeat, we have information about structure and personnel – doctors and others – for only very few. Of the majority, we do not know what went on inside. For the reasons given above, we cannot predict where doctors would have been found. Some references in the texts might be taken to imply that hospital doctors were commonplace. They generalise about them in ways that must have been plausible to the intended

---

[14] Du Cange, 1680, bk. 4, ch. 9.
[15] Janin, 1969, pp. 552-567.
[16] Mentzou-Meimare, 1982.
[17] Van Minnen, 1995.
[18] Phillips, 2001.

audience, who would have been unreceptive if the therapy had not been described in terms that the audience would recognise. For example, in a letter to a friend a learned cleric, Nilus of Ancyra, deployed the image of the hospital physician examining patients and making individual prescriptions in the service of an analogy between somatic and spiritual medicine. The analogy itself was old, but the hospital setting for it was novel. Remarkably, Nilus used this setting already at the end of the fourth century, when Christian charitable institutions such as hospitals had been known for only a few decades[19]. Even such references as this fail, however, to solve the problem of how to judge proportions; fail to shed even indirect light on the mass of small, usually provincial, establishments about which we know nothing beyond the fact of their foundation.

IV

With this sketch of some common ground and this foretaste of controversy in mind, we can turn to considering the optimists' case in more detail. For the optimists of course have a solution to the problem of proportion. They extrapolate from the best hospitals that we know about – measured in terms of recorded medical sophistication – to the more obscure, and postulate that the best documented reveal, if not all the details, then the 'essence' of the more obscure ones. The argument relates only to 'true hospitals', which by definition were concerned with the cure or rehabilitation of the sick, not to the whole spectrum of Byzantine philanthropic foundations. But it makes a strong claim none the less – that houses for the sick mostly had doctors on the staffs and were organized in a highly sophisticated way.

The optimistic case rests above all on one institution, which no study of Byzantine hospitals can ignore and to which we must now devote some attention[20]. In 1136, the Emperor John II Comnenus and his wife Irene

---

[19] Nilus of Ancyra, *Letter* III.33, in Migne, 1857-1866, vol. 79, col. 397; see also, in the same vein, *Letter* II.110, in Migne, 1857-1866, vol. 79, col. 248; Miller, 1997, pp. 22-23, 69; Nutton, 1984, pp. 9-10; Temkin, 1991, pp. 176-177; Horden, 2004.

[20] For what follows the principal source is Gautier, 1974, with introduction, full references to earlier literature, text, and French translation. The section of concern here, on the hospital, is pp. 82/83-112/113, which is the basis of Miller, 1997, ch. 2 and *passim*. The *typikon* has been translated into English (Thomas and Constantinides Hero, 2000). The Pantokrator *typikon* is no. 28 and the section on the hospital begins at cl. 36. All subsequent references to the Pantokrator and other *typika* are to these Dumbarton Oaks translations, by text number and clause. The translation gives details of original-text editions as well as commentary and recent bibliography.

I

established in Constantinople, jointly, though perhaps on Irene's initiative, the monastery of Christ the Saviour, Pantokrator (Ruler of All). It was built on a prominent hill in the north-central part of the City, overlooking the Golden Horn, and incorporated three already existing churches. Transformed into a mosque after the Ottoman conquest, the three churches still stand, extremely dilapidated, as the Zeyrek Camii. Somewhere in an area of 250 square metres stretching broadly northwards from the churches (now rendered inaccessible to archaeology by the bulldozer and the developer) lay those establishments in which any historian of medieval medicine and charity is bound to take an interest. For information about them we have to turn to the monastery's *typikon* or foundation charter.

The obvious disadvantage of using this extensive text is that it tells us how things were intended to be, not how they were. None the less we must start by looking at the medical aspirations expressed. The Pantokrator was to be not only a monastery but a hospital and philanthropic centre. Its *xenon* was intended to provide for the sick and injured, both men and women; to offer them clean beds, adequate food, round-the-clock nursing, and regular medical attention. There were to be 50 beds in normal use, and these (contrary to what medieval hospital historians would expect) were clearly for only one patient each. The beds were grouped in five *ordinoi*, which I do not think we should necessarily envisage as separate wards (although I would prefer not to commit myself to a definite view of the hospital's layout).

In the first section were 10 beds for men suffering from wounds or fractures: in effect the surgical area, with its own hearth. Three other *ordinoi*, for men, shared a (probably central) hearth. The first had eight beds and dealt with eye or intestinal or other acute disorders. The other two, of ten beds each, were also for men – suffering from presumably chronic diseases. The last of the five *ordinoi* had twelve beds and its own hearth, and it was reserved for women.

Fifty beds in all for fifty patients. But there was to be an extra bed in each *ordinos* in case of unusual demand, whether in terms of numbers or the seriousness of a particular case. Also, there were six beds with mattresses that had a hole in for those who could not move or were taking purgatives.

A grand total, then, of 61 beds. The hospital was not the only welfare institution planned for the Pantokrator complex. There was a *gerokomeion* (old people's home) for 24 men, both the aged and those so debilitated that they could not look after themselves. If one of these became seriously ill, he might be transferred to the hospital for the duration of his illness. The second institution ancillary to the hospital was to be a small one for those afflicted with the *hiera nosos* (sacred disease) – leprosy, rather then epilepsy as has sometimes been supposed[21]. This was separate from the main complex, partly so that patients in the hospital should not be infected. We are told virtually nothing about its organization, however. The number of lepers that it was to contain is not stipulated. The third ancillary institution was in effect an out-patient clinic or dispensary, and again little can be said other than that anyone could, it seems, call in for advice or treatment; apart from indicating its staff, the *typikon* takes its workings very much for granted.

After a survey of the principal institutions, I turn to their personnel. The sick were, by the standards of any age, to be looked after impressively well – and not only in terms of material comfort. Each of the five sections of the hospital had two *iatroi*. In the sections for men, these *iatroi* were assisted by three *hypourgoi embathmoi* (titular assistants), two *perissoi* (lesser or supernumerary) *hypourgoi* and two *hyperetai* (or servitors). The two physicians of the women's section were aided by a *iatraina* or female physician (who was, incidentally, paid only a half of her male colleagues' salary). And, taking the women's ward overall, we can see that twelve women were to be cared for by twelve medical or nursing functionaries. In sum, fifty patients were to enjoy the direct attention of over sixty doctors and subordinates. But there was also the outpatient clinic, served by four doctors, two of them surgeons, and these four had eight assistants. Among the *iatroi* there was a hierarchy of genuinely Byzantine sophistication, up which it was possible to work one's way.

Two doctors enjoyed the distinctive title of *protomenutes* ('chief physician' or 'leading diagnostician'; not 'first of the month' as it has nonsensically been translated up to now)[22]. These were not the only physicians involved in the Pantokrator complex. The *typikon* is clear that there were to be two *primmikerioi* (a Byzantine term for various kinds of high-ranking official)[23] who outranked even the *protomenutai*. In alternating month-long shifts, they were to monitor daily the progress and hear the complaints of each inpatient, and they also oversaw the treatment of serious cases in the outpatient clinic. The total numbers just given create a slightly deceptive impression, however. The doctors in each *ordinos* also worked monthly shifts, so that there was only one physician (two in the outpatient section) on duty at any one time. When on duty the doctors were to make their rounds once a day (twice daily from May to September, with the second visit in the evening). The rest of the time, including the night shift, the *hypourgoi* were in charge.

---

[21] Philipsborn, 1963.
[22] Criscuolo, 1996, p. 114; Gautier, 1974, p. 85, line 945, reads 'protomenites'.
[23] Bury, 1911, p. 122; Oikonomides, 1972.

I

Beyond all these medical attendants, mention must be allowed to a variety of other staff – a *didaskalos* hired to instruct the 'children of doctors' (which just means 'doctors'[24]), a surgeon specializing in hernias, four pharmacists, and so on. Add all these and the doctors together and the figure is of the order of 100 – a very high staff-patient ratio indeed.

Altogether the Pantokrator *typikon* is an astonishing document, and the aspect of it that is most astonishing is the number of doctors envisaged as attached to the hospital that it describes. Those doctors are the sticking point of all attempts to interpret this foundation. If there were not so many *iatroi*, we would not, I think, find the other provisions of the imperial couple so striking; we could in effect dismiss the hospital as really a heavily-staffed nursing home. The senior personnel, moreover, are to be no workaday physicians. The founders expect that they might be tempted outside the city to attend members of the ruling elite, and even the emperor's relatives. 'In general we forbid any of the doctors to carry out additional work'[25]. Modern commentators have assumed that this restriction should apply only during the months when the doctors are on duty because their annual stipend from the hospital was scarcely a living wage and would have had to be complemented by the profits of six months' private practice[26]. But that is not what the text actually stipulates. So it may be that the emperor was planning to employ only those physicians who had already made their fortunes and could afford to demonstrate their philanthropy in his, or his successors', service. On either interpretation the leading physicians in attendance on the Pantokrator patients were to be distinguished as well as plentiful.

V

Why? Before we look, as others have done, to the wider context for answer, it is important for a moment to try to analyse the text on its own terms. To some extent this helps us to understand the founders' train of thought as they planned their monastic establishment[27]. For example: fifty monks were to perform the liturgy; fifty clergy were allocated to the Church of the Virgin; fifty sick people were to be sheltered in the hospital; and the core staff for the five wards numbers – slightly unfortunately for the tidy-

[24] Kazhdan, 1984, pp. 46, 48.
[25] Thomas and Constantinides Hero, 2000, no. 28, cl. 54.
[26] Miller, 1997, p. xiii; Thomas and Constantinides Hero, 2000, no. 28, p. 734.
[27] Congdon, 1996; Horden, 2005.

minded historian – forty-nine (although of course not all were on duty at any one time)[28]. The broad similarity in strength of the monks, clergy, patients, and medical carers reflects their common task as intercessors for the emperor and his family. The *typikon* is, it should be stressed, essentially a liturgical document and its medical provisions should all be read in that light. The sick and leprous are to be looked after so as to encourage them to intercede on the emperor's behalf with all the more fervour. The physicians are at all times to act in the knowledge that they must render account to Christ the Pantokrator for their actions. 'For our Master accepts as his own what is done for each of the least of the brothers [as in Matthew XXV.40] and measures out rewards in proportion to our good deeds'[29].

The theological approach to the *typikon* will take us only part of the way towards an explanation of its contents. It would apply to all monastic hospitals of the period. And yet the level of medical provision in the main Pantokrator hospital – two doctors and several attendants per ward – is unparalleled in the explicit documentation now available to us. Admittedly the pool of evidence is not large. The most detailed information usually comes from monastic *typika*, even though hospitals attached to secular churches may have been the more common. So our archive is unbalanced. Still, it is all we have to go on and must be used. There survive some 60 *typika* and similar texts recording monastic foundations. Only thirty or so of these include any reference to charity and health care[30]. A number of founders planned that their monasteries should offer food and lodging to the poor or to wayfarers. Others looked primarily to the needs of sick monks. Yet, apart from the Pantokrator, only three other documented religious houses were to maintain a public hospital (as a distinct from an infirmary for monks) with designated medical personnel[31].

None of these is quite comparable to the Pantokrator in scale or staff. The mid-twelfth-century *typikon* of the monastery of the Mother of God *Kosmosoteira*, founded by John II's younger brother Isaac, provides for 36 elderly patients treated by just one doctor[32]. The charter of San Salvatore in Norman Messina – a royal foundation but inaugurated by Greek monks – refers to both a hospital and a hospice but no mention is made of doctors[33]. Only the

---

[28] Thomas and Constantinides Hero, 2000, no. 28, cls 19, 30.
[29] Ibid., no. 28, cl. 42.
[30] Volk, 1983.
[31] Kislinger, 1987, n. 44.
[32] Thomas and Constantinides Hero, 2000, no. 29, cl. 70
[33] Ibid., no. 26, cl. 8.

I

thirteenth-century Lips convent in Constantinople approaches the Pantokrator in intensity of medicalisation. There was to be a twelve-bed hospital for women staffed by three doctors, an assistant, a nurse, a pharmacist, two apothecaries, six attendants, and a bloodletter[34]. That outperforms the Pantokrator women's ward in staff-patient ratio. But it is an isolated analogue (and imitation?) from a later age. In neither the Lips nor the Pantokrator *typikon* do the founders betray any hint that they are requesting novelty. Yet the very fact that they felt the need to list personnel in detail, while others were content with generalities and presumably left particular arrangements to the abbot or hospital director, might suggest that the levels of staffing envisaged in the two hospitals were unusual enough to require specification. In the case of the Pantokrator there is an additional telling discrepancy: between the precision with which the hospital's staff is recorded and the much briefer and generally less helpful references to the other parts of the philanthropic complex, such as the leprosarium[35] and the outpatient facility.

Comparison with other documented hospitals of the period thus only strengthens our intuition that the Pantokrator *typikon* is an extraordinary document for its time. Let us try a different approach to the question of why this hospital was so medicalised: an approach from the history of medicine rather than that of hospitals. One facet of the context within which the *typikon* might become intelligible is that 'lordship over the professional classes' to which Paul Magdalino has referred in his study of the Empire in the twelfth century[36]. He is discussing the nobility as a whole, but the phenomenon therefore embraces the emperor's lordship as well. And its scope might surely be extended from the imperial bureaucracy, the armed forces, and the Church (all of which Magadalino mentions) to the 'professional class' of doctors. The emperor, we may conjecture, is setting up involvement with the Pantokrator hospital as one major avenue to his continued patronage.

In taking this interest in medicine he was responding to and enhancing the relatively new status and prominence enjoyed by certain doctors in Comnenian court and aristocratic circles. By the beginning of the twelfth century, Alexander Khazdan has suggested[37], doctors become quite frequent recipients of the letters of which texts survive (much more so than can be accounted for by positing a change in epistolographic fashion). The doctors

[34] Ibid., no. 39, cls. 50, 51.
[35] Kislinger, 1992.
[36] Magdalino, 1993, p. 220.
[37] Khazdan, 1984, pp. 46, 48; see also Timplalexi, 2002.

are very much part of the court's intellectual and social world. One Comnenian emperor, Manuel I, was himself skilled in medicine. A physician is even named in the list of those to be commemorated in the Pantokrator Church: Nicetas 'the first', presumably another leading physician or *protomenutes*. Theodore Prodromus, John II's court poet, satirised the bunglers, including a dentist who broke his aching tooth with an instrument that would have done justice to an elephant. But he also paid tribute to a few men of outstanding skill, among them Nicholas Kallikles, physician to Alexius I. We can thus discern in the 'high profile' achieved by a few doctors at least one reason why they, and some of their colleagues, should have been seen as a necessary adornment of the Pantokrator complex[38].

Thus far, intentions. Monastic typika are no more than statements of intent. They do not seem to have had a set form. And that is indicative of their essential quality: unlike a *diatheke* (will) they were not binding; they exerted moral rather than legal force on those whom they favoured[39]. Even an imperial *typikon* may be evidence more of aspiration than of achievement. Some of the imperial couple's stipulations – not to do with the hospital – were demonstrably being ignored within a few years of the monastery's foundation[40]. The text was drawn up in 1136. John II was away from the city on campaign for almost all his remaining years, until he was killed in a hunting accident in Cilicia in 1143[41]. That is presumably why the only evidence we have that describes the Pantokrator's charitable facilities gives much of the credit for them to the Empress Irene. These few texts make it clear that some kind of impressive medical institution (a *iatreion*, so they call it) was actually built[42]. An anonymous poem may even attest a Pantokrator hospital patient – the emperor's daughter-in-law, no less[43]. But none of this material fully confirms the scale of medical provision foreseen in the *typikon*[44]. It simply adds the Pantokrator to the ranks of 'doctored' hospitals that are attested in general references in texts of the period. Nor is there any evidence that the

---

[38] Kazhdan, 1984.
[39] Galatariotou, 1987, pp. 83, 88; Angold, 1993.
[40] Jeffreys and Jeffreys, 1994.
[41] Angold, 2002, pp. 187-189.
[42] Volk, 1983, pp. 189-192; Miller, 1997, pp. xix-xxi.
[43] Jeffreys and Jeffreys, 1994, p. 198; Miller, 1997, p. xxi.
[44] *Pace* Miller, 1997, p. xix, the fact that the Pantokrator hospital was praised in an encomiastic biography of its empress-founder as 'almost' or 'virtually' (*schedon*) the most outstanding hospital of its time and of preceding times, does not prove that other large hospitals were even more highly medicalised. Surely no encomium would have admitted such precisely qualified praise.

hospital or *iatreion* lasted for very long, perhaps because such a large and complex staff proved impossible to sustain. Whereas the monastery as a whole endured as long as the Byzantine Empire itself, there is no evidence that medicine was practised there after about 1150. That is why Ewald Kislinger has described this hospital as 'ein trügerisches Ideal'[45].

VI

If the Pantokrator was a hospital without much of a future (an assertion which not even the optimists have contested) what of its past? Into what tradition can it be inserted so as to make it more comprehensible? One tradition, which the pessimists prefer, is the Islamic. If the Pantokrator hospital was unique to Byzantium perhaps it reflected Islamic influence. The Islamic hospital, as distinct from the Christian hospital within the 'land of Islam', was a relatively new creation in the time of John II Comnenus. Only ten or eleven hospital foundations are attested before the year 1000 CE. Seven of them were in Baghdad, three in Iran, one (perhaps) in old Cairo. Only from the eleventh century onwards did the Islamic 'hospital idea' spread to Mesopotamia, Syria and westwards around the Mediterranean[46]. These were highly elaborate foundations, staffed by physicians, sometimes associated with medical education, prominent in the medical scholarship of their time – conforming in fact very nicely to the optimistic image of the Byzantine hospital. According to Ibn Jubayr, who undertook the *hajj* from Andalusia in the late twelfth century, the Adudi *bimaristan* (house of the sick) in Baghdad was like a large palace and the chief physicians examined the patients twice a week. He was similarly complimentary about the Nuri hospital in Damascus and another one in Cairo that had a separate women's section. He also remarked that he had seen imitations of such hospitals in the Crusader states, through which he travelled on his return journey[47]. Were the Byzantine Greeks just as imitative? Is this a key to understanding the Pantokrator? The lines of cultural communication were certainly open. There was a sizeable Muslim mercantile presence in Constantinople – witness the mosque opened in the early eleventh century and reportedly still crowded with worshippers at the end of the twelfth[48].

---

[45] Kislinger, 1987.
[46] Conrad, unpublished; Horden 2005a, pp. 369-70.
[47] Broadhurst, 1952, pp. 43-4, 234-5, 296.
[48] Note also the doctor Abram 'the Saracen', perhaps active in a Constantinopolitan hospital, referred to below, p. 61. Reinert, 1998; Kazhdan and Wharton Epstein, 1985, p. 175.

The Islamic perspective may be important for understanding the degree of medicalisation that the Pantokrator evinced. But there is no need to seek precedents for other aspects of the foundation outside the Empire. Separate wards, *leprosaria, gerokomeia,* the presence of different grades of doctors and surgeons, distributions to the transient poor at the monastery gate, clean bedding, large numbers of beds – all can be documented for Byzantium, many of them in imperial foundations. This is what the 'optimistic' case builds on.

> [T]he Pantocrator Xenon operated fully within the tradition of Constantinopolitan hospitals [...] In the complex rules governing the Pantocrator Xenon, the typikon does not employ a single novel term or introduce a single new feature of hospital organization. Every term the typikon has selected, every title ascribed to members of the medical staff, and every detail of daily regime can be documented in sources describing earlier Byzantine xenones[49].

'Every' term, detail, or title: that may, perhaps, be asserting a little too much. The 'pessimist' should, however, readily concede that there is no shortage of possible precedents for details of the Pantokrator. There had after all been large and lavish philanthropic complexes in Byzantium since the 'Basileias' of Caesarea in the later fourth century[50]. One problem is that we seldom find evidence of a sufficient number of them together in any one establishment for us to conclude that the establishment was like the Pantokrator and could have served as a model for it. Another problem is that the evidence of hospitals with some features analogous to those of the Pantokrator is widely scattered across time and space. For example: the hospitals of late antique Hermopolis in Egypt were staffed by *hypourgoi*, as in the Pantokrator[51]. Again, according to a seventh-century collection of miracle stories, the Sampson *xenon* in Constantinople had surgical facilities and an eye clinic (much as the Pantokrator would some four centuries later), and the Christodotes hospital was staffed by *archiatroi* and (once more) *hypourgoi*[52]. We shall come back to the *archiatroi* below. Here it can be noted that while, in

---

[49] Miller, 1997, p. xxii.
[50] For more immediate precedents see Magdalino, 1993, pp. 115-117; also Patlagean, 1987; Angold, 1995, pp. 308-310.
[51] Van Minnen, 1995, p. 164.
[52] Crisafulli and Nesbit, 1997, miracles 21, 22.

I

Modern Greek, *hypourgos* means 'cabinet minister', in ancient and late antique usage it is simply 'servant' or 'assistant'. It had no specifically medical connotations and tells us nothing about hospital organisation. As for those surgical and ophthalmic wards, it has never been contested that a few hospitals (mostly in the capital) were medically specialised and sophisticated. The question that remains is whether these diverse references, and others that we shall encounter below, can be spliced together into a tradition as solid and as relatively unchanging as the optimists would prefer.

If they cannot, then not only this facet of the optimistic argument but a subordinate one must also be called into question. It concerns Byzantine hospitals as centres of medical excellence in a wider sense.

VII

Great claims have been made:

> By the eleventh and twelfth centuries they [Byzantine hospitals] had become the *principal theatres of the Byzantine medical profession*, providing both *specialized treatment* to hospital patients and walk-in clinical services to the general population. Moreover, by that time these xenones were also providing *instruction in the theory and practice of medicine to those who wished to become physicians*[53]. [italics added]

An 'optimistic' judgement indeed. Let us first question the 'specialized treatment' attributed to these hospitals. Apart from the brief descriptions in *typika* and other texts already considered, we have only the evidence of medical manuscripts. If the claim just quoted has any validity, there ought to be codicological evidence to support it.

David Bennett has recently surveyed the manuscripts and texts relevant to Byzantine hospitals, in an as yet unpublished discussion that supersedes all others in both scope and thoroughness[54]. I am very grateful to him for permission to summarise and disseminate his main findings.

First, the texts in question. There are five or six of these (depending on how one counts a text that has at some point been divided into two by its copyists).

A. 'Prescriptions and classifications [of fever?] of the great hospitals, of the kind that doctors prescribe from experience for healing, especially for patients in the hospitals.' Such is the title of one version of a compilation of treatments (parts of which, including the heading, variously appear in at least

---

[53] Miller, 1997, p. xi.
[54] Bennett, 2003. Cfr. also Miller, 1997, ch. 9.

four other manuscripts). The compilation is divided under sixteen very miscellaneous headings and dates from (very approximately) 1050. It is found in the fourteenth-century Vatican MS. gr. 292. Three other manuscripts (B, D, and E below) also preserve these 'prescriptions and classifications' in varying degrees but sometimes without the titular ascription to hospitals.

B. Vat. gr. 299 is an anthology of medical writings dating from the later fourteenth-century. It contains, within a long concluding medical compilation (c. 180,000 words), five remedies ascribed to three named physicians of the Mangana hospital in Constantinople, founded in the mid-eleventh century[55], and one other remedy ascribed to a named, but otherwise unknown doctor, for whom no institutional affiliation is given. The named hospital physicians are: (a) Stephanos, *archiatros* and *aktuarios*; (b) Abram 'the Saracen', *aktuarios* and *basilikos archiatros*; and (c) Theodore, *iatros* at the Mangana. (We shall have to come back to the possible significance of the title *archiatros*.) There are six other passages ascribed only to the Mangana hospital (with no physician named). These are dispersed over about a half of the compilation but form only a tiny proportion of the whole. A further six passages in the same remedy collection correspond to parts of the collection in Vat. gr. 292 (A, above) in which they are derived from 'the great hospitals'.

C. The fifteenth-century Paris MS. gr. 2194 includes six remedies ascribed to Michael, *aktuarios* of the otherwise undocumented Mauraganos hospital (perhaps a mirage: Mauraganos could be the man's surname). These six remedies are found in a text headed, in a hand that differs from that of the copyist, 'dynameron xenonikon dia peiras' ('on the potency of hospital prescriptions found by experience'). (That text is succeeded by another similar brief collection entitled, even more simply, 'xenonika'.) Apparently, none of the hospital-related material found here survives in any other manuscript.

D. The Vienna MS. med. gr. 48, from the late thirteenth century, has a text attributed in its title to Romanos, *koubouklesios* of the Great Church (Hagia Sophia) and *protomenutes* of the imperial Myrelaion Hospital (in an anticipation of the Pantokrator to add to those mentioned earlier). Fragments of this text survive in only two other manuscripts. The title *koubouklesios* disappeared after the tenth century; the Myrelaion hospital was re-founded by the Emperor Romanus Lecapenus in the mid-tenth century[56]; Romanos the *koubouklesios* cannot be dated any more precisely.

---

[55] Miller, 1997, pp. 149-50; Lemerle, 1977, pp. 273-283.
[56] Miller, 1997, pp. 113-14.

I

E. Romanos's text is actually only the first half of a much longer work. Its second half survives separately under a different author's name, as the *Apotherapeutike* of one Theophilos, in which the material is said to be drawn from hospital books ('xenonikon biblon'). (*Apotherapeutike* is an odd term: its sense is clear enough but its exact translation hard).

Both these two parts – Romanos's and Theophilos's – contain passages similar to those of Vat. gr. 292 (A, above) where the hospital treatments are attributed to the Mangana hospital, but here (in D and E) the hospital ascription is lacking.

F. MS Laur. 7. 19, of the thirteenth to fourteenth centuries, is a collection mainly of theological works. Like nine other manuscripts, it contains a text (mostly but not always the same text) with the title: 'Therapeutic medicines set in order according to the defined procedure of the *xenon*'. This is a short piece of some 2,750 words, which in none of its versions lives up to the orderliness implied in its title. It includes abbreviated versions of remedies recorded in four other manuscripts under the name of an otherwise unknown John *archiatros*, in one other manuscript under that of Galen, and in a sixth, under both names.

Overall, then, five or six texts, known to us from eighteen manuscripts, have hospital connections made explicit in their titles or their contents. To them can be added two manuscripts (Paris gr. 2315 and 2510) that were copied for hospitals, a manuscript (Scorialensis Y. III. 14) dedicated to a hospital by George, its scribe (all three of these from the fourteenth century), and perhaps three or four others that may at some stage have been owned by a hospital, including such luxury products as the 'Niketas codex' and the 'Vienna Dioscorides'[57].

These figures should set against the estimated aggregate of 2,200 medical manuscripts surviving in European libraries[58]. The numbers of hospital manuscripts could of course be inflated a little. Many that once existed will have succumbed to ordinary wear and tear, let alone the Fourth Crusade or the Ottoman onslaught. As the examples above show, hospital material can survive without its title. And more hospital texts doubtless remain to be discovered, hiding behind misleading or inadequate catalogue entries. Yet there are limits to the number of hypothetical manuscripts that can plausibly be introduced. For, as the above examples also show, material can gain as well as lose its *xenon* ascription in the unpredictable course of copying and re-copying.

---

[57] Bennett, 2003, Appendix V, pp. 440-441.
[58] Touwaide, 1992.

However we exercise the imagination, then, the number of hospital manuscripts that were produced in Byzantium must remain a very small proportion – a fraction of one per cent – of the entirety of medical writing. We are dealing with a tiny and unique corpus, as far as the Byzantine Middle Ages are concerned[59].

Two points of a more positive kind ought to be made none the less. The first is the sheer longevity of the tradition of hospital writing. What survive are mostly later medieval copies of ninth-to-eleventh-century texts. And some of the *xenon* remedies continued to be copied in the sixteenth century. Given the cost of the materials and the skills required for the making of the least pretentious Greek codex, this longevity is a tribute to the perceived value of *xenon* remedies. (That is especially true of those in Vat. gr. 292, which recur in several other contexts.).

The second point is an amplification of that. It relates to the considerable stature that must have attached to *xenon* remedies and treatments as well as *xenon* doctors (with or without some grandiose title). This is a medical world in which texts mutate with each copying, and bits of them detach themselves and (as it were) wander among the stemmata. A title, if there is one, becomes an assertion of value rather than a certificate of authenticity. Witness the remedies which are now given to a hospital, now to John *archiatros*, now to Galen. What matters in the present context is not which (if any) of those ascriptions is the right one. Nor is it whether a given remedy generally originated, or was used, in a hospital. What is significant, rather, is that, at some stage in the remedy's manuscript career, someone thought that the hospital ascription was an appropriate measure of value. A hospital remedy is as good – so the manuscripts imply – as one supplied by Galen. A *xenon archiatros* is as good an authority as any of the other possible names that might be attached to a treatment. And this is so even in the later medieval period when there were fewer Byzantine hospitals and it is far from clear that even the 'great ones' continued to function after the Latin conquest ended[60]. By the same token, hospital texts – when they are labelled as such – keep very good company in the medical anthologies that have preserved them. They can be found associated with all the 'big names' from Hippocrates to John 'Aktuarios', one of the last of the stellar Byzantine physicians. This is perhaps the strongest part of the optimists' case.

---

[59] Bennett, 2003, p. 441.
[60] Miller, 1997, pp. xvi-xviii; Miller, 1999. Here Miller produces arresting new evidence of doctors active in late Byzantine hospitals in the capital.

I

On the other hand, in qualification, we should ask what sort of medicine seems to have constituted the tradition. First, there is nothing distinctive about it. There is no generic difference between remedies and treatments ascribed to hospitals in the manuscripts and those which are either anonymous or appear under an illustrious name. That is one reason why a remedy can gain as well as lose the hospital ascription as copies of it multiply.

Hospital medicine is not only indistinguishable from that of 'mainstream' remedy collections. It is, ipso facto, what might be called 'low-level' medicine – at least as it presents itself to us in the texts. This is not medicine underpinned by philosophy. There is virtually no humoral theory, no semiology, little quantification of ingredients. It resembles the written medicine characteristic of the early Middle Ages in Europe: the doctor's experience had to supply the gaps and elisions in the manuscript record. One might be reminded by it of certain treatments or techniques; one could not learn these from scratch simply by reading such unhelpful stuff. There is a stark contrast between this material and the syllabus-based, theoretically articulate, educationally-orientated university medicine of the high and later Middle Ages in Europe[61].

VIII

This contrast must have implications for the optimistic thesis that Byzantine hospitals were centres of medical excellence in the practice and teaching of medicine and in the copying and accumulating of medical texts. Miller has contended (a) that from the sixth century onwards the formerly city-funded *archiatroi* ('public physicians' originally) were transferred to *xenon* service by the Emperor Justinian (or transferred themselves); (b) that from then on hospitals developed as centres of medical training; and (c) accordingly, that scriptoria and libraries were regularly attached to them[62].

This is surely extreme optimism[63]. First, it is inherently implausible that civic physicians could be transferred to hospital service and would obediently stay there – for centuries. The administrative and financial arrangements that might have made such reorganisation effective are wholly obscure and probably could never have been implemented. The legislation in question does not survive, most likely because it was never enacted. Moreover there is some specific evidence that no great transformation in the position of *archiatroi* occurred during Justinian's reign. The will of an *archiatros* of Antinoöpolis in

---

[61] Siraisi, 1990, ch. 3, is a convenient summary.
[62] Miller, 1997, pp. xxii-v, 48-9; Miller, 1999, pp. 328-330.
[63] Bennett, 2003, pp. 66-72.

Egypt datable to 570 shows him as having been in charge of a hospital all his life, like his father (also an *archiatros*) before him. Yet he is still also receiving a sizeable annual salary as a public physician. So not only has this public physician *not* been deprived of his civic livelihood, even after Justinian's death five years previously: his father's association with the hospital takes us some way back into that emperor's reign, perhaps as much as four decades. That does not leave much time for the supposed transfer from civic to hospital duties[64]. Agreed, there was no incompatibility between service as a public physician and involvement with a hospital. Equally, there was no necessary association between the two activities.

The text which has been taken as proxy evidence of the supposed redeployment of the *archiatroi* is drawn from a venomous indictment of Justinian's regime (unpublishable during the emperor's lifetime) by his erstwhile panegyrist Procopius. The details are unverifiable and in any case refer to the withdrawal of public subsidy from teachers and *iatroi*. There is no mention of hospital service[65]. That can be inferred – somewhat boldly – only from the conjunction of *archiatroi* and hospitals in later evidence. But such a conjunction, though frequent, and represented in the texts noted above, does not inevitably imply a 'system'[66], and it is far from exclusive[67]. Moreover, there are no *archiatroi* mentioned in the Pantokrator *typikon*. The theory that they were at the centre of hospital life thus has to be modified so as to allow their title to be replaced by that of *protomenutes*. But if titles can change in that way, and if other titles in the florid vocabulary of Byzantine officialdom also changed meaning over time, we cannot be sure that *archiatros* in the fourteenth century meant the same as it did in the twelfth or the seventh[68]. The circumstantial evidence – the way it is used in the surviving texts – suggests that the term lost its original civic associations and quickly became an honorific

---

[64] Van Minnen, 1995, pp. 164-5.
[65] Procopius, *Secret History* (*Anecdota*), XXVI.5-8, ed. and trans. Dewing, 1935, pp. 302-303, with Nutton, 1986, p. 219; Bennett, 2003, pp. 67-68. See also Allan, 1990, p. 457.
[66] Miller, 1990, p. 115, cites an anecdote in the seventh-century (d. circa 701) writer Anastasius of Sinai, about 'a certain *archiatros*' of the late sixth century, who had the oversight of a particular hospital – as if this showed that all hospitals were thus superintended: Anastasius, *Homilia in Sextum Psalmum*, in Migne, 1857-1866, vol. 89, cols 1112-1113.
[67] Miller, 1997, p. 174, for example recruits the medical writer John 'the Archiatros' (about whose career virtually nothing is known) to the ranks of hospital physicians, first on the circular argument that *archiatroi* are always to be found in hospital settings, and second, on the tenuous ground that some of John's medical writing was later incorporated in a hospital manuscript.
[68] Nutton, 1977, pp. 210-12.

equivalent of the modern 'consultant': a learned expert but not by any means necessarily a hospital physician.

The evidence for hospital schools, scriptoria and libraries is even more fragile. The only attested hospital medical school is that of the Pantokrator, and we know nothing more about it than that it was proposed in the *typikon*. There is a hitherto unnoticed reference in MS Vat. gr. 299, f. 422v, to instruction in phlebotomy within a hospital[69]. But that is best seen as evidence of exactly the kind of clinical training that we might expect. It is hardly a sign of institutionalised medical education. Finally, John Argyropoulos, one of the great figures of late Byzantine medicine, is depicted in a miniature as giving a lecture in front of a *xenon* and is recorded as having taught somewhere within the monastery to which that *xenon* was attached[70].

And that is all that can be said. Of the libraries and scriptoria there is no trace beyond the few manuscripts reviewed above, and the latter bespeak only the ascription of remedies to hospitals and the presence of medical texts within them. Again there is no sign of the firm institutional continuity that the optimists discern.

The most telling argument against the optimistic view may, however, be the 'low level' of the contents of these hospital texts. A tradition in which the best doctors taught in hospitals and built up medical libraries surely ought to have generated a literature that was durable enough to survive *with its provenance clear from its texts*, and that resembles the stable, theoretically-informed university texts of high medieval Europe far more than do the disorderly, mutable, a-theoretical materials that have come down to us. These actually have far more of an *early* medieval appearance, so little do they attest a strong educational tradition.

IX

I have sought to assess the degree to which Byzantine hospitals were medicalised by trying to inject a sense of proportion into the continuing debate between the optimists and the pessimists. How many hospitals are known to have had doctors? What is the likely ratio of that figure to the total number of therapeutic institutions documented? How far can we extrapolate from the details of the Pantokrator? What fraction of surviving medical manuscripts can be associated with hospitals? How do we square the paucity of these manuscripts with the status that some of them accord to hospital remedies?

---

[69] Bennett, 2003, p. 84.
[70] Živojinović, 1975.

The only safe overall conclusion seems to be that at various times some hospitals, especially in the capital, were sophisticated in their organisation and highly medicalised. But such hospitals may have been few. The evidence is neither clear nor plentiful enough to warrant optimistic generalisation.

To arrive at that conclusion I have naturally focused on the presence or absence of doctors and on the tools and institutions of their craft – texts, libraries, scriptoria, schools. But is this the appropriate focus? To put it another way: what difference did the presence of doctors make? We have seen plentiful signs that the medicine dispensed in hospitals was 'low-level'. We might conjecture that perhaps nurses or *hypourgoi* could have administered it just as effectively. But that begs the question of what distinguished a doctor from an assistant – of what exactly a doctor was or was perceived to be.

In the case of some of the hospitals we have encountered, the attainments of the doctors whose involvement was envisaged or actually secured is fairly clear. The *primmikerioi, archiatroi*, and the like were obviously highly esteemed and learned. A patient who accepted the premises of Hippocratic-Galenic medicine should rationally have preferred their attentions to those of a raw junior. Yet it would be a mistake to infer from that the presence in Byzantium of a clearly stratified and demarcated medical profession. There was a gild of doctors in tenth-century Constantinople[71]. But we do not know when it originated, how long it lasted, or what its scope was. Did it exercise a monopoly, and if so how effectively? Did it have any regional counterparts? The evidence is silent.

One text has been adduced as evidence of a rigorous system of licensing by some chief physician, who would offer the successful candidate a *symbolon* or diploma of some kind. But this text is no official record; it is part of a synodal decree by the Patriarch Leo Stypes, a contemporary of the Emperor John II[72]. He is justifying the condemnation of an errant theologian by recourse to the old analogy between the healing of the soul and that of the body: neither is to be left to the unqualified. But the analogy is forced: the god-like examination of the would-be physician that he describes obviously suits his Christian comparison. Nothing more of a historical nature can be inferred from it than that the president of a medical gild, a senior physician or *archiatros*, was believed by the patriarch somehow to acknowledge professional standing. And even if some more ambitious system of licensing physicians had actually

---

[71] Nutton, 1977, pp. 211-212.
[72] Grumel, 1949.

been set up, all the comparative evidence we have from medieval Europe suggests that many physicians either evaded, or gained exemption from, its control. Beyond the 'great hospitals' in the capital, I suspect, the doctors who sometimes worked in hospitals were accredited – earned their designation *iatros* – through the approbation of their patients rather than of their superiors. So when we notice that a hospital was, in this sense, medicalised, we are registering local, informal, 'lay' judgements, not the application of some widely-acknowledged touchstone of excellence. As in classical antiquity so in medieval Byzantium: the secret of medical success was to persuade others to take one at one's own estimation. Medicine remained a career open to talent[73].

Local lay opinion might have had priorities of quite other kinds. A second respect in which the attendance of doctors in Byzantine hospitals may not have been as crucial as the debate about them has suggested derives from the religious character of Byzantine philanthropic establishments. I touched on this above. To close, I wish simply to give the subject additional emphasis[74].

I can do this by means of a puzzling anecdote. Around 1070, only two generations before the imperial dream of the Pantokrator, the great Persian mystic al-Hujwiri set down the following description of hospital practice in Byzantium:

> It is well known that in the hospitals of Rum they have invented a wonderful thing which they call *angalyun*; the Greeks call anything that is very marvellous by this name, for example the Gospel and the Books of Mani. The word signifies 'promulgation of a decree'. This *angalyun* resembles the gut strings [of a musical instrument]. The sick are brought to it two days a week and are forced to listen while it is being played, for a length of time proportionate to the malady from which they suffer; then they are taken away. If it is desired to kill anyone, he is kept there for a longer period until he dies… Physicians and others may listen continually to the *angalyun* without being affected in any way, because it is consistent with their temperament[75].

We are not quite sure where Hujwiri was writing. It was either somewhere in Iraq, or in Lahore, whither he was taken in captivity and where he ended his days within a few years after 1072. His account appears unexpectedly towards the end of a treatise on Sufi mysticism. He intends to illustrate the potentially

---

[73] Nutton, 1985; Nutton, 2004, p. 248.
[74] Horden, 2001; Horden, forthcoming.
[75] Nicholson, 1936, ch. 24, pp. 407-408. Modified, with the kind assistance of Emilie Savage-Smith.

dangerous effects of music on the uninitiated (here, the patients). Hujwiri had travelled all around the Middle East, including Syria. He could have seen Christian charitable institutions within the 'land of Islam' or received reports of Byzantine ones from travellers. There was, moreover, no need for him to invent such a striking example to make his point. As the remainder of his chapter on *sama* (listening) shows, he had many anecdotes from closer to home at his disposal.

None the less, for all its specious authenticity the vignette is deeply puzzling. The *angalyun*, which clearly derives from the Greek *euaggelion* (gospel), appears to have been Hujwiri's coinage. In Persian it is silk of changing colour, a species of brocade so called because of the type of material in which Eastern Christians wrapped their gospel books; but that hardly illuminates Hujwiri's usage. Nor is there anything in the patristic or Byzantine definition of *euaggelion* that could have prompted the assimilation of 'gospel' to 'decree' and, yet more improbably, to the books of Mani and instrumental 'gut strings'. Yet the anecdote can, as I have tried to show elsewhere, be given a context of sorts – in the conception of the hospital less as a place where either doctors cured or nurses cared, more as an environment in which therapy could come from a variety of sources: for example, from the singing of the divine liturgy[76].

In the writings of St Basil, who founded the first clearly medicalised Byzantine hospital, medical analogies are easy to find. In particular the 'psychotherapeutic' effects of psalmody are described in his homilies on the Psalms and in his correspondence. 'A Psalm is a tranquillity of soul... it settles one's tumultuous and seething thoughts. It mollifies the soul's wrath and chastens its recalcitrance'; 'the consolation of hymns favours the soul with a state of happiness and freedom from care'[77], and so on: sentiments that can be given either a theological or a medical gloss – or both simultaneously. Basil knows all the anecdotes bequeathed by antiquity about the power of music – a power also shown, and to exemplary effect, by the Biblical King David:

> The passions born of illiberality and baseness of spirit are naturally occasioned by this sort of music. But we must pursue that other kind, which is better and leads to the better, and which, as they say, was used by David, that author of sacred songs, to soothe the king in his madness[78].

---

[76] Rawcliffe, 1999a.
[77] Basil, *Homilia in Psalmum*, I.2, trans. McKinnon, 1987, no. 131, p. 65; *Epistulae* II.2, trans. McKinnon, 1987, no. 138, p. 68.
[78] Basil, *Ad adulescentes* 7, trans. McKinnon, 1987, no. 140, p. 69; I Samuel XVI.23.

I

Historians will be better placed to understand the medicalisation of Byzantine hospitals when they have understood the significance for medical history not only of the *archiatros* but also of the Psalm – and even of the *angalyun*.

BIBLIOGRAPHY

Allan Nigel, 1990, 'Hospice to hospital in the Near East: an instance of continuity and change in late antiquity', *Bulletin of the History of Medicine*, 64, 446-462.

Angòld Michael, 1993, 'Were Byzantine monastic *typika* literature?'. In: Beaton Roderick. and Roueché Charlotte (eds), *The making of Byzantine history: studies dedicated to Donald M. Nicol*, Aldershot, Ashgate, 46-70.

Angold Michael., 1995, *Church and society in Byzantium under the Comneni, 1081-1261*, Cambridge, Cambridge University Press.

Angold Michael, 2002, *The Byzantine Empire 1025-1204*, 2nd ed., Harlow: Longman.

Bennett David.C., 2003, *Xenonika: medical texts associated with 'Xenones' in the late Byzantine period*, University of London PhD thesis.

Brown Peter, 2002, *Poverty and leadership in the later Roman Empire*, Hanover, NH, and London, University Press of New England.

I

Broadhurst Roland J.C., (trans), 1952, *The travels of Ibn Jubayr*, London, Jonathan Cape.

Bury John B., 1911, *The imperial administrative system in the ninth century* (British Academy supplemental papers 1), London, British Academy.

Congdon Eleanor A., 1996, 'Imperial commemoration and ritual in the *typikon* of the Monastery of the Pantokrator', *Revue des études byzantines*, 54, 161-199.

Conrad Lawrence I., [unpublished], 'The institution of the hospital in medieval Islam: ideals and realities'.

Constantelos Demetrios J., 1991, *Byzantine philanthropy and social welfare*, 2nd rev. ed., New Rochelle, NY, Caratzas.

Constantelos Demetrios J., 1992, *Poverty, society and philanthropy in the later mediaeval Greek world*, New Rochelle, NY, Caratzas.

Crisafulli Virgil S. and Nesbit John W. (ed. and trans), 1997, *The miracles of St. Artemios*, Leiden, New York and Köln, Brill.

Criscuolo Ugo, 1996, 'Pour le texte du médecin Romanos'. In: Garzya Antonio (sous la direction de), *Histoire et ecdotique des textes médicaux grecs. Actes du colloque international Paris 24-26 mai 1994*, Naples, M. D'Auria, 113-131.

Dewing Henry B., 1935 (ed. and trans), *Procopius, The Anecdota or Secret History* (Loeb classical library), Cambridge, MA, and London, Harvard University Press.

du Cange Charles D., 1680, *Historia Byzantina, vol. 2: Constantinopolis christiana*, Paris, Louis Billaire.

Galatariotou Catia, 1987, 'Byzantine *ktetorika typika*: a comparative survey', *Revue des études Byzantines*, 45, 77-138.

Gautier Paul, 1974, 'Le typikon du Christ Sauveur Pantokrator', *Revue des études Byzantines*, 32, 1-145.

Grumel Venance, 1949, 'La profession médicale à Byzance à l'époque des Comnènes', *Revue des études Byzantines*, 7, 42-46.

Holman Susan R., 2001, *The hungry are dying: beggars and bishops in Roman Cappadocia*, Oxford and New York, Oxford University Press.

Horden Peregrine, 1988, 'A discipline of relevance: the historiography of the later medieval hospital', *Social History of Medicine*, 1, 359-374.

Horden Peregrine, 2000, 'The millennium bug: health and medicine around the year 1000', *Social History of Medicine*, 13, 201-219.

Horden Peregrine, 2001, 'Religion as medicine: music in medieval hospitals'. In: Biller P. and Ziegler J. (eds), *Religion and medicine in the Middle Ages*, York, Boydell, 135-153.

Horden Peregrine, 2004, 'The Christian hospital in late antiquity: break or bridge?'. In: Steger F. and Jankrift K.P. (herausgegeben von), *Gesundheit– Krankheit: Kulturtransfer medizinischen Wissens von der Spätantike bis in die frühe*

I

Neuzeit, Beihefte zum Archiv für Kulturgeschichte 55, Köln, Weimar and Wien, Böhlau, 2004, 2-24.

Horden Peregrine, 2005, 'Memoria, salvation, and other motives of Byzantine philanthropists'. In: Borgolte M. (herausgegeben von), *Stiftungen in Christentum, Judentum und Islam vor der Moderne*, Berlin, Akademie Verlag, 2005, 137-146.

Horden Peregrine, 2005a, 'The earliest hospitals in Byzantium, Western Europe, and Islam', *Journal of Interdisciplinary History*, 35, 361-389.

Horden Peregrine, 2006, 'A non-natural environment: medicine without doctors and the medieval European hospital'. In: Bowers B. (ed.), *The medieval hospital and medical practice*, Aldershot, Ashgate, 133-45.

Janin Raymond, 19 9, *La géographie ecclésiastique de l'empire byzantin, première partie, 3: Les églises et les monastères*, 2nd ed., Paris, Institute français d'études byzantines.

Jeffreys Elizabeth M., 1994, 'Immortality in the Pantocrator?', *Byzantion*, 64, 193-201.

Kazhdan Aleksandr P., 1984, 'The image of the medical doctor in Byzantine literature of the tenth to twelfth centuries', *Dumbarton Oaks Papers*, 38, 43-51.

Kazhdan Aleksandr P. and Wharton Epstein Ann, 1985, *Change in Byzantine culture in the eleventh and twelfth centuries*, Berkeley, University of California Press.

Kislinger Ewald, 1987, 'Der Pantokrator-Xenon, ein trügerisches Ideal?', *Jahrbuch der Österreichischen Byzantinistik*, 37, 173-179.

Kislinger Ewald, 1992, 'Zur Lage der Leproserie des Pantokrator-Typikon', *Jahrbuch der Österreichischen Byzantinistik*, 42, 171-175.

Lemerle Paul, 1977, *Cinq études sur le XIe siècle byzantin*, Paris, Presses universitaires de France.

Magdalino Paul, 1993, *The Empire of Manuel I Komnenos, 1143-1180*, Cambridge, Cambridge University Press.

McKinnon James W.. (trans), 1987, *Music in early Christian literature*, Cambridge, Cambridge University Press.

Mentzou-Meimare Konstantina, 1982, 'Eparchiaka evage hidrymata mechri tou telous tes eikonomachias', *Byzantina*, 11, 243-308.

Migne Jacques-P. (ed.), 1857-1866, *Patrologia cursus completus, series Graeca*, Paris.

Miller Timothy S., 1990, 'The Sampson hospital of Constantinople', *Byzantinische Forschungen*, 15, 101-135.

Miller Timothy S., 1997, *The birth of the hospital in the Byzantine Empire*, 2nd rev. edn, Baltimore, Johns Hopkins University Press.

Miller Timothy S., 1999, 'Byzantine physicians and their hospitals', *Medicina nei secoli*, 11, 323-335.

Miller Timothy S., 2003, *Orphans of Byzantium*, Washington DC: Catholic University of America Press.

Nicholson Reynold A. (trans), 1936, [Hujwiri, *Kashf al-mahjub*] *The oldest Persian treatise on Sufiism* [sic], 2nd ed., London, Luzac.

Nutton Vivian, 1977, '*Archiatri* and the medical profession in antiquity', *Papers of the British School at Rome*, 45, 191-226.

Nutton Vivian, 1984, 'From Galen to Alexander: aspects of medicine and medical practice in late antiquity', *Dumbarton Oaks Papers*, 38, 1-14.

Nutton Vivian, 1985, 'Murders and miracles: lay attitudes to medicine in classical antiquity'. In: Porter Roy (ed.), *Patients and practitioners*, Cambridge, Cambridge University Press, 23-53.

Nutton Vivian,1986, [review of first edn of Miller (1997)], *Medical History*, 30, 218-221.

Nutton Vivian, unpublished, 'Hospitals in antiquity'.

Nutton Vivian, 2004, *Ancient medicine*, New York and London, Routledge.

Oikonomides Nicolas, 1972, *Les listes de préséance byzantines des IXe et Xe siècles*, Paris, Éditions du Centre National de la Recherche Scientifique.

Orme Nicholas and Webster Margaret, 1995, *The English hospital 1070-1570*, New Haven and London, Yale University Press.

Park Katharine. and Henderson John, 1991, 'The first hospital among Christians: The Ospedale di Santa Maria Nuova in early-sixteenth century Florence', *Medical History*, 35, 164-188.

Patlagean Evelyne, 1987, 'Les donateurs, les moines at les pauvres dans quelques documents byzantins des XIe et XIIe siècles'. In: Dubois Henri, Hocquet Jean-C., and Vauchez André (sous la direction de), *Horizons marins, itinéraires spirituels (Ve-XVIIIe siècles)*, 2 vols, Paris, Publications de la Sorbonne, vol.1, 223-231.

Phillips Ellie, 2001, *Charitable institutions in Norfolk and Suffolk*, University of East Anglia PhD thesis.

Philipsborn Alexandre, 1963, "ΙΕΡΑ ΝΟΣΟΣ und die Spezial-Anstalt des Pantokrator-Krankenhauses', *Byzantion*, 33, 223-230.

Pournaropoulos Georgios C., 1960, 'Hospital and social welfare institutions in the medieval Greek empire (Byzantium)', In: *XVIIe Congrès international d'histoire de la médecine*, Athens, The Congress, 1, 378-380.

Rawcliffe Carole, 1999, *Medicine for the soul: the life, death and resurrection of an English medieval hospital. St Giles's, Norwich, c. 1249-1550*, Thrupp, Sutton.

Rawcliffe Carole, 1999a, 'Medicine for the soul: the medieval English hospital and the quest for spiritual health'. In: Hinnels J.R. and Porter R. (eds), *Religion, health and suffering*, London and New York, Kegan Paul International, 316-338.

I

Reinert Stephen W., 1998, 'The Muslim presence in Constantinople, 9th-15th centuries: some preliminary observations'. In: Ahrweiler H. and Laiou A.E. (eds), *Studies on the internal diaspora of the Byzantine Empire*, Washington DC, Dumbarton Oaks, 125-150.

Siraisi Nancy G., 1990, *Medieval and renaissance medicine: an introduction to knowledge and practice*, Chicago and London, University of Chicago Press.

Temkin Owsei, 1991, *Hippocrates in a world of Pagans and Christians*, Baltimore and London, Johns Hopkins University Press.

Thomas John and Constantinides Hero Angela (eds), 2000, *Byzantine monastic foundation documents: a complete translation of the surviving founders' 'typika' and testaments*, 5 vols, Washington DC, Dumbarton Oaks; and at <www.doaks.org/etexts.html>.

Timplalexi Paraskevi, 2002, *Medizinisches in der byzantinischen Epistolographie (1100-1453)*, Frankfurt a. M. and Oxford, Peter Lang.

Touwaide Alain, 1992, 'The corpus of Greek medical manuscripts: a computerized inventory and catalogue'. In: Stevens W.M. (ed.), *Bibliographic access to medieval and renaissance manuscripts: a survey of computerized data bases and information services*, New York, Haworth Press, 75-92.

Van Dam Raymond, 2002, *Kingdom of snow: Roman rule and Greek culture in Cappadocia*, Philadelphia, University of Pennsylvania Press.

van Minnen Peter, 1995, 'Medical care in late antiquity'. In: van der Eijk Philip J., Horstmanshoff Manfred H. F. J., and Schrijvers P.H. (eds), *Ancient medicine in its socio-cultural context*, 2 vols, Amsterdam and Atlanta, Rodopi, vol. 1, 153-169.

Volk Robert, 1983, *Gesundheitswesen und Wohltätigkeit im Spiegel der Byzantinischen Klostertypika* (Miscellanea byzantina monacensia 28), München, Institut für Byzantinistik und neugriechische Philologie der Universität München.

Živojinović Mirjana, 1975, 'Bolnica Kralja Milutina u Carigradu', *Zbornik radova Vizantološkog Instituta*, 16, 105-17.

II

THE CONFRATERNITIES OF BYZANTIUM

'THE medieval drive to association'. That phrase comes from a monograph by Susan Reynolds. It is to be found in a chapter on guilds and confraternities. And it is representative of the quasi-biological vocabulary to which historians of those institutions seem especially prone.[1] How appropriate is this talk of drives? What, in this context, is the force of 'medieval'? My ultimate purpose is to address those questions from a Byzantine perspective; to ask in effect whether evidence of confraternities from the eastern Roman empire between approximately 400 and the Ottoman conquest will sustain talk of a Byzantine 'drive to association'. The enquiry is, however, worth a preliminary approach on a broader front. This is partly because the historiography of European confraternities shapes the questions that must be put to the Byzantine sources. It is also because, unusually, a Byzantine perspective may illuminate problems arising from the western material. Finally it is because the comparative history of confraternities may, by implication, have a modest contribution to make to the larger question of the differences between eastern and western Christianity. Much energy has been expended on accounting for the 'parting of the ways' – less, perhaps, on measuring the distance between them.[2]

I begin, then, with Europe, particularly with later medieval Europe. For it was, of course, during the later Middle Ages that large, highly formal confraternities proliferated in the West – to the point where there would have been around a hundred in any

---

[1] Reynolds, *Kingdoms and Communities in Western Europe 900–1300* (Oxford 1984) cap 3 (to which I am generally indebted) at p. 77. Cf John Bossy, *Christianity in the West 1400–1700* (Oxford 1985) p. 58; Denys Hay, *The Church in Italy in the Fifteenth Century* (Cambridge 1977) p. 66.

[2] Cf Peter Brown, 'Eastern and Western Christendom in Late Antiquity: A Parting of the Ways', *SCH* 13 (1976) pp. 1–24.

major city, and where aggregate membership could have represented as much as a fifth of the total population.[3] It may be tempting to imagine that only the expression of some obscure but powerful instinct – a drive to association – could lie behind such an apparently unique phenomenon. The strength of the temptation is, moreover, likely to reflect the difficulty of arriving at an alternative general analysis. Most attempts to explain the efflorescence of confraternities are of the functionalist variety. Some of them come close to circularity of argument. They assert that confraternities satisfied many important lay needs – ascetic, convivial, political and so on.[4] But often the only substantial evidence of those needs is that of the confraternities themselves. Other functional explanations at least avoid merely inferring cause from effect. Yet they lack chronological specificity. They do not tell us why these particular needs were met at this particular time.

Confraternities were, for instance, 'of course an artificial kin group': they embodied the tradition of kinship and compensated for its supposed decline.[5] The difficulty with explanation in these terms is that we can say remarkably little about the strength of kinship in any given period of the Middle Ages.[6] Bonds of kinship are always dissolving whenever historians catch sight of them, be it in the ninth century or the fifteenth.[7] Confraternities have also been thought to reflect a variety of other social changes: a rising age at first marriage, the weakening of parish loyalties, scarcity of resources. Yet, again, none of these phenomena can be assigned

---

[3] Cf in this volume John Henderson, 'Confraternities and the Church in Late-Medieval Florence', of which he kindly sent me a typescript; Susan Brigden, 'Religion and Social Obligation in Early Sixteenth-Century London', *PP* 103 (1984) p. 94; Linda Martz, *Poverty and Welfare in Hapsburg Spain: The Example of Toledo* (Cambridge 1983) p. 159; Bossy, *Christianity*, p. 58.

[4] Gabriel Le Bras, 'Les confréries chrétiennes: problèmes et propositions', *RHDFE* (1940–41) pp. 310–63 remains the best brief survey.

[5] Quotation from Bossy, 'The Counter-Reformation and the People of Catholic Europe', *PP* 47 (1970) p. 58, who is rightly cautious of its implications. Cf Le Bras p. 310.

[6] Cf Bossy, 'Counter-Reformation', p. 55; Jack Goody, *The Development of Marriage and the Family in Europe* (Cambridge 1983).

[7] Cf Jean Devisse, *Hincmar Archevêque de Reims 845–882* (Geneva 1976) 2 p. 878 n 361.

The Confraternities of Byzantium

with any precision to the right period.[8] Another type of explanation, and a final example, is provided by the historical anthropologist. We are told that confraternities created a 'ritual space' wherein escape from the pressures of living in an 'agonistic' society could be symbolically enacted. This account, ultimately perhaps reducible to a truism about peace and order in the midst of chaos, is specifically intended to apply to the confraternities of fifteenth-century Florence. But with minimal adjustment it could surely be applied to other institutions of different types, and from different places and periods.[9] Until we can show that later medieval society was peculiarly agonistic, and its confraternities peculiarly restful, we shall not have advanced very far. The solution may not, in any case, lie with an improved chronology. As Natalie Zemon Davis has written, 'it seems implausible to explain the confraternity... by the special events of the fourteenth and fifteenth centuries'; its history 'might better be related... to the more slowly changing features of life that influence people's sense of community'.[10] It is easier to applaud such an agenda than to comply with it. To do so would involve abandoning the functionalist stance and developing something more elusive: a sense of context. There are, I suggest, two ways forward.

The first I can no more than hint at. It involves viewing later medieval confraternities in their contemporary setting, not as substitutes for, but rather as complements to, numerous other forms of association – trade guilds in particular, sects, youth groups, networks of kinship and the like. A satisfactory integration of so many areas of enquiry will not easily be achieved. The evidence is seldom sufficient. Worse, our abiding image of the Middle Ages may hinder the proper interpretation of what evidence there is. We knew that the significant bonds of society in that 'world we have

---

[8] Bossy, 'Holiness and Society', *PP* 75 (1977) pp. 120–6, discussing *The Pursuit of Holiness in Late Mediaeval and Renaissance Religion*, ed Charles Trinkhaus and Heiko A. Oberman (Leiden 1974). Cf R.M. Smith, 'The Peoples of Tuscany and their Families in the Fifteenth Century: Medieval or Mediterranean?', *Journal of Family History* (1981) pp. 107–16 on marriage age. On parishes compare Henderson, 'Confraternities'; Brigden pp. 94–6.

[9] Ronald F.E. Weissman, *Ritual Brotherhood in Renaissance Florence* (New York and London 1982). Cf Barbara H. Rosenwein, *Rhinoceros Bound: Cluny in the Tenth Century* (Philadelphia 1982), using a similar model.

[10] *The Pursuit of Holiness* pp. 315, 318.

lost' were not only the 'vertical' ones created by king, lord and *paterfamilias*.[11] Yet such a conspectus of medieval 'horizontals' as *Kingdoms and Communities* was none the less a major *desideratum*. It reminded us of how much we knew but had never put together. Still more tellingly, it showed us that horizontal ties were probably as significant in the period before 1300 as during the later Middle Ages.

The second way forward that I propose derives from that assertion of essential continuity across the supposedly trans-formative twelfth century. It involves asking whether the 'medieval drive to association' was genuinely medieval. Historians acknowl-edge that confraternities were 'un fenomeno commune a tutta la cristianità'.[12] They then, however, tend to proceed as if evidence from much before 1200 belonged merely to the prehistory of the subject. It is time that the imbalance was redressed.[13] Broadening the scope of confraternity history in this way does not simply replace a functional explanation with a genetic one. Rather, a necessary chronological dimension is added to the context within which the later medieval proliferation of confraternities may eventu-ally become intelligible. Giving due weight to the early Middle Ages does not commit us to the belief that confraternities remained unchanged throughout. (The rise of the mendicants, for example, and perhaps also the consolidation of the doctrine of purgatory, may have decisively altered the character of confraternal devotion.)[14] But the perspective of the *longue durée* does alert us to the possibility that the similarities between early and later associations are at least as noteworthy as the differences – and that the later developed out of the early ones in a less dramatic way than some have thought.

There may for instance have been a sustained period of growth in the early period just as in the later one: growth in the number, distribution and sophistication of confraternities. The crucial phase would, on this account, have been the century or so preceding the

---

[11] *Pace* Peter Laslett, *The World We Have Lost – Further Explored* (London 1983) pp. 7, 10.

[12] Gilles Gerard Meersseman, *Ordo Fraternitatis*, 3 vols (Rome 1977) 1 p. ix.

[13] I have not seen Meersseman, 'Per la storiografia delle confraternite laicali nell'alto medioevo', *Storiografia e Storia, Studi... Theseider* (Rome 1974) 1 pp. 39–62.

[14] Weissman cap 2; Jacques Le Goff, *The Birth of Purgatory*, ET (London 1984) pp. 326–8.

The Confraternities of Byzantium

Gregorian Reform.[15] It could, however, be wrong to place too much emphasis on periods of expansion. The small cluster of tenth or eleventh-century Italian confraternity statutes that have come down to us may hint at a development both earlier than we think and more precocious than we can know.[16] Nothing about these texts implies the rarity or novelty of the institutions they describe. The hardly larger collection of statutes from tenth and eleventh-century England is a still more eloquent testimony to a vigorous and highly diversified Anglo-Saxon 'drive to association'.[17] It is surely safer to conclude that Anglo-Saxon society was 'rich in gilds'[18] than to suppose the few we know about to have been merely an isolated anticipation of an essentially later medieval state of affairs.

Evidence of trading or artisan associations might be interpreted in the same light. The guild of (possibly) Frisian traders recorded in runic inscriptions from early eleventh-century Sigtuna is not 'quite evidently witness... to a new age'.[19] We now have a greater sense of certain similarities in commercial organization between the late antique Mediterranean and the Dark Age North. It may therefore be possible to reopen the old question of how much early medieval associations inherited from the classical world.[20] Of course between the merchants of Sigtuna and the last known late antique 'professional' corporations in the West – for example the Neapolitan *saponarii* with whom Gregory the Great concerned himself – there stretch centuries for which little evidence survives.[21] Were merchants and artisans therefore unassociative during that period? The problematic *magistri commacini*, a builders' federation

---

[15] R.I. Moore, 'Family, Community and Cult on the Eve of the Gregorian Reform', *TRHS* 30 (1980) pp. 56–7; Robert Fossier, *Enfance de l'Europe Xe-XIIe siècles*, 2 vols (Paris 1982) I pp. 361–2.

[16] Meersseman, *Ordo Fraternitatis*, I pp. 55–65, 95–9.

[17] Benjamin Thorpe, *Diplomatarium Anglicum Aevi Saxonici* (London 1865) pp. 605–17.

[18] Frank Barlow, *The English Church 1000–1066*, 2 ed (London 1979) p. 249. See also pp. 196–8.

[19] Richard Hodges, *Dark Age Economics* (London 1982) pp. 89, 193. Cf Edward James, *The Origins of France* (London 1982) p. 71.

[20] C.R. Whittaker, 'Late Roman Trade and Traders', *Trade in the Ancient Economy*, ed Peter Garnsey *et al.* (London 1983) pp. 163–80.

[21] *MGH Epistolarum* vol 2 pp. 118–19. L. Cracco Ruggini, 'Le associazioni professionali nel mondo romano-bizantino', *SSSpoleto* 18 (1970) pp. 192, 222–4. Cf Fossier I p. 538.

of Lombard Italy, suggest otherwise, if only for the highly Roman-ized Mediterranean.[22]

The search for such continuities has a greater bearing on the history of the early medieval confraternity than might be imagined. For the emphatic lesson of the early sources, 'if one removes the economic spectacles of modern preoccupations, is that economic motives and interests were much less important to fraternities and guilds than historians have generally supposed'.[23] Guilds of artisans or tradesmen might be predominantly devotional and charitable in character; members of the most pious confraternity might have many secular interests in common. The early medieval evidence seldom tells us what the occupations of confraternity members were.[24] Nor does it describe the full range of any given association's purposes. No clear distinction can be drawn between 'professional' and devotional groups – and neither should be neglected by the religious historian. It is best to envisage a spectrum of possibilities: the soberly devotional association at one extreme, the wholly secu-lar trade or craft guild at the other, and a large, undivided central portion where religious, economic and convivial functions are vari-ously but inextricably mixed.

We can then make some sense of the few texts available from the ninth century and before. Some associations are relatively articulate. The *collectae* castigated for excessive drinking by Arch-bishop Hincmar in the ninth century sound like the very model of a later medieval association. Apart from gathering for a glass of wine, they were to come together 'in omni obsequio religionis... videlicet in oblatione, in luminaribus, in oblationibus mutuis, in exsequiis defunctorum, in eleemosynis, et caeteris pietatis officiis'.[25] Of the corporate piety of other Carolingian groups (some perhaps consisting of merchants) we hear nothing.[26] We should not, however, assume that they had none. More partic-ularly, we should not assume that immoderate conviviality was always a legacy of some pre-Christian cult. Assuredly certain pagan

[22] M. Salmi, 'Magistri Comacini o Commàcini', *SSSpoleto* 18 (1970) pp. 409–24.
[23] Reynolds pp. 72–3.
[24] The Paris MS BN Latin 9430 is exceptional. Cf Meersseman 1 pp. 99–108.
[25] *Capitula Presbyteris Data* cap 16, *PL* 125 cols 777–8. Devisse, *Hincmar* 2 pp. 877–8.
[26] References in Reynolds pp. 67–8. I here omit discussion of monastic con-fraternities of prayer.

The Confraternities of Byzantium

ritual feasts of the newly-converted peoples of north-western Europe had to be transformed beyond recognition or suppressed.[27] But it would be odd if there were no antecedent tradition of conviviality and corporate worship within the Christian congregations into which the least objectionable of those feasts could be incorporated. We know far too little about the internal workings of pre-Constantinian communities to trace the origins of such confraternal worship. The long history of common meals, feasts at martyrs' tombs and collective devotions might none the less be thought to have had some influence on the subsequent development of confraternities. There could still be a sense in which the early Church 'apparut... comme une fédération de confréries'.[28] If that were so it would, moreover, naturally be worth asking whether a comparable federation can be discerned in the immediately succeeding period.

And so to Byzantium. The approach there should be that enforced by the western sources. An ample sense of context is needed; enough to give weight to the early Middle Ages, and to the number of confraternities it may have witnessed. The model of a spectrum of possibilities can be carried over and refined. It is a way of reminding ourselves that the purely 'professional' and the purely devotional association are hardly more than Weberian ideal types; that some mixture of secular and religious purposes is characteristic of the majority of guilds and confraternities. It can also be a way of conceptualizing the shifting relation between highly formal associations (such as those of later medieval Europe) and much looser, more nearly spontaneous groupings (of the type that may now seem to have been virtually inevitable throughout the Middle Ages).

That is the required approach. The evidence to satisfy it is not so easily found. Byzantium presents the historian of western confraternities with two paradoxes. First, the earlier evidence is the more plentiful. There is no obvious later medieval proliferation

---

[27] E.g. Bede *HE* i 30; Gregory of Tours, *Liber in gloria confessorum*, cap 2, *MGH SRM* 1 pp. 749–50. Cf Alcuin, *Ep* 290, *MGH Epp Karolini Aevi* 2 p. 448.
[28] Le Bras p. 312. W.H.C. Frend, *Martyrdom and Persecution in the Early Church* (Oxford 1965) pp. 325–6; Ramsay MacMullen, *Christianizing the Roman Empire* (New Haven and London 1984) pp. 90, 104–5; Wayne A. Meeks, *The First Urban Christians* (New Haven and London 1983) caps 5–6; Peter Brown, *The Cult of the Saints* (London 1981) pp. 26–30.

to be accounted for. Second, the social history which ought to provide the necessary context for the continuities and developments that we may uncover is almost wholly lacking. As with the West, part of the problem is an insidious governing image. In a recent survey, for example, Alexander Kazhdan presents *homo byzantinus*, an isolated individual whose attention is monopolized by imperial autocracy.[29] *Homo byzantinus* is, of course, only another ideal type. Yet the notion that Byzantine society was articulated primarily in a 'vertical' direction is one of which we rid ourselves with difficulty. Evidence has after all adhered best to those who exercised authority. One traverses Byzantine society downwards from the top.[30] No more than a few pioneers have managed to make the refractory texts yield worthwhile conclusions about the strength and character of 'horizontal' ties like those of natural and ritual kinship. The everyday religion of the laity remains comparably obscure; it can only be glimpsed indirectly through the media of sermon, icon and saint's life.[31]

With the obvious exception of monasticism, voluntary religious associations in Byzantium have thus been neglected. In 1975 two editors could still find the important question about confraternities novel enough to be worth stating quite simply: 'did Byzantium stand wholly outside the orbit of events which were transforming the religious life of the laity in the cities of its Catholic neighbour Italy?'[32] The relatively well-documented history of Byzantine craft guilds might have formed part of the answer to that question. Yet guilds, like circus factions and other such 'horizontal' associations, have usually been examined only for their 'vertical' significance:

[29] (With Giles Constable) *People and Power in Byzantium* (Washington 1982).

[30] Evelyne Patlagean, *Pauvreté économique et pauvreté sociale à Byzance, 4e–7e siècles* (Paris 1977) shows what can be achieved. Contrast the evidential – and analytical – impoverishment of P.A. Yannopoulos, *La société profane dans l'empire byzantin des VIIe, VIIIe, et IXe siècles* (Louvain 1975) and A.P. Kazhdan and Ann Wharton Epstein, *Change in Byzantine Culture in the Eleventh and Twelfth Centuries* (Berkeley and Los Angeles 1985).

[31] Cf Patlagean's collected papers, *Structures sociales, famille, chrétienté à Byzance, IVe–XIe siècle* (London 1981); *The Byzantine Saint*, Studies supplementary to *Sobornost* 5, ed Sergei Hackel (1981); Peter Brown, 'A Dark Age Crisis: Aspects of the Iconoclastic Controversy', *EHR* 88 (1973) pp. 1–34, a rare perspective on local religion.

[32] J. Nesbitt and J. Wiita, 'A Confraternity of the Comnenian Era', *BZ* 68 (1975) pp. 360–84 at p. 361.

The Confraternities of Byzantium

their relations with the state, their disruptive potential.[33] The insistence of a few western historians is even more timely in the field of Byzantine economic history: 'La corporation est aussi une association religieuse. On a trop longtemps considéré la chapelle, les messes et les processions comme des à-côtés secondaires de la vie des arts'.[34] To establish the chronological extent and possible scale of guild activity in Byzantium would be to bring to light a principal aspect of confraternal religion. I shall therefore consider craft associations first.

'God be praised that I have overcome the task of describing the guilds and confraternities of Constantinople'. So wrote the seventeenth-century traveller Evliya Çelebi, having recounted in lavish detail the thousand and one guilds of Ottoman Istanbul, their numbers, their patrons, the symbols they carried in procession. Among these associations our sympathies surely extend most readily to the fraternity of 'dung-searchers', whose melancholy but rewarding privilege it was to carry dung from the city's streets to the seashore, there to sift it for coins and jewels.[35] We do not know whether there were any Christians in this fraternity. But we do hear of both Christian guilds and at least one guild of mixed Muslim and Christian membership in early Ottoman times.[36] We also know enough about general continuities between Byzantine and Ottoman economies to warrant extrapolating back from Çelebi's depiction and linking it with possible evidence of guild activity in the thirteenth and fourteenth centuries.[37] That evidence implies some degree of continuity with the period before the Latin conquest. It indirectly puts us in touch with the major sources for the earlier history of Byzantine guilds;[38] and these in

---

[33] Cf Alan Cameron, *Circus Factions* (Oxford 1976); Speros Vryonis Jr, 'Byzantine *Demokratia* and the Guilds in the Eleventh Century', *DOP* 17 (1963) pp. 289–314 with bibliography p. 293 n 13. See however Patlagean, *Pauvreté* pp. 228–9.

[34] Jacques Heers, *L'Occident aux XIVe et XVe siècles* (Paris 1963) p. 308.

[35] *Seyâhatnâme* pt 2 cap 80. Standard ed by Neib Asim (Istanbul 1896–1900). I have used the translation by J. von Hammer, *Narrative of Travels in Europe, Asia and Africa* (London 1834–48) vol 1 pt 2 pp. 104 *seq*, at pp. 250, 106.

[36] Vryonis, 'The *Panegyris* of the Byzantine Saint', *The Byzantine Saint*, pp. 196–226 at p. 220; Vryonis, 'Byzantium and Islam', *East European Quarterly*, 2 (1968) pp. 236–7.

[37] N. Oikonomidès, *Hommes d'affaires grecs et latins à Constantinople* (Paris 1979) pp. 108–14.

[38] For all which see Vryonis, '*Demokratia*'.

their turn find a starting point in antiquity. Çelebi's testimony thus takes its place as perhaps the richest – if also the most fanciful – in a sequence of texts distributed over the whole of Byzantine history, showing at the very least that the guilds never died out for long.

From Çelebi, too, we gain our most extensive portrait of Byzantine guilds as primarily sociable and ceremonial associations. The details of the portrait conform to what the much older evidence of the pagan guilds or *collegia* reveals. The *collegia*, indeed, answer exactly to the model of a spectrum already proposed. Cult associations at one extreme shade imperceptibly into groups who habitually celebrate together in a temple; the function of providing burial for members can be found at any point on the spectrum between the sacred and the secular; family cults develop gradually into cult associations; conversely, at the 'economic' end of the spectrum, craft associations may include members not of the same craft out of neighbourliness. At no point on the spectrum is there a clear division between different types: virtually every *collegium* is devotional and convivial in tone.[39] Ancient historians have been at pains to stress this general feature as if it demonstrated a radical difference between ancient and medieval European guilds – wrongly, unless the latter are seen through the 'economic spectacles of modern preoccupations'.[40] Some historians have even envisaged a discontinuity between classical and early Byzantine associations. For this they have blamed the 'dirigiste' government of the fourth to sixth centuries that regulated guilds too closely and engendered among them an emphasis on the pursuit of economic and political advantage that had not previously been apparent.[41] The extent of the discontinuity can, however, be exaggerated. It is not clear that all guilds were transformed into single-minded pressure groups.

[39] The most useful modern works are Ramsay MacMullen, *Roman Social Relations* (New Haven and London 1974) pp. 68–83, and *Paganism in the Roman Empire* (New Haven and London 1981) pp. 12, 36–9; Meeks, *First Urban Christians*, pp. 31–2. On burial clubs see Keith Hopkins, *Death and Renewal* (Cambridge 1983) cap 4 pt 3.

[40] Cf M.I. Finley, *The Ancient Economy* (London 1973) p. 138.

[41] Cf J.H.W.G. Liebeschuetz, *Antioch: City and Imperial Administration in the Later Roman Empire* (Oxford 1972) pp. 219–24, with bibliography on monopolistic and restrictive practices p. 222; Ruggini pp. 146–93; Patlagean, *Pauvreté* p. 175.

The Confraternities of Byzantium

There is no warrant for assuming that they shed their convivial and neighbourly aspects or their functions as burial clubs.[42] And despite the view of most historians that recruitment to the guilds was compulsory for urban craftsmen in the early Byzantine period,[43] the major pieces of evidence are susceptible of alternative interpretation.[44] The guilds probably remained essentially voluntary associations; and they were still such, it seems, in the tenth century when we again catch sight of them.[45] They had by then acquired patron saints; they took part in religious processions; at the *panegyreis* of the saints (religious festivals that, despite ecclesiastical umbrage, inevitably doubled as fairs) they had a festive and devotional role to play.[46]

Of the guilds' charitable activity less can be said. Some glimpses of it do, however, emerge in the evidence of the various groups that ought to be considered alongside them. Take for instance the *argyropratai* – financiers rather than mere silversmiths. Predictably, financiers could amass considerable wealth and power. Many citizens of Constantinople, and presumably elsewhere, became substantially indebted to them.[47] So it is perhaps appropriate that we should find in Antioch a financier turning to the ascetic life and to good works, and joining a manifestly pious confraternity whose other members were of the same lucrative calling.[48] Here we see something like a guild within a guild – for which a western analogy

---

[42] For the urban geography of crafts compare MacMullen, *Roman Social Relations* pp. 71–2 on antiquity with Vryonis, '*Demokratia*' pp. 298–9 on Constantinople c.1000. For Byzantine burial clubs see Patlagean, *Pauvreté* pp. 70, 158.

[43] Cf A.H.M. Jones, *The Later Roman Empire* 3 vols (Oxford 1964) 2 p. 858; Liebeschuetz pp. 219, 221.

[44] Patlagean, *Pauvreté* pp. 169, 173–4 (compare Liebeschuetz p. 223); W.H. Buckler, 'Labour Disputes in the Province of Asia', *Anatolian Studies presented to Sir W.M. Ramsay* (Manchester 1923) pp. 36 *seq*.

[45] Kazhdan and Epstein pp. 39 *seq*; Michael Angold, *The Byzantine Empire 1025–1204*, cap 4; Yannopoulos pp. 161–73 for the seventh to ninth centuries. I gloss over here the question of 'the disappearance and revival of cities' in the latter period: see Cyril Mango, *Byzantium* (London 1980) cap 3. For a different perspective, which makes the proposed continuity of guild life more intelligible, see Hugh Kennedy, 'From *Polis* to *Madina*: Urban Change in Late Antique and Early Islamic Syria', *PP* 106 (1985) pp. 3–27.

[46] Vryonis, '*Demokratia*' p. 302, '*Panegyris*' pp. 213, 220–3.

[47] Jones 2 pp. 863–4; Vryonis, '*Demokratia*' pp. 294–5.

[48] 'L'orfèvre Andronicus et Athanasie son épouse', *Vie et récits de l'abbé Daniel le Scétiote*, ed L. Clugnet, *Revue de l'Orient Chrétien* 5 (1900) pp. 371 *seq*.

is provided by the specifically devotional craft confraternities formed by members of the major guilds in, for example, Renaissance Florence.[49] The trade association was not just a model for voluntary religious groups. The sociability promoted among members of the same profession could directly spawn new, more emphatically devotional, forms of concerted lay activity.

Early Byzantine sources indicate further ways in which professional associations could give rise to charitable groups. Guilds were subject to *munera*, compulsory obligations of various kinds.[50] Some of these were of a distinctly charitable nature, reflecting a wider imperial interest in the needs of the deserving. Shopkeepers in the capital, for example, sustained the scheme that provided free funerals for the entire population; they provided the corps of functionaries known as *dekanoi*.[51] Those in Antioch had to provide monthly assistance to beggars.[52] Against this background we may begin to interpret the activities of that perplexing band, the *parabalani* of early fifth-century Alexandria, who have sometimes been interpreted as forming a confraternity. All we know about them is derived from two passages in the Theodosian Code.[53] 'Parabalanin [sic], qui ad curanda debilium aegra corpora deputantur', had perhaps been behaving too much like the janissaries of the patriarch.[54] Their numbers were thereafter limited and they were to be drawn from the humbler guildsmen who 'pro consuetudine curandi gerunt experientiam' – which had, presumably, been lacking in the past. Much philological and historical energy has been expended on these people.[55] They have been taken as representatives of an inferior grade of the medical profession (otherwise unattested) or a minor order in the Church (which makes no allowance for the connection with guilds); as ambulance-men who brought lepers to hospital or as a group who bathed the poor. An agnostic stance may be wisest. Certainly it is important to resist

---

[49] Cf Weissman pp. 63–5.
[50] Jones 2 pp. 858–9.
[51] Patlagean, *Pauvreté* p. 173.
[52] Libanius, *Oratio* xlvi 21.
[53] XVI ii 42, 43.
[54] *DACL sv* 'Parabalani' (H. Leclercq) col 1575.
[55] W. Schubart, 'Parabalani', *Journal of Egyptian Archaeology* 38 (1952) pp. 97–101 with bibliography; Owsei Temkin, 'Byzantine Medicine: Tradition and Empiricism' *DOP* 16 (1962) p. 112.

The Confraternities of Byzantium

the tendency of historians always to relate charitable activity to doctors and hospitals. Byzantine philanthropy was not nearly so centralized, even when managed by a patriarch.[56] And the *parabalani* may have performed a variety of functions to which neither the laconic imperial legislation nor the etymology of their name is necessarily any guide.[57] What deserves emphasis is that for any student of guild *demokratia* the Alexandrians' behaviour has a familiar ring; also that the emperor's solution to the problem they posed was to regulate their activity by turning it into a kind of *munus*, as if the model of a charitable guild were the obvious one in the circumstances.

The context of these professional associations and their offshoots is a suitable one in which to introduce a Byzantine instance of that perhaps surprising phenomenon, the confraternity consisting entirely of priests. It is not obvious that such associations were ever widespread in Europe; and it would be tempting to assume that they must have been at their most numerous in the early Middle Ages, when diocesan organization was relative weak.[58] From late Anglo-Saxon England there is certainly evidence of five priests' guilds. Legislation apparently presupposes, moreover, that priests were generally organized into fraternities of this kind.[59] There were, though, still at least four confraternities of priests in early modern London, suggesting that the institution had not lost its uses.[60] One of these confraternities, that 'of the Holy and Undivided Trinity of Sixty Priests', is reminiscent of two groups that could be found on later medieval Byzantine Corfu. The first of them functioned in the city. From the reign of Manuel I (if not earlier) until well into the fifteenth century, there was a *universitas* (as it is described in the Latin charter surviving from the Venetian

---

[56] *Pace* the latest general account, Timothy S. Miller, *The Birth of the Hospital in the Byzantine Empire* (Baltimore 1985).

[57] *Papyri Iandanae*, ed J. Hummel (Leipzig 1938) pp. 383–7 no 154 lists those to whom wine should be distributed, probably by a church at Oxyrhynchus, c.600. It seems to include *parabalani* among the minor clerics. We cannot, however, assume a similarity of function between these and the Alexandrian *parabalani*. Cf Miller p. 129 for the analogous case of the *dekanoi*.

[58] Cf Meersseman, *Ordo Fraternitatis*, I pp. 25, 113–35, 154–87.

[59] Barlow, pp. 22–30, 249.

[60] Brigden p. 96 with n 157. Cf Norman P. Tanner, *The Church in Late Medieval Norwich 1370–1532* (Toronto 1984) pp. 75–6 for a further example.

archives) of thirty-two priests, called *oratores*, who enjoyed a number of privileges and exemptions. In the countryside of Corfu there was a similar fraternity known as the *Leutheriotai* (Freemen).[61] They formed a type of caste closely restricted to members of their own families – and for that too there is an English parallel in the 'clerks of St Cuthbert' at Durham.[62]

The charters of these priests' confraternities form a point of transition from the 'professional' to the mainly pious in Byzantine religious associations, and to the one set of confraternity statutes that has survived. Among the *typika* or foundation charters that have come down to us is an informative twelfth-century text.[63] It represents a fresh copy (with a new subscription list) of a lost original dating back to 1048 that is said to have become illegible. It describes a confraternity of twenty clerics and twenty-nine laymen associated with the cult of the Theotokos Naupaktetissa in a monastery of Thebes. The members prayed for one another, their predecessors, the patriarch and others. They functioned as a burial club. And once a month they assembled at the icon of the Theotokos. They carried it in procession, singing hymns the while, to the station elected by the member whose turn it was to look after the image for the month following. There is very little here that a member of a twelfth or thirteenth-century Italian confraternity might have found strange. The *typikon* includes no reference to a common fund for feasting – but then not every Italian confraternity maintained one either.[64] In the West, miraculous altarpieces or wax images of patron saints rather than icons would have been processed around the countryside, but that is the only major difference.[65] The Theban *typikon* is the only one of its kind to survive. But nothing in the text suggests the rarity or novelty of any of its provisions; its uniqueness may simply reflect the accidents of

---

[61] C.N. Sathas, *Documents inédits relatifs à l'histoire de la Grèce au moyen âge*, vol 1 (Paris 1880) pp. 46–51 no 41; I.A. Romanos, *Deltion tes Istorikes kai Ethnologikes Etairias tes Ellados*, vol 2 (1889) pp. 591–608. See also P. Lemerle, 'Trois actes du Despote d'Epire Michel II concernant Corfu', *Hellenika* 4 (1953) pp. 418–23, 425–6. I owe these references to the kindness of Professor D.M. Nicol.

[62] Barlow pp. 229–30.

[63] ed J. Nesbit and J. Wiita in *BZ* 68 (1975) pp. 360–84.

[64] Cf Meersseman, *Ordo Fraternitatis*, 1 pp. 60–5.

[65] Henderson, 'Confraternities and the Church'; Weissman pp. 54–6. Cf R. Janin, 'Les processions religieuses à Byzance', *REB* 24 (1966) pp. 69–88.

The Confraternities of Byzantium

archival preservation. There are no internal grounds for interpreting it as the product of some western influence or of some change in the character of Byzantine society.[66] Other pieces of evidence can, furthermore, be adduced as partial analogues. I here present them in reverse chronological order so that we may work our way back to the early Byzantine period.

Processions of fraternities bearing icons of the Virgin, for instance, seem to have been noted during the later Middle Ages – alas without the vividness of a Çelebi – by foreign witnesses as diverse as Pero Tafur, Clavijo (envoy to the Mongols) and Stephen of Novgorod.[67] Earlier on, Nikephoros Choumnos (c. 1260–1327) noted a group of monks and pious laymen, the *Abramaioi andres*, who met to read the Scriptures and practise charity.[68] An eleventh-century manuscript dealing with events in the 840s tells how an icon of the Virgin had miraculously returned to Constantinople from Rome with the ending of iconoclasm and how a *diakonia adelphon* was formed to help parade it.[69] (It is unfortunately not clear whether these 'brothers' were laymen.) Lastly, the seventh-century *Miracles of Saint Artemius* describe a brotherhood which paid funds into a common treasury for a supply of candles, and met to keep vigil every Saturday night and on feast days in the Constantinopolitan Church of St John Prodromos that contained Artemius's relics.[70]

Serendipity produces no more than these few obscure references dealing mostly with the capital city. But they are sufficient to make the point that voluntary religious groups are evident from a number of centuries between the Arab and the Ottoman conquests. Whether such groups could have been found at every significant shrine, how their numbers and degree of coherence altered over time, and into what sociological context they should be inserted

---

[66] Yet Kazhdan and Wharton Epstein suppose that 'confraternities began to appear in the eleventh century' (*Change in Byzantine Culture* p. 52) and that the location of the Theban confraternity reflects a new 'decentralization' of Byzantine life.
[67] References in Nesbitt-Wiita p. 382 with n 40.
[68] J. Fr. Boissonade, *Anecdota Graeca*, 2 (Paris 1830) pp. 146–7.
[69] E.v. Dobschütz, 'Maria Romaia', *BZ* 12 (1903) p. 202 no 23. Cf Janin p. 71.
[70] P. Maas, 'Artemioskult in Konstantinopel', *Byzantinisch-Neugriechische Jahrbücher* 1 (1920) pp. 377–80. The *Miracles* were edited by A. Papadopoulos-Kerameus in *Varia Graeca Sacra* (St Petersburg 1909) pp. 1–79. See especially *Miracle* 18.

must all remain matters for surmise. So far, at least, no obvious reason has emerged why they should not have been widespread; Byzantine *mentalités* were not against them.

Reference to the *Miracles of Artemius* has transferred the discussion back to what is usually taken as the earliest distinct period in Byzantine history, the one ending in the seventh century. Here the evidence becomes unexpectedly plentiful – in comparison, that is, with the sources of both late Byzantium and early medieval Europe. It is also in many respects better evidence: narrative and circumstantial rather than cursory and legal. In Jerusalem, Antioch, Constantinople, Berytus, Alexandria and smaller towns the size of Oxyrhynchus (in Egypt if no other province) we find, from the mid-fourth century onwards, groups of those 'devoted to the full Christian life with little, perhaps, to mark outwardly any sharp line between them and the rest of the Christian community'.[71] These associations of *philoponoi* (labour-lovers) or *spoudaioi* (zealots) – as they were often known – are what historians of early Byzantium have come to think of as lay confraternities.[72] They were to be found in Monophysite and Chalcedonian areas alike. Taken as a whole, their membership ranged widely in wealth and age. In some places there were separate associations for men and women.[73]

Their recorded attributes and activities are various. In his *Life of Severus of Antioch*, Zacharias Scholasticus enumerates the qualities of an Alexandrian *philoponos* – orthodoxy, humility, chastity, love of his fellows, compassion for the poor.[74] Orthodoxy was demonstrated in prayer, liturgical chanting and the keeping of

[71] Derwas J. Chitty, *The Desert a City* (Oxford 1966) p. 3. S. Pétridès, 'Spoudaei et Philopones', *Echos d'Orient*, 7 (1904) pp. 341–8, to which *DACL sv* 'Confréries' (H. Leclercq) adds little; Ewa Wipszycka, 'Les confréries dans la vie religieuse de l'Egypte chrétienne', *Proceedings of the Twelfth International Congress of Papyrology*, ed Deborah H. Samuel (Toronto 1970) pp. 511–25. See also Miller pp. 124–31, perhaps viewing confraternities too exclusively from the perspective of urban monasticism. Generalizations that follow are largely based on the evidence assembled by Pétridès and Wipszycka, though I cannot always follow their interpretations of it. Full discussion and documentation must be reserved to a forthcoming work.

[72] Zacharias Scholasticus, *Life of Severus* ed M-A. Kugener, *PO* 2 p. 24 shows that *philoponos* was the local Egyptian variant of *spoudaios*, and refers to still other groups of 'companions' who are for obvious reasons virtually untraceable.

[73] The story of 'L'orfèvre Andronicus' (n 48 above) is the clearest evidence.

[74] *PO* 2 p. 12; cf p. 214 (*Life* by John of Beith-Aphthonia).

The Confraternities of Byzantium

vigils, participation in ecclesiastical festivals, ceremonies and processions.[75] We do not find icons being venerated, but that is to be expected at this early date.[76] Otherwise the piety of these confraternities clearly has a good deal in common with that of the later ones already mentioned. In this respect there seems to have been no break in confraternity history during the seventh century: throughout the Byzantine period, as throughout the Middle Ages in the West, some form of lay religious association seems to have been more or less inevitable. Zacharias Scholasticus's mention of humility and chastity points, however, towards the more obviously ascetic character of the early associations – sexual abstinence, avoidance of baths, fasting and so forth. Charity towards others, as distinct from the exclusive, fraternal charity characteristic of the Theban group and of so many western confraternities, is also abundantly documented. We hear much of washing the dead, tending the sick, and distributing money or clothing.[77] Members' conviviality is, in contrast, not mentioned in the sources. We know of the *philoponion* or meeting place that some associations maintained or were given, doubtless next to a shrine, but we do not know that there was feasting inside. That omission may simply reflect the nature of the texts. Members of these confraternities had after all intensified their links with the Church much more than they had severed their ties with the world; there remained a good deal in common between them and the ordinary lay worshipper – especially during the day, since their corporate activities were often nocturnal.[78] They did not, with rare exceptions, attain to the feats of miraculous power that their world had come to expect from

---

[75] Wipszycka pp. 513–15; *Vita Auxentii* (Metaphrastic) *PG* 114 col 1380 *seq*; Cyril of Scythopolis, *Vita Theodosii coenobiarchae*, ed H. Usener (Leipzig 1890) pp. 105–6. The strangest function of the Alexandrian *philoponoi* was to remind the Patriarch John 'the Almoner' that his tomb was unfinished: E. Dawes and N.H. Baynes, *Three Byzantine Saints* (Oxford 1948) pp. 228–9.

[76] Ernst Kitzinger, 'The Cult of Images in the Age before Iconoclasm', *DOP* 8 (1954) pp. 83–149.

[77] Wipszycka p. 513. *Philoponoi* or *spoudaioi* might marry, though perhaps live chastely: 'L'orfèvre Andronicus'; L. Clugnet, 'Vies... d'anachorètes', *Revue de l'Orient Chrétien* 10 (1905) pp. 47–8; Sophronius, *Miracles of SS Cyrus and John*, ed Natalio Fernández Marcos, *Los 'Thaumata' de Sofronio* (Madrid 1975) cap 5 pp. 249–51. Charity: 'L'orfèvre Andronicus'; *Cyrus and John* cap 35 pp. 318–22. See also n 93 below.

[78] *PO* 2 pp. 54–5; 'L'orfèvre Andronicus'.

holy men.[79] They were not monks. Some of them could none the less be said to have 'yielded nothing to monks' in their dedication; membership of a confraternity might be seen as a preparation for becoming a monk; and some confraternities might themselves with the passage of time be converted into monasteries.[80]

It is thus easy to conceive of the *spoudaioi* or *philoponoi* as constituting a 'third order' akin to that of the Mendicants in Italy. They certainly appear with some frequency in the texts as a distinct *tagma* or corps intermediate between clergy (or monks) and laity.[81] And they could on occasion be treated as part of the ecclesiastical hierarchy, at least so far as distributions of wine were concerned.[82] Encountering confraternities thus seemingly integrated into the structure of the Church, we may indeed begin to question whether they should be thought of as voluntary lay associations at all. But it would be wrong to envisage all confraternities of the period as having so formal and dependent a character that they were on the verge of turning into monasteries or minor clerical 'orders'.

Again the model of a spectrum suggests itself. A contrast with the extreme of formality and dependence among known lay groups will help to bring the character of the *philoponoi* and *spoudaioi* into clearer focus. At that extreme can be located the groups that are sometimes, perhaps too hastily, taken as the simple equivalent of the *philoponoi* and *spoudaioi* among the congregations of the Syrian Orient, the *benai* and *benat qeiama*, 'sons and daughters of the covenant'.[83] The term had originally embraced the whole Church. With the end of persecution, growth in the number of converts, and a concomitant decline in standards, the *qeiama* came to designate the group of Christians upon whom 'the task fell to carry on the traditions of ascetic Christianity in the heart of the

---

[79] Though cf John Moschus, *Pratum Spirituale*, cap 176, PG 87 col 3044.
[80] Clugnet, 'Vies... d'anachoretès'; PO 2 p. 54; Wipszycka pp. 518–19; Pétridès pp. 342–3. Length of service in a confraternity: *Pratum Spirituale* cap 61, PG 87 col 2913; *Miracles of Artemius* p. 19.
[81] Cf 'Fragmente einer Schrift des Märtyrerbischofs Petrus von Alexandrien', ed C. Schmidt, *TU* 5.4 (1901) p. 7.
[82] *Papyri Iandanae* (n 57 above); Berlin papyrus published Wipszycka pp. 522–5.
[83] Arthur Vööbus, *History of Asceticism in the Syrian Orient*, vol 1 CSCO *sub* 14 (Louvain 1958) pp. 97 *seq*, vol 2 *sub* 17 (1960) pp. 332 *seq* gives the 'standard' interpretation. For different etymologies see Sebastian Brock, 'Early Syrian Asceticism', *Numen* 20 (1973) pp. 7–8.

The Confraternities of Byzantium

congregations'.[84] In many Syrian churches could thus be found these *tagmata* of men and, less frequently, women who 'shall be continually in the worship service of the church and shall not cease the times of prayer and psalmody night and day'.[85] They assisted in ecclesiastical administration. They acted as nurses in the Church's hospitals and ministered to the poor.[86] In all this they may have resembled the *philoponoi* and *spoudaioi*. But one peculiar feature already emerges in the type of source from which we can learn a good deal about them. The sons and daughters of the covenant emerge most clearly in legislative texts. Their career was nothing if not regulated. Some would have been recruited as children by an itinerant chorepiscopus, who was not above trickery in getting his way with their parents.[87] Adult *benai* could live only with blood relatives or in specially designated dwellings adjacent to the church. They took a vow of virginity, wore distinctive clothes, and were not allowed to wash.[88] Wine and meat were alike prohibited – so much for fraternal conviviality. There is indeed no sign of 'horizontal' ties between members of the *qeiama*. But there are many signs of their strict supervision and maintenance by the Church. It is no surprise to find that ordinands were for preference to be sought among their number.[89]

The sons of the covenant thus represent one clear extreme of 'clericalization' and uniformity in the confraternities of the early Byzantine era; there is more to their coming together than a spontaneous intensification or co-ordination of ordinary lay religiosity. Comparison with them alerts us to the probable heterogeneity and informality which the evidence for *philoponoi* and *spoudaioi* would tend to conceal. Only a few texts hint at the ways in which a confraternity might begin, or might gain in members.

---

[84] Vööbus, *Asceticism*, 2 p. 332.
[85] *Syriac and Arabic Documents regarding Legislation relative to Syrian Asceticism*, ed Vööbus (Stockholm 1960), pt 1 cap 3 no 20.
[86] Vööbus, *Asceticism*, 2 pp. 339–41. Charity: *Vita* of Rabbula of Edessa in *S Ephraemi Syri, Rabulae Episcopi... Opera Selecta*, ed J.J. Overbeck (Oxford 1965) p. 203.
[87] John of Ephesus, *Lives of the Eastern Saints*, cap 16, *PO* 17 pp. 242–3; *The Canons Ascribed to Maruta of Maipherqat*, ed Vööbus, *CSCO* 439 (Louvain 1982) no 26.
[88] Vööbus, *Asceticism*, 2 pp. 336–7.
[89] *Canons Ascribed to Maruta* canon 25.

The more 'zealous' and 'industrious' in a congregation naturally distinguished themselves from the rest and consorted with one another;[90] parents no longer had children to care for and so could devote themselves more fully to extra-familial piety; a Chalcedonian shrine isolated in a Monophysite province needed maintaining and defending; students found the energy and the leisure to respond to the challenge of undiminished paganism; while for the philanthropic in a large poverty-ridden city the pooling of resources had obvious advantages.[91] Much, too, would depend on compelling leadership.[92] (The prime example is the Monophysite Paul of Antioch travelling from city to city, establishing in each a *diakonia* or charitable centre and cajoling rich men into running it.)[93] To all this the encouragement and involvement of clerics or monks was perhaps secondary.

A proper account of such *ad hoc* associations would place them in the context not only of guilds (which have already been examined) but of numerous monastic regimes, changing boundaries between cleric and layman, and the obscure growth of heretical sects.[94] There are no clear limits to what may serve as immediate background. That is one lesson to be derived from a comparative investigation. The other is that we should acknowledge the distant beginnings and essential continuity throughout the Middle Ages of the history of confraternities. 'The medieval drive to association' was indeed pan-medieval. Developments in late antiquity and the early Middle Ages merit longer attention than they have so far received. The confraternities and guilds of the medieval eastern empire were closer to European ones in purpose and structure than

---

[90] Cf *PO* 2 p. 24: 'we found ourselves in the churches with those that one calls *philoponoi*'. References to *spoudaioi laikoi* and such like need not on the other hand always indicate the formation of confraternities. *Spoudaios* and *philoponos* retained their 'non-technical' meanings: cf Athanasius, *Life of Antony*, cap 4, *PG* 28 col 436A for individual *spoudaioi*; Socrates *HE* viii 23. The sixth-century Monophysite philosopher John Philoponos need not ever have belonged to a *philoponion*: that was simply his name (I am grateful to Mr P.M. Fraser for advice here).

[91] 'L'orfèvre Andronicus'; *Cyrus and John* caps 5, 35; *PO* 2 pp. 54–5 – cf W.H.C. Frend, *The Rise of the Monophysite Movement*, 2nd ed (Cambridge 1979) p. 203; Pétridès pp. 346–7; Chitty p. 93. See also n 93 below.

[92] *Cyrus and John* cap 5; *PO* 2 pp. 32–3; *Vita Theodosii* pp. 105–6.

[93] Evidence collected by Patlagean, *Pauvreté*, p. 192.

[94] Heresy: Gilbert Dagron, 'Les moines et la ville', *Travaux et Mémoires*, 4 (1970) pp. 229–76; Patlagean, *Pauvreté*, pp. 134–5.

The Confraternities of Byzantium

might have been thought. And they deserve ample space in any future conspectus – not least because they tell us much about the 'horizontal' aspect of Byzantine society. Whether we adopt the perspective of *la longue durée* or of *histoire totale*, periods of proliferation such as that of the later Middle Ages in the West perhaps come to seem less extraordinary – and certainly less in need of biological summation.[95]

Postscript. Dr Judith Herrin has kindly allowed me to read her unpublished paper presented to the Davis Center in March 1985, 'From Bread and Circuses to Soup and Salvation: the Origins of Byzantine Charity'. She there draws attention to evidence of a group of persecuted Chalcedonians attached to the Anastasis church in Constantinople in the 660s whose members sustained one another through correspondence and appear to have continued the traditions of the *spoudaioi*. See Robert Devréesse, 'La lettre d'Anastase l'apocrisaire . . .', *An Bol* 73 (1955) pp. 5–16.

---

[95] I discussed the topic of confraternities with the late Professor J.M. Wallace-Hadrill only a few days before his sudden death. I take this, the first opportunity of recording a large scholarly indebtedness to him. I am grateful to Mr. P.M. Fraser, Dr John Henderson and Dr Richard Smith for comments on an earlier version of this paper.

III

Ritual and public health in the early medieval city

It would be an error to put ... [public] works in a category by themselves as 'utilitarian' in opposition to 'religious' works such as temples. Temples are just as utilitarian as dams and canals, since they are necessary to prosperity; dams and canals are as ritual as temples, since they are part of the same social system of seeking welfare. If *we* call reservoirs 'utilitarian' it is because *we* believe in their efficacy; *we* do not call temples so because *we* do not believe in their efficacy for the crops.[1]

A temple is as useful as a dam

The following discussion of ritual and public health takes the form of a sermon with two texts. Above is the first text. It comes from *Kings and Councillors*, a monograph, published in 1936, by that neglected pioneer of British social anthropology, Arthur Maurice Hocart. Like Fustel de Coulanges in *The Ancient City*, Hocart set out to trace the origins of social institutions back to archaic ritual. Like Frazer's in *The Golden Bough*, Hocart's key ritual was one that promoted fertility.[2] But Hocart was a greater scholar than Frazer and far more wide-ranging than Fustel. In the quotation above, he is writing about public works in general. So his main point applies *a fortiori* to public health projects. And that main point, to repeat, is: 'temples are just as utilitarian as dams and canals'.

In writing the history of health care, it is clearly important to respect indigenous categories in the way that Hocart demands. If we also employ our own concepts, it must be solely because they permit analytical refinements that help us find our way around the world of the people we are investigating. My second text illustrates how the balance can be struck, while unconsciously

---

[1]   A.M. Hocart, *Kings and Councillors: An Essay in the Comparative Anatomy of Human Society*, first published Cairo, 1936, repr. ed. R. Needham (Chicago and London, 1970), p. 217.

[2]   On Hocart see Needham's long introduction to his edition of *Kings and Councillors*.

echoing Hocart on the significance and efficacy of ritual. In her fine book about charity in early modern Turin, Sandra Cavallo politely chides historians for interpreting plague measures of the sixteenth century simplistically in terms of the broad social and economic *conjoncture* and the workings of the centralised state. A much more local and finely-tuned approach is called for, she argues: first, to the politics of plague prevention; and second, also, to the way in which we try to evaluate the measures taken.

'The elaborate segregation and disinfection measures adopted within cities', Cavallo writes,

> undoubtedly had an important role on the *symbolic* level (based as they were on notions of physical contamination and *purification*), and on the *ritual* level (contributing for example to preserve a sense of community and to discourage anti-social behaviour). But these aspects of the question are yet to be analysed, while most studies of the plague tend instead to look at anti-plague practices from the point of view of the impact they had on the disease itself.[3]

Those are the two texts. The message of the sermon they are intended to introduce is this. In the history of pre-modern – let us say, pre-nineteenth-century – public health measures, sewers and skeletons are not quite enough. A materialist–biological account will clearly capture some of the story. It will tell us about 'public health' as the *object* of policy: public ill health, as it usually turns out. But it will do that only in the narrow terms of biomedicine and demography, ignoring other aspects of the sort that Cavallo mentions, such as purification, or the sense of community. A materialist account will also tell us about the *instruments* of policy: the measures taken to promote collective health and combat epidemics. But it will do that legalistically, in terms only of centrally-framed 'practical' regulations. And these will have been selected for consideration primarily because they conform to our secular and biomedically-inspired notions of what public health promotion involves. My contention in this chapter is that this should not be the whole story. After all, medical historians no longer think that the only question worth asking of a pre-modern drug concerns its biological efficacy. 'Did it work?' deserves – and nowadays usually evokes – a more subtle response. And yet, by contrast, two of the liveliest controversies in the historiography of modern public health have revolved entirely around material questions: I refer to the McKeown debate and the question of whether quarantine measures were the reason why the plague came to an end in Europe.[4] This materialist approach will not, I submit, enable

---

[3]   S. Cavallo, *Charity and Power in Early Modern Italy: Benefactors and their Motives in Turin, 1541–1789* (Cambridge, 1995), pp. 44–5, 47 (quotation, italics added).

[4]   On McKeown and his critics, R.M. Smith, 'Demography and Medicine', in W.F. Bynum and R. Porter (eds), *Companion Encyclopedia of the History of Medicine* (London,

us to understand why pre-modern European public health measures evolved as they did. A broader conception of the topic is called for: one that gives due weight to ritual and symbolism, as we define them; and one that, equally, takes past conceptions of health seriously and does not just Whiggishly seek out foreshadowings of what was to come in the industrial age. The symbolic may be as important as the material. That is, purity and community may be as desirable as health in a biomedical sense. A temple is as useful as a dam.

Plague and piety

Let me now try to illustrate what one chapter in a non-materialist account of public health might look like. It is in the measures to contain the spread of the Black Death in the fourteenth century that general accounts of public health often locate the first stirrings of real modernity.[5] And it is in terms of 'strategies for collective health' that such general accounts often define public health.[6] So let us stay with plague for the moment (other diseases can enter the discussion later), and let us ask what strategies for curtailing the plague epidemics of the early Middle Ages (c. 300–1000) were favoured by those in charge of cities.

There is, unfortunately, no early medieval concept under which these strategies can readily be grouped. *Salus publica*, we know, was not quite what was at stake. As an explicit aim of government, that term possessed too broad a range of essentially political and ethical meanings – focusing on the idea of 'the common good' – to be quite to the point.[7] Was there, however, an unlabelled, implicit notion of a public health measure equivalent in scope and method to those of the later Middle Ages?

> When the bubonic plague was cruelly assailing the population within the walls of the city of Trier, the priest of God [Nicetius] assiduously implored divine mercy for the sheep entrusted to him. Suddenly, in the night, a great noise was heard, like a violent clap of thunder which broke

---

1993), 2, pp. 1663–92. P. Slack, 'The Disappearance of Plague: An Alternative View', *Economic History Review*, 2nd series, 34 (1981), 469–76.

[5] K. Park, 'Medicine and Society in Medieval Europe, 500–1500', in A. Wear (ed.), *Medicine in Society* (Cambridge, 1992), pp. 86–7; D. Porter, 'Public Health', in Bynum and Porter, *Companion Encyclopedia*, 2, pp. 1231–3; *eadem, Health, Civilization and the State: A History of Public Health from Ancient to Modern Times* (London and New York, 1999), p. 31; A.G. Carmichael, 'History of Public Health and Sanitation in the West before 1700', in K.F. Kiple (ed.), *The Cambridge World History of Human Disease* (Cambridge, 1993), p. 197. Cf. G. Rosen, *A History of Public Health*, first published 1958, expanded edn (Baltimore and London, 1993), pp. 41–2.

[6] D. Porter, 'Public Health', p. 1231; compare *eadem, Health*, p. 4.

[7] J.H. Burns (ed.), *The Cambridge History of Medieval Political Thought c. 350–c. 1450* (Cambridge, 1988), pp. 24, 143.

above the bridge over the river, so that one would have thought that the town was going to be split in two. And all the people were lying in their beds, filled with terror and hiding from the coming of death. And one could hear in the midst of the noise a voice clearer than the others, saying 'What must we do, companions? For at one of the gates Bishop Eucherius watches, and at the other Maximin is on the alert. Nicetius is busy in the middle. There is nothing left for us to do except leave the town in their protection.' As soon as this voice had been heard, the malady ceased, and from that moment no-one else died. Thus we cannot doubt that the town had been protected by the power of the bishop.[8]

The author is Gregory, Bishop of Tours, the great hagiographer of Frankish Gaul. He was writing in the 590s, from the personal information of one of Bishop Nicetius's protégés. This man became a distinguished abbot and, according to Gregory, a miracle-worker himself – with a speciality in water management.[9] Nicetius died in 564 or later. Like many bishop-saints of this early phase of the post-Roman West, he had established himself, if a little precariously, as the all-purpose public authority and administrator of his city.[10] In the words of the foremost preacher of the time, he was its 'superinspector'.[11] We cannot know what events gave rise to the miracle story that was passed to Gregory some forty years later. We can be reasonably confident that the epidemic referred to was the wave of bubonic plague which spread across Europe in 543, the year after it first reached and ravaged Constantinople.[12] But that is the limit of our information; and I do not want to speculate, on the basis of this evidence, about what anyone alive in Trier during the plague actually did or thought. It is more important, first, to look at the text itself and then, second, to ask about its presumed purpose.

One major theme in the extract is space. The scene depicted is bounded by the city's walls. The plague rages within those walls. A crisis is reached – a crisis in the strict sense of the turning point of an illness. A clap of thunder

---

[8]   Gregory of Tours, *Life of the Fathers*, 17.4, trans. E. James (Liverpool, 1985), pp. 118–19.

[9]   *Books of Histories* [*History of the Franks*], 10.29. (Primary sources that may for present purposes be consulted in any accessible edition are cited, as here, by standard subdivision of the text rather than by page.) E. Ewig, *Trier im Merowingerreich* (Trier, 1954), pp. 97ff.

[10]   P. Brown, *The Rise of Western Christendom* (Oxford and Cambridge, MA, 1996), ch. 6 for context. P. Horden, 'Disease, Dragons and Saints: The Management of Epidemics in the Dark Ages', in T. Ranger and P. Slack (eds), *Epidemics and Ideas* (Cambridge, 1992), pp. 73–4 for basic references. F. Prinz, 'Die Bischöfliche Stadtherrschaft im Frankenreich vom 5. bis zum 7. Jahrhundert', *Historische Zeitschrift*, 217 (1974), 1–35, also more for sources than for interpretation.

[11]   Caesarius of Arles, *Sermon*, 1.19.

[12]   J.-N. Biraben and J. Le Goff, 'The Plague in the Early Middle Ages', in R. Forster and O. Ranum (eds), *Biology of Man in History* (Baltimore and London, 1975), pp. 48–80 (trans. from *Annales* [November–December 1969], 1484–1510), remains fundamental.

seems to be about to bisect the city by breaking its central bridge. As we would gloss it: under the impact of the epidemic, the city is disintegrating as a social entity. The people are abed, but in a state of panic – the reverse of how dutiful citizens should behave, especially at night. It is easy to see why they are panicking, however. This epidemic is caused by demons, a purposeful, integrated group: their 'spokesman' addresses them as companions. What defeats them are the prayers of Nicetius conjoined with those of two of his predecessors. (This is not a community as sociologists have tried to define it, but one that embraces the dead as well as the living.) All three bishops are strategically placed. Between them they define the key aspects of urban space, its margins and its centre. The dead ones are suitably liminal: they are both present in their tombs in the city and yet absent, in the presence of God, with whom they intercede. They act as gatekeepers. Nicetius, as the central living authority, holds the centre. (By implication, he could even perhaps be 'keeping the bridge'.) The metaphor is, above all, military. The demons of plague lift their progressive occupation of urban space because the city's leaders are too vigilant for them ('Eucherius watches ... Maximin is on the alert'). No reader of Susan Sontag needs to be reminded of how often military metaphors have 'invaded' evocations of disease both literary and scientific.[13] Analogies with the vigilant control of urban space and its boundaries by later health boards would not be entirely fanciful. I suggest that the symbolic equivalence underlying the passage is, however, that of topographical space and social coherence – assaulted, threatened with disintegration, restored.

The conception of health here is more ample than that of biomedicine. In 1946 the World Health Organization famously, and rashly, defined health as 'a state of complete physical, mental and social well-being' – a state seldom attainable outside California. 'Social well-being': it requires no great familiarity with medical anthropology, no subscription to the journal *Culture, Medicine and Psychiatry*, to realise the importance of the social dimension of health. Ill health may quite simply be equated with social dysfunction, as it is, implicitly, by many of the peoples whom anthropologists have studied; or it may be seen as the somatisation, in the individual, of tensions in the family or wider society, a model of social disorder fashioned by and upon the body.[14] Either way, health is no purely personal matter. It is interpersonal: not so much psycho- as socio-somatic.[15]

Health is also spiritual. So Gregory of Tours would have argued. To the WHO definition another dimension should be added: one that partakes of the

---

[13]   S. Sontag, *Aids and its Metaphors*, Penguin edn (London, 1989), pp. 9–11.
[14]   See among a vast anthropological literature, M. Herzfeld, 'Closure as Cure: Tropes in the Exploration of Bodily and Social Disorder', *Current Anthropology*, 27 (1986), 107–20.
[15]   For the relevant historical application of such notions, see R. Van Dam, *Leadership and Community in Late Antique Gaul* (Berkeley and Los Angeles, 1985), pp. 259–60.

mental and the social but goes beyond both. The health of the community that resides in its good internal relations derives ultimately from the relations between the populace and their Maker. The supreme physicians – and therefore the supreme public health promoters – are *Christus medicus*, His healing saints, and confessors as the physicians of individual souls. This is not, of course, to say that all illness was thought to stem from specific, individual sins. Different kinds of aetiology – divine, demonic, natural – might be variously invoked according to context. But the profound connection between the health of the soul and that of the body was held to be inescapable throughout the Middle Ages and, of course, beyond.[16] To the progress or prevention of a plague, the spiritual condition of its likely victims was no irrelevance.[17] In the fourteenth century a learned Spanish physician could analyse 'moral' and 'natural' pestilence side by side, placing them on an equal ontological footing. Until the mid-Victorian age, the English epithet 'pestilent' could mean 'injurious ... to religion, morals, or public peace'.[18]

The remedies for pestilence extended, then, beyond solidarity to collective prayer and penitence. Such I take to be the message of Gregory's little narration quoted above: its intended effects on thought and action. Support your bishop; accept his place in the line of worthies; trust in divine mercy; and above all make yourselves worthy of that mercy. That is what he wants to convey. That is the best prophylactic, the best 'collective strategy' to avert future returns of the epidemic, the way to dispel the demons of a disorder that is at once physical (plague), social (disintegration) and spiritual (sin). A temple is as practical as a dam – and a miracle is as practical as a health board.

Other texts from Gregory's corpus of hagiographies make clear the connection between the demonstration of saintly episcopal power and collective responses to plague. When the same epidemic was threatening Rheims, Gregory reports, the people rushed to the tomb of their dead patron saint, Remigius.[19] They kept vigil, singing hymns and psalms.

> At dawn they searched in a treatise for what was still missing from their request [for protection]. By the revelation of God they discovered how,

---

[16]   J. Agrimi and C. Crisciani, 'Medicina del corpo e medicina dell'anima: note sul sapere del medico fino all'inizio del sec. XIII', *Episteme*, 10 (1976), 5–102; C. Rawcliffe, 'Medicine for the Soul: the Medieval English Hospital and the Quest for Spiritual Health', in J.R. Hinnells and R. Porter (eds) *Religion, Health and Suffering* (London and New York, 1999), pp. 316–38.

[17]   See R. Horrox, *The Black Death* (Manchester and New York, 1994), ch. 3, esp. pp. 97–8 for fourteenth-century parallels.

[18]   J. Arrizabalaga, 'Facing the Black Death: Perceptions and Reactions of University Medical Practitioners', in L. García-Ballester et al. (eds), *Practical Medicine from Salerno to the Black Death* (Cambridge, 1994), pp. 244–5; *OED*, 2nd edn, 'pestilent' 3, with Sontag, *Illness as Metaphor*, Penguin edn (Harmondsworth, 1983), p. 63.

[19]   Gregory, *Glory of the Confessors*, 78, trans. R. Van Dam (Liverpool, 1988), pp. 82–3. See also *Books of Histories*, 9.22.

after first praying, they might fortify the defenses of the city with a still more effective defense.

What was missing from their previous efforts was a (symbolic) appropriation of urban space. They took the saint's funeral shroud and arranged it in the shape of a bier. Carrying crosses and candles, they processed the shroud around the city and also around its suburban villages and any outlying solitary dwellings. Plague approached the edge of the city.

> It advanced all the way to the spot where the relic of the blessed Remigius had gone, and whenever it recognized the boundary that had been set, it did not in any way dare to advance further.

The disease even relinquished places it had previously invaded. There was thus containment as well as prevention – reordering of space, a separation of the sacred and the diseased.

Such collective responses do not merely belong in the literary realm of hagiography. They could rapidly be institutionalised. When plague ravaged the region of Arles, Gallus Bishop of Clermont, Gregory's uncle, interceded for his people. He was, Gregory tells us, assured by an angel that his prayer had been heard and that, while he was alive, no one would succumb to the disease. So, Gregory continues, 'he instituted the prayers called Rogations'.[20] Actually, Gallus seems to have made a special Lenten addition to the cycle of penitential processions that had developed since the fourth century. What had begun as a collective prayer for good harvest – shades of Hocart – could be additionally pressed into service as a remedy for public health hazards and other disasters. Along the Persian Gulf, the Rogation processions of Nestorian bishops had cleared the waters of giant sharks, to the benefit of the local pearl fishers.[21] Plague control was, though, their main health-related purpose in the sixth-century West. In Rome in 590, shortly before Gregory set down the first of the vignettes quoted above, Pope Gregory the Great exhorted the population of the stricken city to contrition. He then divided them up by religious calling – priests, monks, laity and so on – and had each group process from a different church to converge at S. Maria Maggiore. A ritual of penitence and social cohesion combined – not to be thought the less utilitarian or efficacious for the fact that some eighty people reportedly fell dead of plague during the great assembly.[22] Rogations, to follow the verdict of Michael Wallace-Hadrill, 'demonstrated in a dramatic way how the Church could identify local disaster with local sin and provide the remedy in a communal act of propitiation that

---

[20] *Life of the Fathers*, 6.6 (pp. 57–8).
[21] Brown, *Rise of Western Christendom*, p. 173.
[22] Gregory of Tours, *Books of Histories*, 10.1; cf. 9.20.

involved everyone' – not least, it should be added, the rich, who might otherwise have added to the social dislocation by running off (in the words of a preacher, like deserters from an army).[23] Those who shunned the remedy of repentance reportedly found their houses marked with the Greek letter T, or perhaps a cross. Gregory, who provides the report, knew this well from his own family tradition.[24]

So far I have been looking at plague, and at what (following Cavallo) we might label ritual and symbolism in plague control. I have been concentrating on what some might be tempted to think of as a merely religious approach to containing an epidemic. Of course, it is a commonplace of the historiography of plague in later centuries that folk aetiologies, whether learned or lay, had God as the author of pestilence and contrition as its best remedy[25] (even if the connection between the soul's and the body's health was sometimes learnedly 'medicalised' in terms of one of the 'non-naturals').[26] I am arguing, however, for a slightly different approach to religious responses.

First (Hocart's point about practicality) they have to be treated as part of 'the real thing'. They are not a curious by-way from the main subject of public health. Granted, much of the early medieval evidence for them is literary: hagiographical vignettes. Yet literary representations – it hardly needs stating in these 'post-postmodern' days – have their own interest, value and potency. And at the time of their first hearing, they were widely held to represent genuine events. Moreover, these events were not from some age of miracles in a golden past, but, in Gregory's own case, sometimes quite recent 'family affairs'. Nor did the texts just celebrate past achievements. They furnished the attentive with models for both collective and individual action in averting future epidemics.

Second, the collective aspect needs to be given more emphasis than is usually the case with plague historians' glancing references to processions. The ritual procedures reviewed above were (ideally) corporate strategies for collective health that operated in a complex way, under a suitably broad definition of well-being. What they demonstrate is not miraculous power operating in, as it were, a blinding flash but, rather, certain *techniques* for the reconfiguration of urban space. And these techniques are often shown being deployed at the instigation of a particular style of urban leadership – one which in vigour and comprehensiveness bears comparison with that of any Renaissance health board.

---

[23] J.M. Wallace-Hadrill, *The Frankish Church* (Oxford, 1983), p. 11. Brown, *Rise of Western Christendom*, p. 63. Caesarius, *Sermon* 133.

[24] *Glory of the Martyrs*, 50, trans. Van Dam (Liverpool, 1988), 76; *Books of Histories*, 4.5.

[25] For example Horrox, *Black Death*.

[26] Arrizabalaga, 'Facing the Black Death', p. 280.

Finally, since historians tend to associate religious responses to public health with periods of crisis, it should be added that none of the foregoing arguments relates exclusively to plague epidemics. Other less threatening diseases were supposed to have been effaced by dramatic gestures made at the centre of things. Gregory's was a time in which the conversion of the Western barbarians to Catholic Christianity was recent and patchy. So he illustrates the potential effect of conversion on the collective health of a whole population. The leprosy of heresy was no mere metaphor.[27] When the King of the Suevi (in Galicia) and his household accepted Catholic baptism,

> the people were freed from loathsome leprosy, and all ill people were cured; to the present day the disease of leprosy has never appeared on anyone there.[28]

As for still less threatening, characteristically endemic disease, I have suggested elsewhere that bishops who are figured in hagiography as taming dragons should perhaps be understood as symbolically facing up to the challenge of malaria.[29]

Sacraments and pollutions

All such spectacular and literally space-saving 'miracles of public health' (as I dare to call them) were, in many respects, simply occasional magnifications of commonplace rituals that, in the Christian urban communities of the early medieval West, were meant to involve everyone and to promote collective well-being. I shall pass them rapidly in review before focusing on what may have been a still more basic level of 'public health' activity by the church: countering pollution.

There were festivals of saints and martyrs – 'rituals of consensus', social healing, as processions were also intended to be.[30] Preparation to join in such festivals could involve an examination of conscience that had strong implications for somatic health. 'Woe is me,' reportedly lamented a blind

---

[27] See R.I. Moore, 'Heresy as Disease', in D.W. Lourdaux and D. Verhelst (eds), *The Concept of Heresy in the Middle Ages* (Louvain, 1976), pp. 1–11.

[28] *Virtuti Martini*, 1.11, trans. Van Dam, *Saints and their Miracles in Late Antique Gaul* (Princeton, 1993), p. 213.

[29] 'Disease, Dragons and Saints'. See now also P. Squatriti, 'Water, Nature and Culture in Early Medieval Lucca', *Early Medieval Europe*, 4 (1995), 21–40, similarly drawing a connection between hagiography and environmental management.

[30] P. Brown, *The Cult of the Saints* (London, 1981), pp. 99–100. See also W.E. Klingshirn, *Caesarius of Arles: The Making of a Christian Community in Late Antique Gaul* (Cambridge, 1994), ch. 7.

III

woman unable to participate on such an occasion, 'who does not deserve to see this festival with the rest of the congregation, because I have been blinded by my sins!'[31] Prayer restored her sight and enabled her to set off for church. At the festivals themselves, possessions were not simply publicised but perhaps actually induced, and exorcisms were achieved, as the troubled worked through whatever dysfunctions were being somatised into demons within.[32]

More common than great miracles and repeated festivals were the sacraments. Indeed, to the question of what preventive public health measures would have been seen by the élites of Gregory's time as the truly essential, the most far-reaching, one tempting answer would be: baptism and the Eucharist. In these, individual and collective responsibilities merged. Baptism was the equivalent of childhood inoculation: the means to forgiveness of original sin and an exorcism, a rebirth into health.[33] The Eucharist, for both the congregation of observers and the smaller number of actual communicants, was, like the saint's festival which periodically framed it, a ritual of social integration.[34] Presence at it could bring obviously beneficial results: Gregory's mother had saved their household from plague by attending mass.[35]

The last sacrament to be mentioned in this brief review is penance. Gregory's was a time when an ancient system of public one-off penance for very serious sins was just beginning to give way to a private, repeatable, more nuanced transaction between confessor and penitent – a transaction concerning venial sins. The sins might be punished by minor (though not trivial) penances, according to a tariff set out in a penitential. Penitentials are first evident in Ireland but were soon exported to Britain and the Continent. As a body of texts, they bear witness to an attempt by early medieval churches to regulate a significant number of the daily thoughts and activities of priests themselves, as well as of monks and other laity.[36] Penitentials deal with Catholic devotion, paganism and magic; also with the deadly sins, not least those of the stomach and the loins. No systematic or evenly-distributed system of control was ever possible or envisaged. None the less this material does manifest, if only partially and indirectly, what can be seen as corporate priestly concerns for communal health – health under a variety of descriptions. The common way of

---

[31]   *Virtuti Martini*, 2.28, trans. Van Dam, 243.
[32]   Compare Brown, *Cult of the Saints*, p. 111.
[33]   A. Angenendt, 'Der Taufritus im frühen Mittelalter', *Settimane Spoleto*, 33 (1985), 275–321; H.A. Kelly, *The Devil at Baptism* (Ithaca, 1985); P. Cramer, *Baptism and Change in the Early Middle Ages c. 200–c. 1150* (Cambridge, 1993), pp. 136ff.
[34]   Van Dam, *Saints and their Miracles*, p. 93; Klingshirn, *Caesarius*, pp. 155–8.
[35]   *Glory of the Martyrs*, 50, trans. Van Dam, 76; *Books of Histories*, 4.5.
[36]   Brown, *Rise of Western Christendom*, pp. 158–61. A.J. Frantzen, *The Literature of Penance in Anglo-Saxon England* (New Brunswick, 1983).

characterising penitentials as setting out 'health-giving medicine for souls' was, like the leprosy of heresy, far from metaphoric.[37]

On a modern definition of health, the dietary prescriptions that are dotted around the penitential corpus have been seen as promoting hygiene in food preparation. ('If anyone accidentally touches food with unwashed hands ...', as one canon begins.)[38] Other canons which attempt to promote moderation and propriety in matters of alcohol as well as food, in sex and the expression of anger, could be seen as encouraging bodily health, as well as helping reduce that sinfulness which is the harbinger of epidemics. But that is not the reason why penitentials should be important to historians of early medieval public health. Their significance is that they remind us again of the need to relativise the measures we are considering – relativise them to local conceptions of health and well-being. On the question of diet, for instance, what is evident in these sources is not hygiene but 'ethno-hygiene', and of a perhaps unsettling kind. After all, the canon just quoted about touching food with unwashed hands excuses the omission if it was unintentional – just as it goes on to excuse allowing a mouse to touch the food. Such dietary and seemingly hygienic prescriptions can no more be accounted for in modern biological or medical terms than can those of Leviticus. Rather than hygiene, these penitentials aim to promote purity and the avoidance of pollution. Their enemy is not so much dirt as uncleanness.

Now this is not the usual stuff of public health historiography. Narratives conventionally concentrate on those areas in which a pre-modern conception of miasma or corrupt air coincides quite neatly with our contemporary notions of the sources of environmental pollution: sullied water, human and animal waste, and so on. Yet a broader or perhaps different conception of pollution is evoked by these penitential texts: certainly an elusive one. Despite the best efforts of philologists and anthropologists, it remains an 'umbrella' term. We feebly differentiate it from its material equivalent by labelling it 'ritual pollution'; an unsatisfactory solution, because the ritual aspect often seems to subsume the material.[39] For all its ambiguity the term 'pollution' does, however, adequately

---

[37]   *Penitential of Cummean*, prologue, trans. J.T. McNeill and H.M. Gamer, *Medieval Handbooks of Penance*, first published 1938 (repr. New York, 1965), p. 99. For details of editions and further references supporting much of what follows see R. Meens, 'Pollution in the Early Middle Ages: The Case of the Food Regulations in Penitentials', *Early Medieval Europe*, 4 (1995), 3–19. Also *idem*, 'The Frequency and Nature of Early Medieval Penance', in P. Biller and A.J. Minnis (eds), *Handling Sin: Confession in the Middle Ages* (York, 1998), pp. 35–61.

[38]   *Penitential of Theodore*, 7.7 (McNeill and Gamer, p. 191).

[39]   M. Douglas, *Purity and Danger: An Analysis of the Concepts of Pollution and Taboo* (London, 1966), enjoys a higher reputation among historians than among anthropologists. See further R. Parker, *Miasma: Pollution and Purification in Early Greek Religion* (Oxford, 1983); A.S. Meigs, 'A Papuan Perspective on Pollution', *Man*, n.s. 13 (1978), 304–18; Meens, 'Pollution'.

reflect the vocabulary of the Latin texts.[40] It refers to a cluster of acts or states which are characteristically dangerous – and often contagious too. And these acts and states (we can generalise) have the property of being fully intelligible as pollutants only in religious and cosmological terms, even when they are described in a quasi-medical way.

As a further illustration: members of some of the congregations in which the penitentials were applied seem to have regarded the consumption of urine and excrement, scabs, lice, blood and semen as beneficial to health.[41] But in punishing such beliefs – which are by no means without their analogues in other periods and places – the confessors were far from combating superstition with hygienic rationalism.[42] Rather, they were trying to replace one set of pollution ideas with another. A canon in an Anglo-Saxon penitential states: 'the hare may be eaten, and it is good for dysentery; and its gall is to be mixed with pepper for [the relief of] pain'.[43] The medical advantage is paraded, but the ulterior motive is to encourage the view that the hare – despite Leviticus 11.6 – is a 'clean' animal. In similar spirit, the next canon in the same collection allows the consumption of the honey of homicidal bees (although the bees themselves should be killed). Pollution is contagious but not that contagious, or at least not in that particular fashion.[44] On the other hand, the meat of the offspring of an animal that has been party to bestiality should be strenuously avoided. In that case the pollution, a Lamarckian inheritance, remains powerful. Again, by way of final example, to drink the 'leavings' of a dog is obviously dirty, polluting – but no more or less so than to drink those of a thief or a man guilty of incest.[45]

So far I have stressed 'ritual pollution' for two main reasons. First, the concept gives us a view of public health from the receiving end – a view that avoids anachronistic 'biologism'. It shows ritual as being crucial to an understanding of public health *objectives*, as well as measures. Second, it introduces the church at work in a decentralised, indeed uncoordinated manner, promoting 'socio-somatic' well-being. And this, I submit, constitutes a level of activity beneath (or beyond) the church's other sacramental interventions in collective ill-health, as well as those more dramatic miracles wrought by virtuoso bishops with which I began. But pollution can be a useful heading in other ways, too. Its history hints at still further levels of activity – harder to document, scarcely institutionalised, but equally relevant to an assessment of

---

[40] Meens, 'Pollution', p. 23.
[41] Ibid., pp. 12–13.
[42] H. von Staden, 'Women and Dirt', *Helios*, 19 (1992), 7–30 (classical); Parker, *Miasma*, pp. 231, 233–4 (late antique).
[43] *Penitential of Theodore*, 11.5 (p. 208).
[44] Meens, 'Pollution', pp. 6, 12–13.
[45] *Old Irish Penitential*, 17 (p. 159).

urban health and of means of enhancing it in the early Middle Ages. Moreover the concept will, later, provide a way of bringing material considerations back into the picture without distorting their early medieval significance.[46]

Let us explore that sub-institutional level a little further. The theme common to the different types of activity that I have tried to identify is the demarcation and management of space in the city: topographical space, as in those miracles; social space in church festivals; ritual space (for want of a more sensitive term) in the penitentials, involving the separation of the clean from the unclean, the sacred from the polluted. I suggest that church leaders might be thought of as attempting, through subtle adjustments as much as through grand gestures or regulations, to harmonise topographical and ritual space.

They can be seen to do so in three ways: firstly, in the charitable foundations and outdoor relief services that they established or administered for the benefit of the very poor.[47] Of course, the nursing and sustenance provided might have been just sufficient in aggregate to affect the overall health of the urban population – health defined in its modern sense. But the activities in question should also, perhaps, be seen in terms of the management of pollution. At least some of the poor were, I hypothesise, seen as polluted and contagious because of their immorality, their contacts with criminals and animals, the unclean food upon which they, of necessity, sometimes depended,[48] and their diseases (not least leprosy, towards which attitudes could be as hard in this period as in the thirteenth century).[49] They needed purification or, where that was impossible, a certain amount of segregation – not in a draconian anticipation of *renfermement*, but through the allocation of particular urban spaces, in shrines, hospitals, bishops' houses and the like.[50]

Beliefs in the pollution of death, secondly, had to be managed in a different way. To summarise crudely a lengthy and complex process, we could say that the Church turned the topography inherited from the ancient city, not only inside out but also, more pertinently in this context, *outside* in. On one influential argument, it turned the city inside out through the emphasis it gave

---

[46]   On the dangers of 'medical materialism' in interpreting pollution beliefs, Douglas, *Purity and Danger*, pp. 29–32, Parker, *Miasma*, pp. 57–8, and Meens, 'Pollution', p. 5, are salutary.

[47]   See for example T. Sternberg, *Orientalium More Secutus: Räume und Institutionen der Caritas des 5. bis 7. Jahrhunderts in Gallien* (Münster, 1991).

[48]   P. Bonnassie, 'Consommation d'aliments immondes et cannibalisme de survie dans l'Occident du Haut Moyen Age', *Annales* (September–October 1989), 1035–56.

[49]   The extreme instance, not yet adequately explained, is the Lombard Edict of Rothar, cap. 176.

[50]   For comparison with the central Middle Ages see R. Gilchrist, 'Christian Bodies and Souls: The Archaeology of Life and Death in Later Medieval Hospitals', in S. Bassett (ed.), *Death in Towns: Urban Responses to the Dying and the Dead 100–1600* (Leicester, 1992), pp. 112–15.

to religious festivals associated with suburban or peripheral shrines.[51] It turned the city outside in through the admission of intramural burials – burials in the space that ancient society had studiously kept free of their pollution. On this front, it was not the contagion itself that had to be countered but beliefs about its source.[52]

With the third kind of pollution that belongs in this context, the task was the converse. Recognition of a new kind of defilement had to be encouraged: that of an only recently and unevenly suppressed paganism. Demons now embodied the uncleanness lurking in the remains of the cult sites of the old religion. New rules of avoidance and containment were needed if possession was not to become epidemic. Congregations had to be taught how to negotiate a fresh and highly threatening demonic geography.[53]

The case for materialism

In the foregoing, it will seem as if I have done little more than endorse George Rosen's brief account of my topic in his history of public health.

> In the West during the earlier medieval period ... health problems were for the most part considered and dealt with in magical and religious terms ... prayer, penitence and the invocation of saints were the means employed to deal with health problems ... Whatever knowledge concerning health and hygiene survived was ... applied in the hygienic arrangements and regulations of the monastic communities.[54]

Rosen was writing in the 1950s, under the entirely pardonable influence of what now seems like a Dark-Age view of the Dark Ages, as sunk irremediably in superstition and seriously deficient in rational medicine. Of course, early medieval medicine nowadays receives a fuller and more understanding press.[55] And I hope to have shown that religious approaches to public health should be treated with equal sympathy. There are, however, two more substantial points to register in protest at a pessimistic view of the period which, under this

---

[51]   Brown, *Cult of the Saints*, pp. 4–8.
[52]   J. Harries, 'Death and the Dead in the Late Roman West', in Bassett, *Death in Towns*, pp. 57–9.
[53]   Brown, *Cult of the Saints*, p. 125; Klingshirn, *Caesarius of Arles*, ch. 6. For the notion of a demonic geography see references in Horden, 'Responses to Possession and Insanity in the Earlier Byzantine World', *Social History of Medicine*, 6 (1993), 182–3.
[54]   Rosen, *History of Public Health*, pp. 28–9.
[55]   See M.L. Cameron, *Anglo-Saxon Medicine* (Cambridge, 1993), for an extreme defence of the rationality of 'Dark-Age' therapeutics. Contrast F. Wallis, 'The Experience of the Book: Manuscripts, Texts and the Role of Epistemology in Early Medieval Medicine', in D. Bates (ed.), *Knowledge and the Scholarly Medical Traditions* (Cambridge, 1995), pp. 101–26.

heading of public health, survives essentially unaltered in more recent accounts.[56]

First, even on the materialist definition of what constitutes the history of public health, the early Middle Ages were not the dispiriting blank they are still often taken to have been. That is, between the glories of the Roman aqueduct and the environmental regulations of the thirteenth-century Italian communes (regulations that have plausibly been connected to the revival of Roman law) something *did* happen. Monasteries were no more the only centres of hygiene than they were the only guardians of classical culture. There is another article to be written on public health measures that would be the obverse of this one. It could place ritual and symbolism in the background and concentrate, as I have not done, on more familiar tasks: the management of drainage, water supply, perhaps even sewerage, and the oversight of food supply, as well as the provision of nursing services already mentioned.[57] It would also give some space to plague control measures – measures of a sort that would not have been out of place in the later Middle Ages, and that involved an attempt to check the spread of an epidemic by prohibiting movement between fairs.[58] Once again, the primary responsibility for all such measures lay with bishops. To revert to my opening example: besides miraculously warding off plague, Nicetius of Trier was active in poor relief, a pioneering viticulturalist, and above all a great builder – not only of churches but of a castle, its water led by conduits which also turned a mill.[59] Not exactly public health, but enterprises not very far removed from it in terms of techniques and resources. In the following century, the seventh, Desiderius of Cahors was one bishop known to have been asked to set up checkpoints to stop pestiferous merchants (presumably thought to be carrying the disease in their personal miasma). He also wrote to Gallus of Clermont, a successor to that Gallus mentioned above, asking for the loan of specialist craftsmen who could make the wooden tubing necessary for his city's refurbished water supply.[60] Correspondence about such matters seldom comes down to us from this period. It survives only when its presumed literary merits earn it a place in a 'published' letter collection. So it is reasonable to envisage such activity as having been much more frequent than its surviving attestations.

---

[56] Carmichael, 'History of Public Health', p. 193, still privileging clean monasteries. See also Porter, *Health*, pp. 22–3 on the early Middle Ages, discussing only hospitals.

[57] Add to references in n. 10 above: B. Ward-Perkins, *From Classical Antiquity to the Middle Ages: Urban Public Building in Northern and Central Italy* (Oxford, 1984), ch. 7 (water and water supply), esp. e.g. p. 134, sewers and drainage in early medieval Pavia. Compare Squatriti, *Water and Society in Early Medieval Italy, AD 400–1000* (Cambridge, 1998), ch. 2.

[58] J. Durliat, 'Les attributions civiles des évêques mérovingiens: l'exemple de Didier, évêque de Cahors (630–655)', *Annales du Midi*, 91 (1979), 238–9, 244.

[59] Venantius Fortunatus, *Carmina*, 3.11–12.

[60] Durliat, 'Attributions', pp. 242–4.

Did the material activity somehow give rise to the hagiographical miracles? Do the miracles symbolically condense a range of more mundane performances? There may be other ways of putting it. Perhaps if we could draw up a balance sheet of all the relevant connections between 'literature' and 'life', then the net influence might have been exerted in an unexpected direction. That is, the conceptual world of the early medieval hagiography might have been the model for, and stimulus to, the practicalities. A similar possibility has, after all, been entertained by students of anti-plague strategies of the *later* Middle Ages. European readiness to seek a cause, and thus a remedy, for epidemics has been attributed to the connection widely made between illness and sin. And it has been contrasted with the predominant Muslim view of plague as 'a martyrdom and a mercy', a view much less likely to engender public health measures.[61] The problem with this particular theological interpretation of the European response to the Black Death is that positing a link between sin and epidemic was hardly an invention of Europeans in the later Middle Ages. It can be found as far back as pre-classical antiquity and so cannot be used to explain particular fourteenth-century developments.[62] It is not wholly absent from Islamic interpretations of plague.[63] Nor, finally, are public health concerns of a materialist kind alien to the Muslim tradition.[64] But those are 'local difficulties': they do not invalidate the argument's general character, which is to give religious culture an important role in the explanation of medical history.

In this context, whatever causal connections we posit, during the early Middle Ages the miraculous and the mundane, the ritual and the practical, the theological and the material are best seen as lying on a continuum – as blended ingredients in the 'medical pluralism' of public health.[65] They are no more easily separable as categories than are ritual pollution and biomedical dirt. The church had to deal with miasma in whatever form it took, whether from a pagan sanctuary or a stagnant pool, an unclean animal or a blocked drain. Here is a description of how its bishops might have operated:

---

[61] Slack and Ranger, *Epidemics and Ideas*, p. 17, with ch. 4 (Lawrence Conrad). Cf. R. Palmer, 'The Church, Leprosy and Plague in Medieval and Early Modern Europe', *Studies in Church History*, 19 (1982), 94ff; M.W. Dols, 'The Comparative Communal Responses to the Black Death in Muslim and Christian Societies', *Viator*, 5 (1974), 275ff.

[62] Parker, *Miasma*, p. 236.

[63] M. Dols, *The Black Death in the Middle East* (Princeton, 1977), pp. 114–15.

[64] L.I. Conrad, 'The Plague in the Early Medieval Near East' (unpublished PhD thesis, Princeton 1981), 392ff; *idem*, 'Die Pest und ihr soziales Umfeld im Nahen Osten des frühen Mittelalters', *Der Islam*, 73 (1996), 85–9, with references; S. Hamarneh, 'Origins and Functions of the *Hisbah* System in Islam and its Impact on the Health Professions', *Sudhoffs Archiv*, 48 (1964), 157–73.

[65] See Slack, 'Introduction', in Slack and Ranger, *Epidemics and Ideas*, p. 11, for parallels with Far Eastern history.

Authority for the control of health was in the hands of a set of leaders which included chiefs, healers and local patriarchs. These controlled the conditions of health in several different ways. First, they were responsible for controlling the kinds of deviance which were thought to threaten communal health ... Diviners identified witches, and chiefs eliminated them ... Patriarchs ... drove out or killed polluted individuals whose presence threatened the survival of local kinship groups. These included twins, and also people with smallpox who were sent out of the village into isolation ... The same triad of healing specialists, chiefs and patriarchs regulated the use of irrigation channels, burial of the dead ... and the location of sites for human waste ... Those with authority also organized rites for communal well-being, to prevent famine, epidemics and damaging wars.[66]

The setting is Tanzania towards the end of the nineteenth century. Here, again, is a mixture of the ritual and the practical, the material and the symbolic. *Mutatis mutandis*, it describes exactly the sort of context I envisage for the hagiographies previously cited.

Autres temps

My second point in defence of the 'ritualist' approach to the history of public health is that its scope is, or ought to be, much wider than the early Middle Ages. Now historians of religion generally, it hardly needs stating, have never failed to notice that numerous deities, saints, seers or other figures (such as the scapegoat) have been seen as instrumental in protecting the health of the city, either by averting disease or by dispelling it when it has arrived, through miracle, sacrifice or purification. Nor have such historians ignored the ways in which city populations have variously found a 'strategy for collective health' in seeking to appease their divinities through invocations or processions.[67] What is lacking, I think, is a general willingness to integrate such topics from the history of religion more fully into that of public health as it is usually

---

[66] S. Feierman, quoted in Ranger and Slack, *Epidemics and Ideas*, pp. 247–8. See also S. Feierman, 'Struggles for Control: The Social Roots of Health and Healing in Modern Africa', *African Studies Review*, 28 (1985), 117–18; G. Waite, 'Public Health in Pre-Colonial East-Central Africa', in S. Feierman and J.M. Janzen (eds), *The Social Basis of Health and Healing in Africa* (Berkeley, Los Angles and Oxford, 1992), pp. 212–31, on rainmaking and sorcery control.

[67] See from among a vast potential bibliography, Parker, *Miasma*, pp. 7–8. E. Kearns, 'Saving the City', in O. Murray and S. Price (eds), *The Greek City* (Oxford, 1990), pp. 323–44, esp. pp. 335–6 on the scapegoat; Palmer, 'The Church, Leprosy and Plague'; P. Burke, *The Historical Anthropology of Early Modern Italy* (Cambridge, 1987), pp. 210–11.

conceived. The example set by some early modernists has not been widely followed.[68]

The last part of this chapter, therefore, strays chronologically outside the early Middle Ages to offer some partial indication of how we might proceed. The theme remains the intersection of 'material' and 'ritual' conceptions of public health, especially as they bear on the perception or management of urban space.

One obvious body of evidence to investigate is biblical and Talmudic. Indeed, this argument against medical materialism would have been easier to frame if its examples had been drawn from Jewish history. So many Jewish communities, from biblical times onward, seem to have adopted centrally directed and enforced collective 'health' policies. These included not only well-known preventive measures such as ritual hygiene, dietary observance, and the proper disposal of the dead, all of them the legal responsibility of every individual – and all of them measures which have stoutly resisted materialist interpretation. The policies also embraced a subtle range of responses to pestilence.[69] According to the Book of Numbers (16.46–8), for example, during the epidemic that followed the rebellion of Korah, Aaron (at Moses' command) took fire from the altar onto his censer and added incense, as an atonement. He then ran into the middle of the congregation. In a manner that resonates with the hagiography cited above, he stood as a symbolic barrier between the living and the dead (meaning, perhaps, the healthy and the infected). The plague was stayed. In the Mishnah and Talmud – to draw a simplified composite picture – an epidemic was defined in a precise and sophisticated manner in terms of a certain mortality rate. Its presence was to be reported to the sages, 'community leaders'. The shofar was to be blown, to warn the population but also, perhaps, to call upon the Lord for help. A public fast was to be ordained. Non-religious responses were also permissible, flight among them.

Rather than pursue the better-known rabbinic material, let me take one instance of what might be seen as a preventive health measure that has been brought to light only relatively recently, from the fringes of the ancient Jewish world. The text in question comes from the Dead Sea Scrolls famously deposited by that ascetic Jewish sect widely (though not uncontroversially)

---

[68]   For example, numerous works by Carlo Cipolla; Palmer and Burke as in previous note.

[69]   What follows is based on the classic, J. Preuss, *Biblical and Talmudic Medicine*, first published 1911, trans. F. Rosner (repr. Northvale, NJ, and London, 1993); J. Neusner, *A History of the Mishnaic Law of Purities* (Leiden, 1974–77); and N. Zilber and S. Kottek, 'Pestilence in Bible and Talmud: Some Aspects related to Public Health', *Koroth*, 9 (1985), 249–61, and 151–3. For *Numbers*, see M. Douglas, *The Doctrine of Defilement in the Book of Numbers*, Journal for the Study of the Old Testament Supplement Series 158 (Sheffield, 1993), ch. 7. For the key medieval figure see F. Rosner, 'Moses Maimonides and Preventive Medicine', *Journal of the History of Medicine and Allied Sciences*, 51 (1996), 318.

identified with the Essenes. One discourse has been deciphered about the necessity of destroying a house in which mildew has appeared. It was written in code, which is hardly to be expected of a public health measure. But the provisional specialist hypothesis is that texts of this kind were early drafts of fundamental teachings, prepared for the *Maskil* or Guardian of the community as a preliminary to being fully authorised as doctrine. Medical materialists have already picked up the scent, identifying the mildew with the potentially lethal contaminant *Stachybotrys atra*, and interpreting that in turn as the cause of the Tenth Plague of Egypt. It remains to be seen whether the explanation lies here or – more likely given the discourse's apparent descent from Leviticus (14.34–53) – in the realm of religious history.[70]

My next examples are Roman, and that might seem otiose. For the major cities of the empire, Rome itself especially, are given an honourable place in all outline histories of pre-modern public health, for their aqueducts, baths, lavatories and sewers.[71] On a crude biological scale it is, of course, easy to cut such achievements down to size. Rome, it turns out, was no more or less hygienic and healthy than any other pre-industrial metropolis.[72] And no one has demonstrated this better than Alex Scobie. But, in the present 'non-biological' context, what deserves most emphasis in his rightly influential paper is the following comment:

> There was no legal obligation for a homeowner to connect his dwelling to a public street sewer … Extant Roman law is silent on the question of where domestic latrines were to be situated and how they were to be constructed. *The Romans were legally more concerned about the intramural burial of the dead than they were about the disposal of human and animal wastes within the city.*[73]

The relevant point is not that the much-vaunted public sewers had only a limited effect on the population as a whole. (If connected to too many dwellings the sewers would stink and might back up; and in any case human manure was too valuable to be flushed away.) The point is rather that, in the

---

[70]   S.J. Pfann, paper read to 1997 Jerusalem Qumran conference; *New York Times*, 27 July and 1 August 1997.
[71]   See also J. Scarborough, 'Roman Medicine and Public Health', in T. Ogawa (ed.), *Public Health* (Tokyo, 1981), pp. 33–74. A.T. Hodge, *Roman Aqueducts and Water Supply* (London, 1992). Cf. E.J. Gowers, 'The Anatomy of Rome from Capitol to Cloaca', *Journal of Roman Studies*, 85 (1995), 23–32.
[72]   For demographic analysis see B.D. Shaw, 'Seasons of Death: Aspects of Mortality in Imperial Rome', *Journal of Roman Studies*, 86 (1996), 100–138.
[73]   A. Scobie, 'Slums, Sanitation and Mortality in the Roman World', *Klio*, 68 (1986), 399–433, at 409, my italics. See, however, R. Laurence, 'Writing the Roman Metropolis', in H.M. Parkins (ed.), *Roman Urbanism: Beyond the Consumer City* (London, 1997), pp. 11–14, for some criticism of Scobie's method and his anachronistic standards of hygiene.

eyes of the legislators, the 'ritual' pollution of the dead – the human waste in the form of corpses given intramural burial – was of greater moment than the material pollution of the living: human waste in the form of excrement. Excrement could after all be medicinal as well as good for agriculture; bodies were dangerous, and remained so until the empire had been Christianised.

Analogous points can be made about that other focus of Rome's presumed achievement in public hygiene, the baths. Among the deities most frequently represented in the statuary of ancient *thermae* were Asclepius and Hygieia. And baths were, indeed, seen as salubrious. That is why the sick came to them, probably in considerable numbers.[74] The Emperor Hadrian reportedly ordered that the sick alone should use the baths before the eighth hour, ostensibly to separate them from the healthy.[75] But he did not, it seems, prohibit the sick from also bathing *after* the eighth hour and thus mixing with the healthy; and before this measure, if it was ever actually taken, both had presumably used the baths simultaneously. The physician Celsus advised resort to the public baths for the cure of a range of ailments, including worms, dysentery, gonorrhoea, psoriasis and bowel troubles. When it came to infected wounds, though, he counselled caution. One should avoid treating these in the baths – out of concern not for other bathers, but for the patient. The bath water, Celsus says, renders a wound dirty.[76]

Such was Roman ethno-hygiene. On materialist criteria, the Romans cannot be rated very highly. Once again, a far greater danger than biological infection was perceived, a danger of an immaterial kind. The bath could be the setting of magical practices – curses and love charms alike might be thrown into the water. The bath was also the haunt of the souls of the dead and of demons.[77] The apocryphal Acts of John includes the story of a demon that religiously (as one might say) strangled a young bather of either sex three times a year. Similar stories of demons who torture or kill bathers are to be found in the hagiography of Gregory of Tours: Christianised versions of a very ancient theme.

Like human waste, then, baths belong as much to the topography of ritual pollution and supernatural danger as they do to that of somatic health. And it was the former topography that preoccupied the elites of ancient cities. The aedile, the foremost of several Roman officials some of whose functions loosely corresponded to those of modern public health inspectors, was more concerned with the city's morals than with its drains.

---

[74] Scobie, 'Slums', 425.
[75] *Historia Augusta*, Life of Hadrian, 22.7.
[76] Celsus, *de Medicina*, 5.26.28C.
[77] For references supporting what follows, K.M.D. Dunbabin, *'Baiarum Grata Voluptas*: Pleasures and Dangers of the Baths', *Proceedings of the British School at Rome*, n.s. 44 (1989), 35–7.

> The tide of ordure that laps at the feet of Roman civilization is
> simultaneously physical ... and moral. The aediles maintained symbolic
> as well as literal purity.[78]

The haunts of pleasure – places for drinking, eating, and commercial sex – not
blocked sewers or leaking aqueducts, are the places that, as Seneca has it, 'fear
the aedile'.[79] And, on Andrew Wallace-Hadrill's seductive reconstruction, the
power of élite ideology could translate into a progressive zoning of a city such
as Pompeii (and by implication others less well known) so that immoral and
thus polluting occupations were excluded from the city's dignified public
spaces. In such a moral topography the bath – abode of Venus as well as
Hygieia – held a suitably ambiguous position. In Pompeii,

> the façade of the Stabian baths looks nobly onto that part of the Via
> dell'Abbondanza which seems to have a special status; the back entrance
> leads within a few yards to the biggest brothel in town.[80]

Such means of purifying urban space were not the preserve of antiquity and the
Middle Ages. 'With the onset of a terrible epidemic ... the ... senate passed
two decrees intended to clear particular quarters of the city of the beggars
infesting them.' The first decree seemed wholly dedicated to placating the
deity's wrath, of which the epidemic was an unmistakable sign. 'It strove to
create three regions of special holiness, like powerhouses of piety spaced at
intervals across the city.' The senate was Venetian, not Roman; the year,
1630.[81] The three regions lay respectively around the doge's chapel – St Mark's
– the symbolic centre of the city; around the church of San Rocco, the relevant
patron saint; and around the cathedral of San Pietro di Castello.

> In all three holy places the sacrament was to be exposed for adoration
> and to be accompanied at intervals around the immediate neighbourhood,
> as though its effluvia were being sent forth to combat the insidious force
> of the plague.[82]

---

[78]   A. Wallace-Hadrill, 'Public Honour and Private Shame: The Urban Texture of
Pompeii', in T.J. Cornell and K. Lomas (eds), *Urban Society in Roman Italy* (London, 1995),
p. 51. See also R. Laurence, *Roman Pompeii: Space and Society* (London and New York,
1994), ch. 5. On aediles and public health, O.F. Robinson, *Ancient Rome: City Planning and
Administration* (London, 1992), pp. 118–26.

[79]   *On the Truly Happy Life*, 7.3.

[80]   Wallace-Hadrill, 'Public Honour', p. 55.

[81]   B. Pullan, 'Plague and Perceptions of the Poor in Early Modern Italy', in Slack and
Ranger, *Epidemics and Ideas*, pp. 101–2. For 'moral sanitation' as a medieval response to
plague, in Venice and Florence, see A.G. Carmichael, *Plague and the Poor in Renaissance
Florence* (Cambridge, 1986), pp. 98–9, 125.

[82]   Pullan, 'Plague', p. 102.

The boards of magistrates charged with suppressing blasphemy, gambling and other forms of loose living were reminded to do their duty. And, as decreed, the polluting poor were moved on.

Conclusion: secularisation?

All this happened at a time when public health officials and priests had already often come into conflict in Renaissance Italian cities, chiefly on the question of whether the spiritual benefits of processions outweighed the enhanced risk of contagion.[83] So it might seem that, although ritual remained integral to public health in early modern Venice, there had been a good deal of secularisation in perceptions of the subject since classical times. Snapshots of the history of processions across a millennium could be offered as supporting evidence. First exposure: when Pope Gregory the Great ordained a procession in sixth-century Rome, the fact that eighty participants dropped dead was apparently in no way to his discredit. Rather than suggesting that processions enhanced contagion, it proved the urgent necessity for them. Second exposure: when the Black Death reached Avignon, some 750 years later, Pope Clement VI showed himself a true medical pluralist. He banned processions of flagellants, but not on medical grounds; rather, because of their revolutionary zeal. The pope granted indulgences to clergy ministering to the dying, and he instituted a special mass to implore an end to the epidemic. Severe measures were, however, also taken to limit contagion, and physicians were hired to care for the sick.[84] In 1630, by contrast, the year of those Venetian purifications – third exposure – Pope Urban VIII (the one who set the Inquisition on Galileo) responded to a torrent of clerical complaints about secular interference in processions and liturgies by excommunicating the entire Florentine health office.[85] The medical and the religious conceptions of public health were by then distinguishable, as they do not seem to have been in antiquity or for much of the Middle Ages.

Even without the benefit of such snapshots, the history of public health in the West has conventionally been conceived in terms of a sequence of more or less progressive stages. Stage one: Rome, setting the standard. Stage two: the environmental regulations of European cities from 1250 or even earlier (sometimes prompting the suggestion that health as a public good was a

---

[83]   Palmer, 'The Church, Leprosy and Plague', pp. 95–9; J. Henderson, 'The Black Death in Florence: Medical and Communal Responses', in Bassett, *Death in Towns*, p. 144.

[84]   G. Mollat, *The Popes at Avignon 1305–1378* (London, 1963), pp. 40–41.

[85]   C.M. Cipolla, *Faith, Reason and the Plague* (Sussex, 1979), p. 6.

novelty at the time).[86] Stage three: the segregation of lepers. Stage four: the secularist plague measures of the Italian city-states. Stage five: Enlightened medical 'police'. Then, stimulated by industrialisation, stage six: modern public health, the concept and the administrative category with which we are still familiar.

It could appear that adding the religious dimension to this account of the origins of modern social hygiene would leave the overall evolution intact. The gap in the narrative between the Roman empire and the Italian city-states would be reassuringly filled. And the medieval to early modern phase of the story would then be one not so much of development *ex nihilo* but instead, perhaps, of a slow 'separation of powers', a process which the history of plague measures has been taken to illustrate vividly.[87] Sophisticating the narrative in this way obviously has much to be said in its favour. Yet is doing so quite enough? According to legend, the ancient philosopher Empedocles had the course of two rivers altered to purify a third one, the emanations from which were poisoning the citizens of Selinus. His success was so complete that the citizens acclaimed him as a god – to confirm them in which he leapt, alas fatally, into the flames of Mount Etna.[88] The legend anticipates Hocart. In the beginning, it seems to say, public health is very much to do with the sacred; its officials seem god-like. Yet public health is also depicted in the very practical terms of civil engineering, pretensions to real divinity being dramatically punctured. The religious and the material are already intertwined.

Ancient anecdotes such as that one, no less than the other sources that I have been looking at – Jewish, Roman, Frankish and Venetian – imply that the story of public health cannot altogether be told in simple linear terms. Its religious and ritual aspects resist being confined to the earlier Middle Ages. They do not belong exclusively to a gloomy interlude in a chronicle of otherwise growing enlightenment. They are evident at the story's very beginning. And recent clinical studies suggest that secularism has not yet quite triumphed. Apparently 'religion is good for you', both mentally and physically; one controlled experiment even found that the prayer of others may benefit hospitalised heart patients unaware of the intercession. Like historians, perhaps, 'public health

---

[86]   L. García-Ballester, 'Changes in the *Regimina Sanitatis*: the Role of the Jewish Physicians', in S. Campbell et al. (eds), *Health, Disease and Healing in Medieval Culture* (Basingstoke and London, 1992), p. 120; R.E. Zupko and R.A. Laures, *Straws in the Wind: Medieval Urban Environmental Law – The Case of Northern Italy* (Boulder, CO, and Oxford, 1996).

[87]   Arrizabalaga, 'Facing the Black Death', pp. 250–51.

[88]   Diogenes Laertius, *Lives of the Eminent Philosophers*, 8.70. For context, J. Bidez, *La Biographie d'Empédocle* (Ghent, 1894, repr. 1973).

professionals will have to re-examine long-held assumptions regarding the appropriate roles of science and faith in matters of health'.[89]

[89]   For an introduction to the now substantial literature on the 'epidemiology of religion' see J.S. Levin et al., 'Religious Involvement, Health Outcomes, and Public Health Practice', *Current Issues in Public Health*, 2 (1996), 220–25; my final quotation is from p. 223. Also valuable is J. Gartner, 'Religious Commitment, Mental Health, and Prosocial Behavior: a Review of the Empirical Literature', in E.P. Shafranske (ed.), *Religion and the Clinical Practice of Psychology* (Washington, DC, 1996), pp. 187–214.

IV

Religion as Medicine:
Music in Medieval Hospitals[1]

Around the time that the Normans were settling into their newly-conquered kingdom, and Archbishop Lanfranc was establishing the earliest hospital for the poor in England,[2] the revered Persian mystic, al-Hujwiri, set down the following description of hospital practice in Byzantium:

> It is well known that in the hospitals of Rum they have invented a wonderful thing which they call *angalyun*; the Greeks call anything that is very marvellous by this name, for example the Gospel and the Books of Mani. The word signifies 'promulgation of a decree'. This *angalyun* resembles the gut strings [of a musical instrument]. The sick are brought to it two days a week and are forced to listen while it is being played, for a length of time proportionate to the malady from which they suffer; then they are taken away. If it is desired to kill anyone, he is kept there for a longer period until he dies . . . [euthanasia?] Physicians and others may listen continually to the *angalyun* without being affected in any way, because it is consistent with their temperament.[3]

Hujwiri was writing either somewhere in Iraq, or in Lahore, whither he was taken in captivity and where he ended his days within a few years after 1072.[4] His account appears unexpectedly towards the end of a treatise on Sufi mysticism. He purposes to illustrate the potentially dangerous effects of music on the uninitiated (here the patients; the physicians are the adepts). Hujwiri had travelled all around the Middle East, including Syria. He could have seen Christian charitable institutions within the 'land of Islam' or

---

[1] This paper was read in draft, to its lasting benefit, by Carole Rawcliffe and John Henderson, who both also allowed me to profit from their forthcoming publications. Emilie Savage-Smith gave unstinting assistance with Arabic. Rebecca Flemming advised authoritatively about late Antique Galenism. Surviving errors and perversities are, of course, my own.
[2] As distinct from a monastic infirmary. See A. Meaney, 'The Practice of Medicine in England about the Year 1000', in *The Year 1000*, pp. 221–37; N. Orme and M. Webster, *The English Hospital 1070–1570* (New Haven and London, 1995), pp. 19–23.
[3] Hujwiri, *Kashf al-mahjub*, abridged trans. R. A. Nicholson, *The Oldest Persian Treatise on Sufiism*, E. J. W. Gibb Memorial Series 17, 2nd edn (London, 1935), ch. 24, pp. 407–8 (modified, with the kind assistance of Emilie Savage-Smith).
[4] See also Dols, *Majnun*, p. 170.

received reports of Byzantine ones from travellers. There was, moreover, no need for him to invent such a striking example to make his point. As the remainder of his chapter on *sama'* (listening) shows, he had many anecdotes from closer to home at his disposal.

None the less, for all its specious authenticity the vignette is puzzling. The *angalyun*, which clearly derives from the Greek *euaggelion* (gospel), appears to have been Hujwiri's coinage.[5] In Persian dictionaries it is defined as silk of changing colour, a species of brocade so called because of the type of material in which Eastern Christians wrapped their gospel books; but that hardly illuminates Hujwiri's usage.[6] Nor is there anything in the patristic or Byzantine definition of *euaggelion* which could have prompted the assimilation of 'gospel' to 'decree' and, yet more improbably, to the books of Mani and instrumental 'gut strings'.[7] Some hint of what prompted this semantic virtuosity may emerge later on. For the moment, I should simply like to use Hujwiri's vignette as a way of opening up and delimiting a field of investigation. Whatever the veracity of his sources, Hujwiri conveys the perception that there was, in Byzantium, some affinity between cultic practice, prescribing for patients (the 'decree'?), and music – between religion and medicine. Still more to my point, he locates this affinity within a hospital.

This paper is about religion as medicine. It is, therefore, not about medicine as a metaphor within religious discourse, or the theology implicit in medical ideology, or the relations between churchmen and doctors.[8] It looks at a domain in which the distinction between medicine and religion is difficult, a domain to which terms such as 'ambiguity' and 'overlap' are more appropriate than 'tension', the detection of which has driven much of the subject's historiography.[9] To exemplify this ambiguous domain, the paper offers a broad-brush depiction of the use of music in medieval hospitals. It compares the three medical traditions that derived from that of Classical Antiquity – Islamic, Byzantine, and western European, with the emphasis on the last of the three – not from the vantage point of musicology or religious history so much as from that of a theory in which religion can, sometimes, be perceived as medicinal.[10]

---

[5] There is no entry for it in *A Greek and Arabic Lexicon: Materials for a Dictionary of the Medieval Translations from Greek into Arabic*, ed. G. Endress and D. Gutas (Leiden 1992–).

[6] F. Johnson, *Dictionary: Persian, Arabic, and English* (London, 1852), p. 179; F. Steingass, *Persian–English Dictionary* (London, 1892), p. 115, both s.v. *anqalyun*. See also L. Ibsen al Faruqi, *An Annotated Glossary of Arabic Musical Terms* (Westport, CT, 1981), p. 4. I owe these references to Emilie Savage-Smith.

[7] *A Greek Patristic Lexicon*, ed. G. W. H. Lampe (Oxford, 1961), and *Greek Lexicon of the Roman and Byzantine Periods*, ed. E. A. Sophocles (Boston, 1870), s.v. *euaggelion*.

[8] Cf. for example Ziegler, *Medicine and Religion*.

[9] Amundsen, *Medicine, Society, and Faith*.

[10] I have drawn encouragement from ethnographic accounts of medico-religious healthcare systems to which music is central: e.g. S. M. Friedson, 'Dancing the Disease: Music and Trance in Tumbuka Healing', in *Musical Healing in Cultural Contexts*, ed. P. Gouk (Aldershot, 2000), pp. 67–84.

I

Until recently, that project would have kicked against the pricks. Medical historians have understandably identified their subject more or less with the history of doctors – elite 'dead white male' doctors at that. Such men were responsible for most of the evidence of medical thought and practice that survives from the Middle Ages. Through it, they speak to us of their zeal for Aristotelian learning, their concern for professional respectability, and their growing authority in matters previously left to the determination of laymen, such as the diagnosis of leprosy or sanctity.[11] Of course, the cultural and social history of medical scholasticism is an essential topic for medievalists.[12] But its pursuit should not entail that we view the medieval medical world solely in the way that the scholastics' literary legacy invites. Partly as a result of the accomplishments paraded in that legacy, partly (I assume) because of our own inescapable awareness of how modern biomedicine proceeds, we tend to privilege diagnosis and active treatment over prognosis and regimen.[13] It takes an effort of will, not to mention considerable patience in searching the evidence, for a medical historian to offer a narrative of a medieval doctor whose skill lay in doing nothing but making predictions – and in facilitating a 'good death'.[14] A second temptation of the scholastic legacy against which we should guard is to take the university physicians always at their own self-estimation, as the only healers who really mattered. If, as Hugh Trevor-Roper once urged, we roll back the linoleum of time and observe the teeming life that lies beneath, then we begin to detect the activity of numerous female healers – the first and largest casualty of scholasticism triumphant, as well as of contemporary chauvinism more generally.[15] A range of empirics then becomes noticeable: healers by no means necessarily unlettered.[16] Finally, we catch sight of nurses and others attending the sick: men and women whose exertions were so demeaned by university-type physicians, and who are, for that and related reasons, so poorly documented, that only lately has their medieval history begun to be written.[17]

[11] M. R. McVaugh, *Medicine before the Plague: Practitioners and their Patients in the Crown of Aragon, 1285–1345* (Cambridge, 1993), pp. 218–25; Ziegler, 'Practitioners and Saints'.

[12] See now Jacquart, *Médecine médiévale*.

[13] *Western Medical Thought* is unusual among recent synopses in devoting a chapter to regimen.

[14] F. Getz, *Medicine in the English Middle Ages* (Princeton, 1998), pp. 3–4, on the last illness of Archbishop Hubert Walter and his 'non-treatment' by Gilbertus Anglicus as reported by Ralph of Coggeshall, *Chronicon Anglicanum*, ed. J. Stevenson, RS 66 (London, 1875), pp. 156–9.

[15] Green, 'Documenting'.

[16] K. Park, 'Stones, Bones and Hernias: Surgical Specialists in Fourteenth- and Fifteenth-Century Italy', in *Medicine from the Black Death to the French Disease*, ed. R. French et al. (Cambridge, 1998), pp. 110–30.

[17] Rawcliffe, 'Hospital Nurses'.

The topic of nursing naturally brings me back to hospitals. Here anti-scholastic revisionism is still more inchoate. Attention has largely been absorbed by whether or not hospitals had doctors on their staffs. Florence carries off the prize for precocity; England trails in last, with the Savoy hospital.[18] Medicalization of this kind – medicalization in the literal sense of the arrival of *medici* – is presented as the one development that really mattered. It is also presented, for the most part, as a development *ex nihilo*, on the assumption that nothing else preceding it was really medicine. Medicalization becomes, indeed, the leitmotif of an implicit teleological narrative – of the victory of cure over care, of doctors over nurses, and (again) of treatment over regimen.

The work of Carole Rawcliffe and John Henderson, on English and Florentine hospitals respectively, subverts this teleology: so, at least, I read the fruits of their research.[19] Contrast the hospital of Santa Maria Nuova with that of St Giles, Norwich (the 'Great Hospital' as it became after the Reformation). Santa Maria Nuova had its retained corps of physicians who admitted only patients with acute but not life-threatening conditions and discharged them rapidly. St Giles helped the chronically sick and elderly to live out their days in minimum pain. The contrast could hardly be starker. The future of hospitals seems to lie on one side, the Tuscan side; their past on the other, in East Anglia. Yet this contrast, as Rawcliffe and Henderson remind us, is surprisingly superficial. More importantly, both hospitals were religious institutions, with liturgy at their heart.[20] Patients in both lay within sight of the sacrament on the altar. In both, their daily life was punctuated far more deeply by the monastic 'hours' than by the 'ward round'. Exposure to the host, even without reception;[21] regular confession[22] (without which the

[18] K. Park and J. Henderson, '"The First Hospital among Christians": The Ospedale di Santa Maria Nuova in Early Sixteenth-Century Florence', *Medical History* 35 (1991), 164–88; *The Hospital in History*, ed. L. Granshaw and R. Porter (London and New York, 1989), chs. 1–3.

[19] Rawcliffe, 'Medicine for the Soul' and *Medicine for the Soul*; J. Henderson, 'Splendide case di cura: spedali, medicina ed assistenza a Firenze nel trecento', in *Ospedali e città: L'Italia del Centro-Nord, XIII–XVI secolo*, ed. A. J. Grieco and L. Sandri (Florence, 1997), pp. 15–50. I am grateful to Dr Henderson for allowing me to read some of the typescript of his *The Renaissance Hospital* (forthcoming).

[20] Rawcliffe, *Medicine for the Soul*, ch. 4 and 'The Eighth Comfortable Work: Education and the Medieval English Hospital', in *The Church and Learning in Late Medieval Society*, ed. J. Stratford and C. Barron (Stamford, forthcoming), generously shown to me in typescript by the author. Henderson, 'Splendide case', p. 48; Saunier, *'Le pauvre malade'*, ch. 3. I am also indebted to forthcoming work by Christopher Page on hospitals' collections of liturgical music.

[21] K. Thomas, *Religion and the Decline of Magic*, Penguin edn (Harmondsworth, 1973), pp. 36, 39; Rawcliffe, 'Medicine for the Soul', p. 319.

[22] Saunier, *'Le pauvre malade'*, pp. 112–13; F. Kudlien, 'Beichte und Heilung', *Medizinhistorisches Journal* 13 (1978), 1–14. In the sixteenth century Alvise Luisini claimed that physicians could detect objective physical improvements in patients who had confessed one day previously. The psychological freedom from anxiety which the confession produced led directly to better health, including the remission of fever.

hospital would be contaminated by sin);[23] the proximity of relics, their power absorbed either in a single dramatic moment or more slowly and osmotically;[24] contemplation of devotional pictures with their appropriate symbolism of the sure avenue to health;[25] the prayers and Christian magic of nurses;[26] the pleasing ambience of gardens and (sometimes) water courses:[27] all these possible features of hospital life, mentioned by Rawcliffe and Henderson and a few like-minded students of medieval hospitals, erode the starkness of the contrast between England and Italy. They suggest to me a characterization of the hospital less in terms of the presence or absence of doctors and more as a 'total therapeutic environment'.

It is within this approach that I locate my focus on hospital music. I want to use that topic to push the analyses offered by Rawcliffe and Henderson further, and in two directions. One direction is medieval: it leads to the background theory of this environmental view of hospital therapy. The other is modern: conceptual in a different way. It is an attempt to break down the dualism that still seems to order our thinking about such matters as the role of the Mass in the promotion of well-being. We speak of *medicina sacramentalis* or 'medicine of the soul' as against secular medicine; we juxtapose *medicina del corpo e medicina dell'anima*, in a manner which, although apparently justified by many medieval texts, is surely too Cartesian to be without anachronism.[28] The subtext we mistakenly attribute to such binary categorization is, first, that 'sacramental medicine' ministers only to the soul

See R. Palmer, 'The Church, Leprosy and Plague in Medieval and Early Modern Europe', SCH 19 (1982), 79–99 (p. 86), citing [A.] Luisini, *Tractatus de confessione a die decubitus instituenda* (Venice, 1563), pp. 74–5. See also Ralph of Coggeshall, *Chronicon Anglicanum*, ed. Stevenson, p. 158, on the therapeutic effect of the final confession of Hubert Walter.

[23] A composition between St John's Hospital, Bruges, and its chaplain stressed that the latter must meet his obligation to confess each patient on arrival: if just one sin 'slipped through', the whole house would be imperilled: E. van der Elst, *L'Hôpital Saint-Jean de Bruges de 1188 à 1500* (Bruges, 1975), pp. 61–2, a reference I owe to Carole Rawcliffe.

[24] Rawcliffe, 'Medicine for the Soul', p. 325; Orme and Webster, *The English Hospital*, p. 56; Saunier, 'Le pauvre malade', pp. 114–17.

[25] R. A. Koch, 'Flower Symbolism in the Portinari Altarpiece', *Art Bulletin* 46 (1964), 76–7, a reference I owe to John Henderson. See also A. Hayum, *The Isenheim Altarpiece: God's Medicine and the Painter's Vision* (Princeton, 1989); Thomas, *Religion*, p. 29; M.-L. Windemuth, *Das Hospital als Träger der Armenfürsorge im Mittelalter*, Sudhoffs Archiv, Beiheft 36 (Stuttgart, 1995).

[26] Rawcliffe, 'Medicine for the Soul', p. 323.

[27] Rawcliffe, 'Hospital Nurses', pp. 58–9; R. Gilchrist, *Contemplation and Action: The Other Monasticism* (London and New York, 1995), p. 43.

[28] J. Agrimi and C. Crisciani, *Medicina del corpo e medicina dell'anima: note sul sapere del medico fina all'inizio del secolo XIII* (Milan, 1978); Rawcliffe, *Medicine for the Soul*, pp. 160–1. See also Agrimi and Crisciani, 'Charity and Aid', pp. 174–6. Note also the title of Risse, *Mending Bodies, Saving Souls: A History of Hospitals*. For an early, seemingly Cartesian, statement of the theme, see *Acts of Thomas* 95, trans. M. R. James, *The Apocryphal New Testament* (Oxford, 1924), p. 406.

while secular medicine assists only the body; second, that sacramental 'medicine' is not quite 'real' medicine in the familiar (that is, modern) sense – which of course doctors alone can administer. The 'psycho-somaticism' of ancient and medieval thought – *corpus sanum de mente sana* as it might be – is downplayed. Rigorists in medical matters, like St Bernard, might have approved of that.[29] The Fathers gathered at the Fourth Lateran Council (1215) would have been less pleased. For them, famously, 'sickness of the body may sometimes be the result of sin', and spiritual health improves the response to secular medicine, not least because it could banish the pathogenic fear of death.[30]

II

The best evidence in medieval medical history always seems to come from the east. Hospital music-making of expressly therapeutic intent is exemplified for us most fully in the large Islamic hospitals of medieval and Ottoman times. The first surviving discussion of music in hospitals which treats Byzantium as precursor is not Hujwiri's; it is the 'epistle' on music of the 'Brethren of Purity' (*Ikhwan al-Safa'*), a fraternity that flourished in Basra in the second half of the tenth century and dedicated to the pursuit of holiness and truth, especially the truth of (ancient) Greek science.[31] Its members composed a vast encyclopaedia in the form of fifty-two epistles with a summary. That dealing with music asserts that the Greek philosophers

> also invented another melody which they used in the hospitals, at the break of day, and which had the virtue of solacing the pains due to the infirmities and ills suffered by the patient, alleviating their violence and even curing certain sicknesses and infirmities.[32]

The therapeutic power of hospital music came to seem quite uncontroversial. In the mid-eleventh century Sa'id ibn Bakhtishu', of the famous Baghdad medical family, could take it for granted in his treatise on medicine that patients' psychological problems – the quieting of their nerves – would be

---

[29] Bernard of Clairvaux, *The Steps of Humility*, trans. G. B. Birch (Cambridge, MA, 1942), pp. 58–60, cited by Ziegler, *Medicine and Religion*, p. 225 n. 34.

[30] Canon 22, trans. N. Tanner, *Decrees of the Ecumenical Councils*, 2 vols. (Washington, DC, 1990), I, 245–6.

[31] A. Shiloah, 'Jewish and Muslim Traditions of Music Therapy', in *Music as Medicine: The History of Music Therapy since Antiquity*, ed. P. Horden (Aldershot, 2000), pp. 69–83 (pp. 73–4, 80–1), and *Music in the World of Islam: A Socio-Cultural Study* (Aldershot, 1995), pp. 50–1; Dols, *Majnun*, pp. 170–1.

[32] 'The Epistle on Music of the Ikwan al-Safa', trans. A. Shiloah, *Documentation and Studies 3: Department of Musicology and the Chaim Rosenberg School of Jewish Studies* (Tel Aviv, 1978), pp. 16–17, repr. in Shiloah, *The Dimension of Music in Islamic and Jewish Culture*, CS393 (Aldershot, 1993), article III.

addressed in hospitals by the performance of, among other things, entertaining song.[33]

Those are generalized testimonies, prescriptive in character. There is, though, some medieval evidence of music in specific foundations. One of the designated expenditures at the Mansuri hospital in Cairo, founded by the Sultan al-Mansur in 1284, was for troupes of musicians who would entertain the patients daily. At the hospital founded at the behest of the Mamluk sultan, al-Nasir, in Aleppo in 1354, music was played in the courtyards for the benefit of the inmates.[34] For a more detailed account of such performances and their therapeutic rationale, however, we have to wait until Ottoman times and the report of the noted seventeenth-century traveller, Evliya Chelebi.[35] Musicians, he tells us, were employed at the hospital of Muhammad II (d. 1481) to amuse the sick and, especially, to cure the insane patients. At the Nuri hospital in Damascus, which Evliya visited in 1648, concerts were reportedly given thrice daily. At the Edirne hospital established by Bayezid II, three singers and seven musicians visited the hospital three times a week.[36] We should not assume from pronouncements in modern synopses, about the hostility to music of orthodox Islam, that these hospital performances can never have been religious in character.[37]

It is all reminiscent of the intense musical life of some asylums in eighteenth- and nineteenth-century Europe.[38] We should be careful, though, not to splice scattered references in partisan accounts too tightly together and make of them a hospital tradition. Music therapy of this lavish and expensive kind may have been the prerogative of the wealthiest patients and could, overall, have been very occasional, no matter what Evliya says. Of the application of music therapy as a regular element in the physician's armoury we have no direct evidence. The oldest and largest collection of case histories from the Islamic Middle East, that compiled by students of Rhazes (al-Razi) in the early tenth century, makes no mention of the use of music.[39] Rhazes was successively director of two hospitals, in Rayy and Baghdad; and, if his casebook reflects his hospital practice at all, then the fullest evocation we have of hospital medicine would contradict several of the references just assembled.

The Islamic material is important here because it illustrates not so much a

[33] *Über die Heilung der Krankheiten der Seele und des Körpers*, ed. and trans. F. Klein-Franke (Beirut, 1977), fol. 74b (trans. p. 57, modified Savage-Smith).

[34] Dols, *Majnun*, pp. 121, 171.

[35] Shiloah, 'Jewish and Muslim Traditions of Music Therapy', p. 75.

[36] Dols, *Majnun*, pp. 171, 173.

[37] Shiloah, *Music in the World of Islam*, ch. 4; J. C. Bürgel, *The Feather of Simurgh: The 'Licit Magic' of the Arts in Medieval Islam* (New York and London, 1988), ch. 4. See also Dols, *Majnun*, p. 172.

[38] C. Kramer, 'Music as Cause and Cure of Illness in Nineteenth-Century Europe', in *Music as Medicine*, pp. 338–52 (pp. 348–9).

[39] C. Álvarez-Millán, 'Practice versus Theory: Tenth-Century Case Histories from the Islamic Middle East', in *The Year 1000*, pp. 293–306.

solid tradition as a 'horizon of expectation', a cultural possibility. Medieval Islamic scholars seized on the full range of Antiquity's theoretical legacy concerning music therapy: a collection of anecdotes attributing astonishing feats to Pythagoras and other sages, a theory of the educative ethos of particular types of music; the cosmological explanation of musical healing in terms of an 'attunement' of the individual to the 'harmony of the spheres' through the intermediary of *musica instrumentalis*. All this was taken up and elaborated into a comprehensive alignment of zodiacal signs, planets, tones, elements, and bodily humours.[40] One can see why Hujwiri, and also the Brethren of Purity,[41] should have held Greek – and presumably, by extension, Byzantine – example dear. According to Ibn Abi Usaybi'ah, the first medical men were the Greeks who invented the reed pipe and healed body and soul with their playing.[42] The debt to Galen above all, but also to Rufus of Ephesus, ensured that much attention would be given in Islam to 'psychiatry', a therapy directed at the mind because the mind affected the body.[43] In the increasingly available insane wards in hospitals, physical restraint (often of a brutish kind) was thus counterbalanced by music, fountains – and even alcohol.[44] Orthodox wariness of music and dancing was quietly overridden by this Galenic enthusiasm for the creation of a therapeutic environment.

On the basis of scattered passages in Galen and Hippocrates (the latter known largely through Galen's commentary), medieval Islamic physicians developed a conception of health which was to be crucial to the recommendation of music as medicine for centuries to come.[45] Its briefest exposition can be found in the work later known to Western medicine as the *Isagoge* [*Introduction*] of Johannitius (Hunayn ibn Ishaq; died *c.* 877), an Arabic synopsis so convenient that, in partial Latin translation, it was widely diffused across medieval Europe.[46] This text distinguishes between the 'naturals' (chiefly the four elements, qualities such as hot or moist, and the four humours), the 'contra-naturals' (disease, its causes and 'sequels'), and the 'non-naturals'. The last are the pertinent ones. They are the determinants of health. They include air and the environment, eating and drinking, exercise and baths,

[40] M. West, 'Music Therapy in Antiquity', and P. Horden, 'Commentary on Part II, with a Note on the Early Middle Ages', both in *Music as Medicine*, pp. 51–68, 103–8 (pp. 103–4); Shiloah, 'Jewish and Muslim Traditions of Music Therapy'.
[41] Shiloah, 'Jewish and Muslim Traditions of Music Therapy', p. 74.
[42] Dols, *Majnun*, p. 166.
[43] C. Burnett, '"Spiritual Medicine": Music and Healing in Islam and its Influence in Western Medicine', in *Musical Healing in Cultural Contexts*, ed. Gouk, pp. 85–91 (pp. 85–6); Dols, *Majnun*, chs. 1–3.
[44] Dols, *Majnun*, pp. 119–35, 165–73.
[45] Burnett, '"Spiritual Medicine"', pp. 89–90; W. F. Kümmel, *Musik und Medizin: Ihre Wechselbeziehungen in Theorie und Praxis von 800 bis 1800*, Freiburger Beiträge zur Wissenschafts- und Universitätsgeschichte 2 (Munich, 1977).
[46] 'Johannicius, Isagoge ad Techne Galieni', ed. G. Maurach in *Sudhoffs Archiv für Geschichte der Medizin* 62 (1978), 148–74.

sleep, coitus, and the 'passions [or 'accidents'] of the soul'.[47] Johannitius writes:

> Sundry affections of the mind produce an effect within the body, such as those which bring the natural heat from the interior of the body to the outer parts or the surface of the skin. Sometimes this happens suddenly, as with anger; sometimes gently and slowly, as with delight and joy . . . some affections disturb the natural energy both internal and external, as, for instance, with grief.[48]

Those sentences represent the conceptual gateway through which music comes into medicine – under the heading of 'delight and joy'. Music – of the appropriate ethos – can manipulate the accidents of the soul, emotions such as joy, or the workings of the imagination. It can mitigate those feelings that, through their impact on the humours, cause disease, and strengthen those that prevent it. The *Isagoge* is the fount of a whole tradition in Islamic medical writing of discussing 'soul medicine', psychosomatic therapy as we might call it, in terms of the regulation of this particular non-natural.[49]

III

The accidents of the soul as an ingredient in health formed, then, an idea with a future. That future in Islamic medicine is not to the point here. The future of its translated, Latin, version will be. Before I come to it, however, I want to consider whether the non-naturals in their full Islamic glory were essential to the therapeutic role in medieval hospitals which I envisage for religious music. Was the Islamic 'medicalization' of the emotions an essential precondition? Or could a vulgarized form of late Antique Galenism serve almost as well? For answer I turn back to early Byzantium. This is partly to enquire further into what might have prompted Hujwiri's misconception about Byzantine therapy, but mainly to look more generally at the beginnings of another hospital tradition and the role of medicine and music within it.

The first major philanthropic foundation in Byzantium was that of St Basil, called the Basileias by later church historians.[50] This 'new city', as it was

---

[47] For the non-naturals, see G. Olson, *Literature as Recreation in the Later Middle Ages* (Ithaca and London, 1982), pp. 40–4; L. García-Ballester, 'On the Origin of the "Six Non-Natural Things" in Galen', in *Galen und das Hellenistische Erbe*, ed. J. Kollesch and D. Nickel, Sudhoffs Archiv, Beiheft 32 (1993), pp. 105–15; P. Gil-Sotres, 'Modelo téorico y observación clínica: las pasiones del alma en la psicología medica medieval', in *Comprendre et maîtriser la nature au Moyen Age: mélanges d'histoire des sciences offerts à Guy Beaujouan* (Geneva, 1994), pp. 181–204; H. Mikkeli, *Hygiene in the Early Modern Medical Tradition* (Helsinki, 1999).

[48] *Sourcebook of Medieval Science*, pp. 708–9.

[49] Burnett, ' "Spiritual Medicine" ', pp. 88–9.

[50] Sozomen, *Historia ecclesiastica* VI.xxxiv.9; p. 291. For what follows see the summary accounts of P. Rousseau, *Basil of Caesarea* (Berkeley, Los Angeles and Oxford, 1994),

IV

lauded in the funeral oration pronounced by Gregory of Nazianzus, was a philanthropic 'multiplex' outside Basil's episcopal seat at Caesarea.[51] Gregory describes it as a centre in which disease is studied philosophically (*philosopheitai*); he makes it out to be a school of charity, an academy of compassion. The objects of its compassion were above all lepers, limbless (as they often were) victims of 'social death', expelled from all the forms and arenas of association that characterized the ancient *polis*: family, household, fraternity, assembly, bathhouse, public place, city space generally. They existed in name only since their wasted bodies could no longer individuate them. Only music, in Gregory's interesting recollection, could express their identity. They were – to the extent that the disease's ravages had left them any voice at all – 'masters of pitiful songs'.[52] Basil also lodged the transient poor, almost as unwelcome in the *polis* as were lepers, along with those (presumably) local people whose infirmity necessitated care. In a letter to the governor of Caesarea, in which Basil defended his subversion of the social priorities of the city, he anticipates those who would refuse to equate the history of medicine with the history of doctors. He does not sharply differentiate nursing from medicine: he writes, in that letter, not of doctors (*iatroi*) but of those who are doctoring (*iatrouontai*).[53] But if his physicians were amateurs (in the strict sense) from the monastery, that does not entitle us to envisage them as crass empirics with merely a few herbal panaceas in their arsenal. They had Basil's personal example to guide them into a more theoretical approach.

According to Gregory, Basil's own ill health as well as his philanthropy originally turned him towards medicine. Like Gregory, he had studied the care of the sick and medical treatment: the 'deep structure' of the discipline – 'not as far as it relates to what is visible . . . but as far as it is based on principle [*dogmatikon*] and is philosophical'.[54] We cannot know how much actual Galen Basil had read. But he presumably absorbed at least the rudiments of Hippocratic–Galenic thinking about the psychosomatic aspect

pp. 139–44; Temkin, *Hippocrates*, pp. 162–4; D. Constantelos, *Byzantine Philanthropy and Social Welfare*, 2nd edn (New Rochelle, NY, 1991), pp. 75–6, 119–20; T. Miller, *The Birth of the Hospital in the Byzantine Empire*, 2nd edn (Baltimore and London, 1997), pp. 85–8; P. van Minnen, 'Medical Care in Late Antiquity', in *Ancient Medicine in its Socio-Cultural Context*, ed. P. J. van der Eijk, H. F. J. Horstmanshoff and P. H. Schrijvers, 2 vols., The Wellcome Institute Series in the History of Medicine, Clio Medica 27–8 (Amsterdam and Atlanta, 1995), I, 153–69 (pp. 157–9). The political circumstances (and the precursors) of Basil's initiative have been re-examined by Peter Brown in his Menahem Stern Lectures (2000), 'Poverty and Leadership in the Later Roman Empire', the text of which he kindly allowed me to read in advance of its delivery.
51 Gregory of Nazianzus, *Oratio* xliii.63; *PG* 36, 577C.
52 *PG* 36, 580B, with Temkin, *Hippocrates*, p. 162.
53 Basil, *Epistulae* 94, in *Saint Basile: Lettres*, ed. Y. Courtonne, 3 vols. (Paris, 1957–66), I, 206.
54 Gregory of Nazianzus, *Oratio* xliii.23 (*PG* 36, 528B), with Temkin *Hippocrates*, ch. 13.

of health, the potentially pathogenic and the beneficial aspects of the 'accidents of the soul'. In the treatise *On the Nature of Man* (another text with a future) by Basil's near contemporary, Nemesius, bishop of Emesa in Syria, a Christianized and Aristotelian Galenism allows a large conceptual space for the physiology of the emotions and for a 'two-way' traffic between soul and body in matters of daily regimen.[55] People become ill, Basil himself wrote, when diverted from their natural state. For they are deprived of health either because of poor regimen (principally but not exclusively food and drink) or because of something morbific. In the same way the soul is made ill – diverted from its natural state – by sin. The medicine of the body is a paradigm for the therapy of the soul. It is a model conceded to us by God.[56] But that does not make the medicine of the soul a mere metaphor. It actually falls within the province of the ideal physician. Such a figure will be ambidextrous: he will not confine his art to healing the body but will seek also the cure of diseases of the soul.[57] Medicine in the relatively narrow sense of dietary prescription, medication and surgery is certainly, for Basil, a model that helps us understand a greater medicine. Yet the imperative that one should place only limited trust in physicians does not entail that medicine is to be conceived as narrowly somatic in scope. This is borne out if we turn to the more conventionally religious aspects of Basil's philanthropic initiative. Basil is, of course, a major figure in the history of Orthodox liturgy as well as in the history of philanthropy. The two aspects of his achievement are, however, seldom if ever considered in tandem or seen as in any way connected.

Presumably there were priests to attend the needy inmates of the Basileias and officiate in its chapel – priests drawn, if nowhere else, from the numbers of those 'doctoring' monks.[58] Like John Chrysostom while patriarch of Constantinople a few decades later, Basil would have founded a hospital with 'pious presbyters' as well as medical attendants.[59] Within his 'new city', the church would have provided a focus to the philanthropic complex comparable to that of a cathedral in a *polis*. In it would have been heard the 'pitiful songs' which were all that the leprous patients had to offer. What effects could have been attributed to the chants of its divine liturgy? Medical analogies are easy to find in Basil's output, but the 'psychotherapeutic' effects of psalmody are also described in his homilies on the Psalms and in his

---

[55] Nemesius, *De natura hominis*, 17–20, ed. M. Morani, Teubner edn (Leipzig, 1987), pp. 75–82; M. Morani, *La tradizione manoscritta del* De natura hominis *di Nemesio* (Milan, 1981); medieval Latin translation in *Nemesius d'Emèse* De natura hominis, ed. G. Verbeke and J. R. Moncho, Corpus Latinum commentariorum in Aristotelem Graecorum, Suppl. 1 (Leiden, 1975).

[56] Basil, *Quod deus non est auctor malorum* 6 (*PG* 31, 344A), with Temkin, *Hippocrates*, pp. 172–3.

[57] Basil, *Epistulae* clxxxix.1; ed. Courtonne, II, 132.

[58] Rousseau, *Basil*, p. 142.

[59] Temkin, *Hippocrates*, p. 164.

correspondence.[60] 'A Psalm is a tranquillity of soul . . . it settles one's tumultuous and seething thoughts. It mollifies the soul's wrath [or even 'passion of the soul': *tes psyches to thumoumenon*] and chastens its recalcitrance'; 'the consolation of hymns favours the soul with a state of happiness and freedom from care', and so on: sentiments that can be given either a theological or a medical gloss – or both simultaneously.[61] Basil knows all the anecdotes bequeathed by antiquity about the power of music – a power also shown, and to exemplary effect, by David:

> The passions born of illiberality and baseness of spirit are naturally occasioned by this sort of music. But we must pursue that other kind, which is better and leads to the better, and which, as they say, was used by David, that author of sacred songs, to soothe the king in his madness.[62]

For the fullest exposition in late Antiquity of the therapeutic benefits of liturgy, however, we have to look, not (for once) eastward but to the west. One of the now more obscure names in the patrology, Niceta, bishop of Remesiana (modern Bela Palanka, east of Niš, in the former Yugoslavia), who died after 414, was well-known in his time, to Paulinus of Nola and to Jerome among others. He 'theologizes' the power of David's singing over the demon in Saul in a way that will resonate throughout the Middle Ages and be repeated in the *Malleus Maleficarum*:

> He subdued the evil spirit which worked in Saul – not because such was the power of his cithara, but because a figure of the cross of Christ was mystically projected by the wood and the stretching of strings.[63]

Yet his other evocations of the possible effects of psalmody seem to blur any distinction between the literal or somatic and the celestial (or analogical) sense of therapy:

---

[60] For context, see P. Weitmann, *Sukzession und Gegenwart: zu theoretischen Äußerungen über bildende Künste und Musik von Basileios bis Hrabanus Maurus* (Wiesbaden, 1997), pp. 14–15; R. Taft, *The Liturgy of the Hours in East and West: The Origins of the Divine Office and its Meaning for Today* (Collegeville, MN, 1986), ch. 2; J. Quasten, *Music and Worship in Pagan and Christian Antiquity* (Washington, DC, 1983), ch. 4.

[61] Basil, *Homilia in psalmum I* 2 (*PG* 29, 212–13), trans. J. McKinnon, *Music in Early Christian Literature* (Cambridge, 1987), no. 131, p. 65; *Epistulae* ii.2, ed. Courtonne, I, 8, trans. McKinnon, no. 138, p. 68.

[62] Basil, *Ad adulescentes* 7 (*PG* 31, 581), trans. McKinnon, no. 140, p. 69. I Samuel 16. 16, 23.

[63] Niceta, *De psalmodiae bono* (*de utilitate hymnorum*) 4, ed. C. Turner, 'Niceta of Remesiana II', *Journal of Theological Studies* 24 (1922), 225–52 (p. 235); trans. McKinnon, no. 304, p. 135. P. Murray Jones, 'Music Therapy in the Later Middle Ages: The Case of Hugo van der Goes', in *Music as Medicine*, pp. 120–44 (p. 127), quoting J. Sprenger and H. Institoris, *Malleus maleficarum*, trans. M. Summers (London, 1928), p. 41.

A psalm consoles the sad, restrains the joyful, tempers the angry [in true Aristotelian-Galenic fashion], refreshes the poor . . . To absolutely all who will take it, the psalm offers an appropriate medicine . . . effective in the cure of disease by reason of its strength . . .[64]

I think we should again be chary of dismissing the medicine there as merely metaphorical.

IV

A fully-fledged conception of the non-naturals, such as was developed in Islam, may not, then, have been necessary for the appreciation of hospital music as a type of therapy. Music, even if it took the rudimentary form only of liturgical chant in a small hospital chapel, could, through its effects on the soul, be medicinal for the body. Such, at least, was the perception. This is as true, I suspect, of the earliest hospitals in Europe as it is of the first Byzantine ones. From the very start they were institutions of psychosomatic religious healing.[65] According to the hagiographer of Caesarius of Arles, this sixth-century Frankish bishop

> had a very great concern for the sick and came to their assistance. He granted them a spacious house, in which they could listen undisturbed to the holy office [being sung] in the basilica. He set up beds and bedding, provided for expenses, and supplied a person to take care of them and heal them.[66]

No great disjunction there between medicine and religion. It may be no coincidence that the preceding paragraph in Caesarius's *Vita* should picture the bishop attempting to prevent the laity from gossiping in church by ordering them 'to learn psalms and hymns by heart and to sing sequences and antiphons in a loud and rhythmic voice'. The subject of liturgical musical participation as an educative measure led the writer by a natural association to the subject of sickness and the liturgical arrangements of Caesarius's hospital.

Centuries later, the theoretical stimulus given to learned medicine in Europe by the diffusion of Latin translations of the Arabic undoubtedly gave the 'passions of the soul' a currency greater than that enjoyed by any related notion

---

[64] Niceta, *De psalmodiae bono* 5, ed. Turner, pp. 235–6, trans. McKinnon, nos. 305–6, pp. 135–6.

[65] T. Sternberg, *Orientalium more secutus: Räume und Institutionen der Caritas des 5. bis 7. Jahrhunderts in Gallien*, Jahrbuch für Antike und Christentum, Ergänzungsband 16 (Münster, 1991), pp. 174–7.

[66] *Vita Caesarii* i.20, and, for what follows, i.19, trans. W. E. Klingshirn, *Caesarius of Arles: Life, Testament, Letters*, Translated Texts for Historians 19 (Liverpool, 1994), p. 18. On liturgy in Merovingian Gaul see Y. Hen, *Culture and Religion in Merovingian Gaul, AD 481–751* (Leiden, 1995), chs. 2–5.

in Caesarius's time. Still, it was not as wide a currency as it might have been. The culture of musical therapy nurtured by Islamic scholar-physicians was not transmitted in all its fullness to the West. No European hospital that I know of employed visiting musicians. No European hospital until the early modern period, and then only that of Santo Spirito in Rome, used non-liturgical music of any kind as a regular diversion for its patients.[67] Sometimes, in monasteries, secular music was indeed permitted as an aid to therapy, but it was unlikely to have been heard in the infirmary. Take for example the thirteenth-century Customary of St Augustine's Abbey, Canterbury:

> In the infirmary, there should be no disturbing clamour at any time, but nor in that same place should there be any music of any musical instrument played openly in general hearing. But, for reasons of greater need, if it be judged very useful for improving someone's condition – as when it happens that any brother be so weak and ill that he greatly needs the sound and harmony of a musical instrument to raise his spirits – that person may be led into the chapel by the *Infirmarius*, or carried there in some manner, so that, the door being closed, a stringed instrument may be sweetly played before him by any brother, or by any reliable and discreet servant, without blame. But great care should always be taken lest music or melody of this kind be heard at any time in the hall of the infirmary or – perish the thought – in the chambers of the brothers.[68]

Of course, if music in the infirmary was prohibited in this way, it had presumably sometimes been played there. One piece of evidence that supplies a possible context for its medicinal use in English monasteries is a passage in the register of Adam of Orleton, bishop of Hereford. This reveals that in 1318 the canons of Wigmore Abbey were diverted with wanton songs (*cantilenis inhonestis*) while being bled. To protect other patients from the pollution of blood, such prophylactic phlebotomy was, however, less likely to have taken place in the main infirmary than in a separate room, or even in a detached 'seyney hall'.[69]

---

[67] Kümmel, *Musik und Medizin*, pp. 260–1; P. de Angelis, *Musica e musicisti nell'Arcispedale di Santo Spirito in Saxia dal Quattrocento all'Ottocento* (Rome, 1950), ch. 6.

[68] *Customary of the Benedictine Monasteries of St. Augustine, Canterbury, and St. Peter, Westminster*, ed. E. M. Thompson, 2 vols., Henry Bradshaw Society 23 and 28 (London, 1902–4), I, 329–30; trans. C. Page, 'Music and Medicine in the Thirteenth Century', in *Music as Medicine*, pp. 109–19 (pp. 110–11).

[69] *Registrum Ade de Orleton*, ed. A. T. Bannister, Canterbury and York Series 5 (London, 1908), p. 102, cited in Page, 'Music and Medicine', p. 118. On monastic infirmary regimen see B. Harvey, *Living and Dying in England 1100–1540: The Monastic Experience* (Oxford, 1993), pp. 91–9, and (also on Westminster Abbey) 'Before and After the Black Death: A Monastic Infirmary in Fourteenth-Century England', in *Death, Sickness and Health in Medieval Society and Culture*, ed. S. J. Ridyard, *Sewanee Medieval Studies* 10 (2000), 5–31; and (most comprehensively, despite its subtitle), C. Rawcliffe, '"On the Threshold of Eternity": Care for the Sick in East Anglian Monasteries', in the forthcoming Festschrift for Norman Scarfe, ed. C. Harper-Bill and C. Rawcliffe, of which the author kindly sent me a typescript.

One possible reason for this comparatively 'low-key' approach to musical therapy may have been that much of the relevant literature in Arabic which could have encouraged such therapy among the learned was simply not translated. Neither the musicological discourses on therapy that correlated astrology, music and humours, nor the treatises on 'soul medicine' found their way into Latin.[70] But commentaries on the *Isagoge* and the like served as partial substitutes. Regimen had a place in European medicine after *c.* 1200 that it simply could not have gained earlier.[71] In the promotion of a health-giving cheerfulness, the benefits of 'wine, women and song' (alongside, incidentally, a 'good read')[72] became widely recognized.

The consequences of that for the European hospital were several. First, nursing was in effect medicalized. I do not mean that nurses became equivalent to physicians; no aspirant doctor would have conceded so much. Rather, since medicine and doctoring were not, despite appearances, coterminous, nursing could be accorded a status within medical theory. The nurses who ensured that their patients enjoyed a refreshing night's rest and (ideally) the peace and quiet of hospital surroundings, or who tended a fragrant herb garden in the hospital precinct, or who removed the source of noxious smells, were all performing tasks that were, in theory, just as much medicine as was phlebotomy, or medication with complex and exotic drugs, or subtle and penetrating diagnosis.[73] The same applied on a more exalted and occasional level. When Christine de Pisan urged the merits of charitable work upon ladies and extolled the benefits of a royal visit she too was thinking medically. The good princess, she wrote, should tour the hospital in her finery with a magnificent retinue because this would raise the spirits of the poor inmates.[74] That was sound medical theory. In the 'non-natural' scheme of things, the most therapeutic emotion was cheerfulness.

A second relevant consequence of this notion of 'emotional hygiene' was that the distinction between secular and sacred became blurred. The context in which an Aristotelian moderation of the non-naturals appears in the medical *consilia* (physicians' letters of advice) of the later Middle Ages is nearly always secular.[75] But occasionally the patient requesting the advice is a religious and then the recommendations are modified. One sick Franciscan was for example advised by Bartholomaeus da Montagnana to avoid strong emotions such as anxiety or those inspired by reading stories of martyrdoms. Yet, in another *consilium*, Bartholomaeus urges the study of moral or

---

[70] Burnett, ' "Spiritual Medicine" ', pp. 87–90.
[71] García-Ballester, '*Artifex factivus sanitatis*'; P. Gil-Sotres, 'The Regimens of Health', in *Western Medical Thought*, pp. 291–318.
[72] Olson, *Literature as Recreation*, ch. 2.
[73] Rawcliffe, 'Hospital Nurses', pp. 49–50.
[74] Christine de Pisan, *The Treasure of the City of Ladies*, trans. S. Lawson (London, 1985), p. 53.
[75] J. Agrimi and C. Crisciani, *Les 'consilia' médicaux*, Typologie des sources du Moyen Age 69 (Turnhout, 1994).

theological narratives, *along with the singing of psalms,* as among the exercises 'that bring delight'.[76]

The non-naturals themselves as it were migrated easily from medical to religious discourses. John Mirfeld (d. 1407), who lived for forty years in rooms in St Bartholomew's Hospital, London, composed a *Breviarium* of excerpts from medical texts for those (such as hospital attendants presumably) without a suitable library.[77] It includes a number of Christian charms (perhaps to be said by nurses) to assist women, which may be a reflection of St Bartholomew's reputation as a harbour for unwed mothers. It also inevitably includes a discussion of the non-naturals, as indispensable to basic hospital know-how. Towards the end of his life Mirfeld prepared a comparable anthology of religious texts, the *Florarium.* In that later work he reproduced the passages on the *regimen sanitatis* that had originally appeared in the *Breviarium.*[78] As a model of self-discipline, a therapeutic or preventive regime would obviously serve in either a medical or a pastoral context. But was the other reason for repeating the regimen that, in quite general terms, it belonged as much to religion as to medicine? It is significant that, according to an inventory of 1448, the London hospital of St Mary Elsing, Cripplegate, included a copy of the *Florarium* in its remarkable library.[79]

'In theory, if less often in practice, the precisely regulated environment of the medieval hospital lent itself especially well to the implementation of a system which integrated earthly and spiritual medicine in a carefully balanced way.'[80] Liturgical music was a part of that integrated system. Of course there had long been votive masses of therapeutic intent, such as the mass in honour of St Sigismund for the relief of fever; but the saint, not the mass, is supposed to be the source of healing.[81] Any mass, however, votive or not, whether sung simply in a hospital chapel, or elaborately in some grander church, could potentially have beneficial effects on the accidents of the soul through the positive emotions that it inspired in its singers or auditors.

Now historians have tended to make undocumented assertions about how beneficial it would have been for patients to have heard sung liturgy regularly. The 'gret criynge and joly chauntynge' which the Reformers castigated in the thrice-daily masses heard in the hospital of St Giles, Norwich, were likely to have been differently perceived in the Middle

[76] Olsen, *Literature as Recreation,* pp. 61–2.

[77] Getz, *Medicine,* pp. 49–50.

[78] P. Horton-Smith Hartley and H. R. Aldridge, *Johannes de Mirfeld of St Bartholomew's, Smithfield: His Life and Works* (Cambridge, 1936), p. 154.

[79] *Londinium Redivivum,* ed. J. P. Malcolm, 4 vols. (London, 1803–7), I, 29, cited by Rawcliffe, 'Eighth Comfortable Work', n. 76.

[80] Rawcliffe, 'Hospital Nurses', p. 54.

[81] F. S. Paxton, 'Liturgy and Healing in an Early Medieval Saint's Cult: The Mass *in honore Sancti Sigismundi* for the Cure of Fevers', *Traditio* 49 (1994), 23–43; A. Angenendt, 'Missa specialis: zugleich ein Beitrag zur Entstehung der Privatmessen', *Frühmittelalterliche Studien* 17 (1983), 153–221.

Ages.[82] 'The soothing and often melodious routine [of the hours] . . . may itself have proved extremely therapeutic.'[83] Is it possible to confirm this intuition? When, around 1500, a local priest left money for masses to be sung every week in the hospital of the Holy Cross, Orléans, 'for the sustenance of the bodies and souls of the poor', what could he have had in mind?[84] His bequest was unusual by that time in that the first-named beneficiary of the mass was the inmate, not the donor. And the living inmate, not the dead one. The priest seems to have envisaged something more than an abbreviation of future purgatory. In hospitals where the services were sung (an important qualification) how might the liturgical music of plainchant or polyphony have affected body and soul?

There is a tradition of theoretical writing which is bread and butter to medieval musicologists but 'caviare to the general' as far as medical historiography is concerned. I should like to end by simply drawing attention to it and urging its integration into our analysis of how a medieval hospital liturgy might, in ideal circumstances, have worked – worked therapy if not wonders.

The anecdotes of ancient feats of musical correction, moral improvement and healing, replayed throughout the European Middle Ages in copies of, and commentaries on, Boethius's *De Musica*, and endorsed by the theory of the non-naturals, ensured that the medicinal power of music became a topos of medieval discussion.[85]

For example, Gerald of Wales, in famous passage in the *Topographia Hiberniae*:

> The sweet harmony of music not only gives pleasure but renders important services. It greatly cheers depressed spirits, smoothes furrowed brows . . . Moreover, music soothes disease and pain. The sounds which strike the ear . . . either heal our ailments or enable us to bear them more readily . . . there are no sufferings which music will not mitigate, and many which it cures.[86]

Or take the *Summa musice*, a manual for teaching boys to sing from plainchant notation, written around 1200 by two authors, one of them probably a *decanus* in Würzburg Cathedral:[87]

---

[82] Rawcliffe, *Medicine for the Soul*, pp. 123–4.
[83] Rawcliffe, 'Medicine for the Soul', p. 317.
[84] Saunier, 'Le pauvre malade', p. 104.
[85] Horden, 'Commentary on Part II', pp. 103–4; C. Page, *The Owl and the Nightingale: Musical Life and Ideas in France 1100–1300* (London, 1989), pp. 29, 139. For context see T. J. McGee, *The Sound of Medieval Song: Ornamentation and Vocal Style According to the Treatises* (Oxford, 1998), and, for the tradition in medieval musicological treatises, L. Zanoncelli, *Sulla estetica di Johannes Tinctoris* (Bologna, 1979), pp. 117–26.
[86] *Giraldus Cambrensis Opera*, ed. J. F. Dimock and J. S. Brewer, RS 21, 8 vols. (London, 1861–91), V, 155–6.
[87] *The 'Summa musice': A Thirteenth-Century Manual for Singers*, ed. and trans. C. Page (Cambridge, 1991), p. 12.

Music has medicinal properties and performs miraculous things. Music cures diseases, especially those which arise from melancholia and sadness. Through music one can be prevented from falling into the loneliness of pain and despair.... Music calms the irascible, gladdens the sorrowful, dissipates anxious thoughts and destroys them. What is greater still, music terrifies evil spirits and banishes them, just as David the string player . . . expelled the demon from King Saul when he was possessed by a devil.[88]

Or consider this, from the *Treatise on the Two-fold Practice of Church Music in Divine Services* by Egidius Carlerius (d. 1472), dean of the cathedral chapter of Cambrai, later a theologian in the Collège de Navarre, Paris, and (in all likelihood) friend of the composer Guillaume du Fay:

Now let us turn our pen to the question as to how harmonious music may be most acceptable to God, and let us reveal how praiseworthy and useful it is in church . . . The first of [music's special claims] is that it is a reflection of heavenly joys . . . the second special claim is that music tempers mental passions [standard anecdotes from Boethius follow] . . . The third special claim is that music calms physical passions. For the first book of Boethius's *De Musica*, referred to earlier, mentions that when some Pythagoreans suffered sleepless nights because of the worries that plagued them, a soft and peaceful slumber crept over them with certain melodies . . . euphonious music has sometimes even cured severe illnesses, and no wonder! . . . The fourth special claim is that music drives away evil spirits. For they cannot endure music in praise of God . . . Let us therefore praise harmonious music that rouses the sleeping and gives hearing to the deaf.[89]

We thus do not have to rely on informed intuition in attributing a potentially therapeutic effect to liturgical music in hospitals. Of course the ancient topoi from which the above quotations descended were by no means all necessarily appreciated in Lanfranc's hospital at Canterbury, with which I began, or indeed in any given hospital among the other, later ones which I have mentioned. That, quite generally, medieval 'hospitals, clinics, and health spas sounded with rhythm and melody'[90] seems unlikely. All I would conjecture is the topoi provided hospital life with a general background of possibility: they brought music therapy within donors', priests', and patients' 'horizon of expectation'. To be sure, the liturgical musical round can numb with boredom. That was recognized in the Middle Ages as it can be today.[91] But chant, whether in New Age or Middle Age guise, can also be

---

[88] 'Summa musice', ed. Page, pp. 55–6 (trans.), 145–6 (text). For the later medieval debate on the power of music over demons see Page, *The Owl and the Nightingale*, pp. 158–60; Jones, 'Music Therapy in the Later Middle Ages', pp. 123–4.

[89] *On the Dignity and Effects of Music: Two Fifteenth-Century Treatises*, ed. and trans. R. Strohm and J. D. Cullington, Institute of Advanced Musical Studies, King's College London, Study Texts 2 (London, 1996), pp. 26–32 (trans.), 42–7 (text).

[90] M. P. Cosman, 'Machaut's Medical Musical World', *Annals of the New York Academy of Sciences* 314 (1978), 1–36 (p. 1).

[91] Page, *The Owl and the Nightingale*, p. 158.

hailed as therapeutic. The hope that amelioration, or even cure, might come through hearing it could contribute to an atmosphere of confidence and trust. And such an atmosphere is crucial to successful medicine of any kind, in any age. Osler would have understood. 'Faith in *St Johns Hopkins*, as we used to call him, an atmosphere of optimism, and cheerful nurses, worked just the same sort of cures as did Aesculapius at Epidaurus . . . The Christian Church began with a mission to the whole man – body as well as soul – and the apostolic ministry of health has never been wholly abandoned.'[92]

---

[92] W. Osler, 'The Faith that Heals', *British Medical Journal* (18 June 1910), I, 1470–2 (p. 1471).

V

A Non-natural Environment: Medicine without Doctors and the Medieval European Hospital

Introduction

Norman Cousins' *Anatomy of an Illness*[1] ought to be required reading for historians of pre-modern medicine. Cousins was diagnosed with a collagen illness, a disease of the connective tissue. He had, especially, ankylosing spondylitis, a disease of the spine which would bring about its disintegration. The prognosis was grave – literally so, and soon. Cousins discharged himself from hospital and moved into a hotel. There, he embarked on a prolonged, and eventually successful, therapy of his own devising. He arranged to be drip-fed massive doses of Vitamin C to build up his resistance. He also watched Marx Brothers videos. "Ten minutes of genuine belly laughter …," he writes, "would give me at least two hours of pain-free sleep."

His experience is an excellent introduction to the topic of this chapter, not so much because he provides a shining example of the power of positive thinking, but more for two other reasons (which are, ultimately, related). First, because his auto-therapy is a clear instance of what can reasonably be called "medicine without doctors." Second, less obviously, because the psychological element in that auto-therapy is so medieval. Norman Cousins would be thoroughly at home with medieval medical theory, particularly that part of it which insists that the right emotions – in essence, good cheer – are essential to the preservation or restoration of health. This theory is as well known to medical historians as it was to medieval physicians. Yet the historians have not always appreciated its implications; and the possible consequences of its vernacular understanding, beyond the medical profession, have been very little explored. What happens if, in a deliberately simplistic way, both the notion of medicine without doctors and the medical theory of the emotions are pushed to their limits? What might taking them both seriously do for an understanding of the medieval hospital? The answer suggested below is that, in the medieval hospital,

---

1 Norman Cousins, *Anatomy of an Illness* (New York, 1979), p. 39. Many Websites are now devoted to laughter as "the best medicine." See also Esther M. Sternberg, *The Balance Within: The Science Connecting Health and the Emotions* (New York, 2000), for the controversial field of psycho-neuro-immunology.

medicine without doctors can achieve its fullest expression. It does so under the influence of a vulgarized form of medical theory. Hence the two exemplary aspects of Norman Cousins' case intersect. The hospital as a non-natural environment is the extreme instance of medicine without doctors.[2]

Passions of the Soul

The origins of the relevant medical theory lie in various passages of Galen,[3] but the theory was first systematically elaborated by Islamic writers.[4] The briefest exposition of the underlying ideas can be found in the work later known to Western medicine as the *Isagoge*, or "Introduction," of Johannitius (Hunayn ibn Ishaq, died *c.* 877). This Arabic synopsis was so convenient that, in a partial Latin translation, it was widely diffused across medieval Europe. Available by the beginning of the twelfth century, it served as an introduction to Galen's *Ars medica* (*Tegni*) and became the first book in the corpus of treatises known as the *Articella*, in effect the basic university medical textbook.[5] Vernacular translations followed during the later Middle Ages.[6]

Hunayn distinguishes between *res naturales*, the *naturals* (chiefly the four elements, qualities such as hot or moist, and the four humors) which are the constituents or faculties of a healthy organism, *res contra naturam*, the *contra-naturals* (disease, its causes and sequelae) which upset that healthy state, and *res non naturales*, the *non-naturals*. The last are the pertinent ones here. Generally six in number (though Johannitius in fact enlarged them through his inclusion of coitus and bathing), they are the determinants of health. In standard medieval form, they include ambient air, food and drink, exercise and rest, sleeping and waking, evacuation and

---

2   This chapter attempts to clarify and develop some of the ideas presented at greater length, but in more tangled form, in "Religion as Medicine: Music in Medieval Hospitals," in *Religion and Medicine in the Middle Ages*, ed. Peter Biller and Joseph Ziegler (Woodbridge, NY, 2001), 135–53. It owes much to John Henderson and Carole Rawcliffe, and to the publications of Faye Getz and Glending Olson. I am also grateful to Caroline Barron, Jonathan Hughes, Jennifer Neville and Sethina Watson for advice on specific matters. The usual exculpation of scholarly creditors is more than usually necessary.

3   Luis García-Ballester, "On the Origin of the 'Six Non-Natural Things' in Galen," in *Galen und das Hellenistische Erbe*, ed. Jutta Kollesch and Diethard Nickel (Stuttgart, 1993), 105–15.

4   Glending Olson, *Literature as Recreation in the Later Middle Ages* (hereafter cited as Olson), (Ithaca, NY, 1982), pp. 40–44; for earlier bibliography, see esp. 41 n. 3; Heikki Mikkeli, *Hygiene in the Early Modern Medical Tradition* (Helsinki, 1999), pp. 9–10; for bibliography, see esp. 10 n. 4, pp. 14–23.

5   See Jon Arrizabalaga, "The Death of a Medieval Text: The *Articella* and the Early Press," in *Medicine from the Black Death to the French Disease*, ed. Roger French et al. (Aldershot, 1998), 185–6, for summary and full bibliography.

6   See Linda Ehrsam Voigts and Patricia Deery Kurtz, *Scientific and Medical Writings in Old and Middle English: An Electronic Reference*, CD-ROM (Ann Arbor, MI, 2000).

V

repletion, and the *passions of the soul*, or *accidents of the soul* (*accidentia animae*) as physicians tended to call them. Hunayn writes of these accidents:

> Sundry affections of the mind produce an effect within the body, such as those which bring the natural heat from the interior of the body to the outer parts or the surface of the skin. Sometimes this happens suddenly, as with anger; sometimes gently and slowly, as with delight and joy ... some affections disturb the natural energy both internal and external, as, for instance, with grief.[7]

So emotions are as important for health as is the state of the body or the condition of the environment, which means that emotions fall within the sphere of medicine. Negative emotions can generate somatic illness; positive ones can counteract it, or keep illness at bay. For Hunayn and his followers, practical medicine divides into three parts, and the regulation of the non-naturals is one of them, alongside surgery and the administration of drugs. The salutary importance of moderating emotions such as joy and sadness was made familiar to the whole medieval audience of medical learning through its inclusion in many medical treatises, theoretical and practical, even surgical ones.[8] It appeared in numerous regimens of health (especially the hundred or so manuscript versions of the *Regimen sanitatis salernitanum*), and was mentioned in even more numerous letters of advice from physicians to better-off patients (*consilia*).[9]

What matters here is neither the learned vocabulary nor the physiological details,[10] but the simple underlying psychosomatic anthropology. That emotions can determine health was appreciated well beyond the circles of university physicians and their patients. But historians have devoted little attention to the matter, and the evidence remains to be collected. All that can be offered are some examples of the sort of material we might look for.

"Because of my worries I got dry pimples and my skin peeled off my bones."[11] So wrote a Jewish inhabitant of medieval Old Cairo, echoing, perhaps unconsciously, Proverbs 17:22, "a cheerful heart is a good medicine, but a downcast spirit dries up

---

7   Edward Grant, trans., *Sourcebook of Medieval Science* (Cambridge, MA, 1974), pp. 708–9.

8   Carole Rawcliffe, "Hospital Nurses and their Work," in *Daily Life in the Middle Ages*, ed. Richard Britnell (Stroud, 1998), 43–64; see esp. 62; Olson, 46.

9   Mikkeli, *Hygiene*, pp. 19–23; Jole Agrimi and Chiara Crisciani, *Les "consilia" médicaux, Typologie des sources du moyen âge*, 69 (Turnhout, 1994); Peter Murray Jones, "Music Therapy in the Later Middle Ages: The Case of Hugo van der Goes," in *Music as Medicine: The History of Music Therapy since Antiquity*, ed. Peregrine Horden (Aldershot, 2000), 134–40.

10   See Pedro Gil-Sotres, "Modelo teórico y observación clínica: las pasiones del alma en la psicología medica medieval," in *Comprendre et maîtriser la nature au Moyen Age: mélanges d'histoire des sciences offerts à Guy Beaujouan* (Geneva, 1994), 181–204.

11   S.D. Goitein, *A Mediterranean Society, Volume 5: The Individual* (Berkeley, CA, 1988), 56.

the bones,"[12] and reminding us thereby of the endorsement that these medical notions must have gained from a range of non-medical sources, and indeed from common sense and observation.[13] Several of the twelfth-century biographies of Thomas Becket describe how the archbishop's pain in his side was caused or aggravated by the anxieties of his trial at Northampton in October 1164.[14] Exchanges about regimen between Francesco di Marco Datini, the fourteenth-century "Merchant of Prato" made famous by Iris Origo, and his physician Lorenzo Sassoli can be followed closely through the abundant surviving correspondence.[15] At one point Maestro Lorenzo writes: "I think the chill you have taken is your own fault, for I am certain that it came to you only because you take your troubles and anxieties as if you were a man of thirty, and this you must not do." And later: "pray tell me how you feel, and that you now take the vexations of your trade more easily. For if you do not, ailments and bodily anguish will be your first profits." Again, in a long letter that was tantamount to a personal regimen, Lorenzo referred specifically to the accidents of the spirit:

> as to [which] ... let me tell you the things of which you must most beware. To get angry and shout at times pleases me, for this will keep up your natural heat; but what displeases me is your being vexed and taking everything so much to heart. For it is this, as the whole of physic teaches, which destroys our body, more than any other cause.

This is the physician speaking, not the patient; and the patient does not seem to be following the repeated advice. Still, one could hardly claim that Francesco remained ignorant of the principles of psychosomatic medicine.

Francesco's near contemporary, Geoffrey Chaucer, is another famous figure who can be called upon here, a medical "layman" who clearly knew his non-naturals. Recall both the author and the knight who are suffering physically from melancholy in *The Book of the Duchess*,[16] or the lovesick Troilus in *Troilus and Criseyde*, and Arcite in the *Knight's Tale* whose "loveres maladye of hereos" is overlaid with more serious mania.[17] But the clearest instance of Chaucer's awareness of the non-naturals

---

12 Revised Standard Version. For the confluence of medicine and theology in the medieval interpretation of such passages, see Beryl Smalley, *The Study of the Bible in the Middle Ages*, 3rd edn (Oxford, 1983), pp. 314–16.

13 And, in the West, from medieval traditions of Stoicism. See Faye Getz, *Medicine in the English Middle Ages* (Princeton, NJ, 1998), p. 85.

14 David Knowles, *The Episcopal Colleagues of Archbishop Thomas Becket* (Cambridge, 1951), App. V; see also Stephen Wilson, *The Magical Universe* (London and New York, 2000), p. 311, wrongly, I believe, aligning such material under "magical influences"; and for another Archbishop of Canterbury prone to stress-related illness, see Eadmer, *Life of St. Anselm*, ed. Richard W. Southern (London, 1962), p. 80.

15 For what follows, see Iris Origo, *The Merchant of Prato* (Harmondsworth, 1963), pp. 306–8.

16 See esp. lines 487–501; Olson, pp. 44, 85–9.

17 Lines 1,373–4. On the physical symptoms, see Mary Frances Wack, *Lovesickness in the Middle Ages: The "Viaticum" and its Commentaries* (Philadelphia, PA, 1990), pp. 63–6,

is the poor but virtuous woman farmer in the *Nun's Priest's Tale* (lines 2,837–9): "Repleccioun ne made hire nevere sik; / Attempree diete was al hir phisik, / And exercise, and hertes suffisaunce"[18] – that is, moderation in the accidents of the soul. Medical theory is used to assert the effectiveness of medicine without doctors.

How representative is Chaucer of educated attitudes in later medieval England? The nature and scale of his contemporary audience is, of course, controversial. The majority of scholars seem, however, to conceive of it as far broader than a coterie or an elite.[19] Moreover, similar echoes of medical psychology emerge in non-fictional material. In the 1430s, for example, Stephen Scrope, member of a cadet branch of a baronial family, wrote to his stepfather Sir John Fastolf accusing him of bringing on Scrope's chronic and disfiguring skin condition by sending him away to school *c.* 1411.[20]

The idea that attention to the emotions could prevent or mitigate illness gained perhaps its widest diffusion from the numerous plague treatises of the post-Black Death period. Like regimens, these were often partly organized according to the non-naturals. Hence many had some advice about the accidents of the soul. As the masters of the Paris medical faculty put it in 1348, in the most influential of these treatises (soon translated into the vernacular), the *Compendium de epidimia*:

> Since bodily infirmity is sometimes related to the accidents of the soul, one should avoid anger, excessive sadness, and anxiety. Be of good hope and resolute mind; make peace with God, for death will be less fearsome as a result. Live in joy and gladness as much as possible, for although joy may sometimes moisten the body, it nevertheless comforts both spirit and heart.[21]

In times of epidemic, given this pathogenicity of the emotions, the fear of disease could easily become the disease of fear – a disease as lethal as plague.[22]

135–9; for context, see Linda Phyllis Austern, "Musical Treatments for Lovesickness: The Early Modern Heritage," in *Music as Medicine*, ed. Peregrine Horden, 213–45

18 Neville Coghill, trans.: "Repletion never left her in disquiet / And all her physic was a temperate diet, / Hard work for exercise and heart's content."

19 John Burrow, *Medieval Writers and Their Work* (Oxford, 1982), Ch. 2; Paul Strohm, *Social Chaucer* (Cambridge, MA and London, 1989), Ch. 3.

20 Jonathan Hughes, "Stephen Scrope and the Circle of Sir John Fastolf: Moral and Intellectual Outlooks," in *Medieval Knighthood IV: Papers from the Fifth Strawberry Hill Conference*, ed. Christopher Harper-Bill and Ruth Harvey (Woodbridge, 1990), 109–46.

21 Olson, trans., p. 169; for context, see 164–74; see also Jon Arrizabalaga, "Facing the Black Death: Perceptions and Reactions of Medical Practitioners," in *Practical Medicine from Salerno to the Black Death*, ed. Luis García-Ballester et al. (Cambridge, 1994), 279–80.

22 David Gentilcore, "The Fear of Disease and the Disease of Fear," in *Fear in Early Modern Society*, ed. William G. Naphy and Penny Roberts (Manchester and New York, 1997), 190–96; Andrew Wear, "Fear, Anxiety and the Plague in Early Modern England," in *Religion, Health and Suffering*, ed. John R. Hinnells and Roy Porter (London and New York, 1999), 339–63: see esp. 51–2 for Van Helmont's argument that the worst cases of plague were *entirely* the product of fear.

Five Steps to the Hospital

Now consider the theme of medicine without doctors from a different angle, one which has less to do with theory and its vernacular transformations and more to do with modern historiography's perceptions. Begin with what is probably a fundamental image of the physician, the image of the *doctor doctoring*, that is, actively intervening in an attempt to restore health through medication or surgery. We can then move away from that image in a sequence of steps so as to prepare the way for another image, that of the medieval hospital as a non-natural environment.

The first step is to recognize that, in treating the sick, medieval healers of all kinds – physicians, apothecaries, empirics, magicians, living holy men, even surgeons – probably said much more than they did. (Dead saints working healing miracles may be the exception.) The interaction between healer and patient might well be imagined, in its verbosity, its domination by question and answer, as more akin to a modern session with a psychotherapist than to an encounter with a practitioner of biomedicine. The analogy is not intended as a full endorsement of David Harley's recent analysis of the "construction" of *all* healing through rhetoric; his strong thesis seems to me to raise more philosophical problems than it offers historical solutions.[23] Undoubtedly, though, the significance of the clinical talking of pre-modern healers has been underestimated by medical historians, partly because it is little documented, partly because our historical imagination is still, on the whole, "infected" by the technological, interventionist, bias of modern biomedicine.

Step two: talk is not necessarily a prelude to action. It is expected that medical rhetoric will focus on diagnosis, and that diagnosis will lead to treatment. But pre-modern healing focussed at least as much on prognosis, on saying what would happen with, or just as likely, without medication. The role of prognosis is easily downplayed. Faye Getz is unusual in opening her recent synopsis of *Medicine in the English Middle Ages* with an account, derived from the chronicler Ralph of Coggeshall, of the last illness of Archbishop Hubert Walter in the summer of 1205.[24] The learned physician in the archbishop's entourage, Gilbertus Anglicus, is portrayed as doing nothing but prognosticate, instructing his patient in the *ars moriendi*. He neither inspects urine nor administers any drug. Instead he advises *medicina sacramentalis*: first confession, then the last rites. "Physical remedies" are taken only when this prescient advice is ignored, and at the behest of another attendant physician. That the archbishop's was an extreme case, a terminal one, should not lead us to think that it was in every other respect exceptional.

Step three: much more of medical doctoring than is now generally acknowledged concerned prevention rather than cure (diet in the pre-modern sense, regimen). But

---

23 David Harley, "Rhetoric and the Social Construction of Illness and Healing," *Social History of Medicine*, 12 (1999), 407–35, with debate in Vol. 13 (2000), 147–51, 535–46.

24 Getz, *Medicine in the English Middle Ages*, pp. 3–4, with Ralph of Coggeshall, *Radulphi de Coggeshall Chronicon Anglicanum*, ed. Joseph Stevenson, Rolls Series 66 (London, 1875), pp. 156–9. See now also Luke Demaitre, "The Art and Science of Prognostication in Early University Medicine," *Bulletin of the History of Medicine*, 77 (2003), 765–88.

V

preventative medicine is the poor relation of medical historiography, just as it is the poor relation of modern therapeutics. Few synopses say much about it. Only one recent scholarly overview of medieval medicine devotes a chapter to the topic.[25] Yet the sheer bulk of the writings about regimen from the Hippocratic corpus to the voluminous dietetic writings of the later Middle Ages bears witness to its importance.[26]

The fourth step is marked by *non*-doctors doctoring. It brings the non-naturals back into the picture. To review: in the first three steps, they were only a background presence. First, the reassuring rhetoric could itself be regarded as therapeutic, whether in modern psychosomatic terms or in pre-modern terms of the effects of emotion on health. Second, even a bleak prognosis can relieve suffering through the clarity and certainty it brings, and with that the chance to prepare properly for death (seizing which chance may make all the difference to one's prospects in eternity). Third, regimen in its medieval form is often structured around the non-naturals: they determine the form the preventative medicinal advice takes.

The right emotions are even more important to the preservation of health than they are to its recovery. The fourth step, however, involves the non-naturals on a broader front, not just the psychological one. If motion and rest, evacuation and repletion, good cheer, sex and other such basics belong to medicine, then the recipients of regimens or medical *consilia* who try (*à la* Norman Cousins) to change their own non-naturals are dealing in medical matters. As the *Salernitan Regimen* put it, in a passage that Chaucer might well have known: *Si tibi deficiant medici, medici tibi fiant / Hec tria: mens leta, requies, moderata dieta* ("If you should lack doctors, these three shall be doctors to you: a joyful mind, rest and a moderate diet").[27]

Those who promote balance of the non-naturals in others are all, in a sense, medical practitioners. Nurses provide the most obvious and the most neglected of examples. This should be stressed, against the weight of received opinion of the medieval medical elite, and even against that of some modern historians attempting sympathetically to recover women's obscured medical activities.[28] It hardly needs stating that many medieval doctors took a dim view of nurses' capabilities, in part so as to enhance patients' perception of their own. They did not apply the theory of the non-naturals impartially. Other countervailing voices therefore deserve amplification. In the Hospital of St Nicholas de Bruille in Tournai, for example, care of the sick was provided by six Augustinian sisters and some novices. The fifteenth-

---

25 Pedro Gil Sotres, "The Regimens of Health," in *Western Medical Thought from Antiquity to the Middle Ages*, ed. Mirko D. Grmek (Cambridge, MA and London, 1998), 291–318.

26 See now G.J. Hardingham, "The Regimen in Late Medieval England" (PhD Thesis, University of Cambridge, 2005).

27 Jones, "Music Therapy," 136.

28 See note 8 above. Contrast the stark separation between nursing and medicine enjoined by Monica H. Green, "Documenting Medieval Women's Medical Practice," in *Practical Medicine from Salerno to the Black Death*, 341.

century Rule of the house gave full weight to the connection between nursing and health. It stipulated that:

> before the sisters take their food, the said sick patients shall be fed in accordance with their infirmities and their wishes, so far as can be arranged and so long as nothing is harmful to their health. As funds allow, they will be diligently supplied with their needs until they regain their health.[29]

Several other rules specified that nurses were to be patient, friendly and cheerful, so as not to depress their patients.[30]

Fifth and final step: under the banner of the non-naturals, the scope of medicine broadens so that it extends beyond the efforts of people (doctors, nurses, autotherapists) to the effects of things. Within the body there lies, of course, the healing power of nature, *vis medicatrix naturae*.[31] But the aspect of medicine without doctors to be emphasized here is environmental. And, like the topic of nursing, this too brings us to the hospital.

Hospital Healing

Much of the attention of medieval hospital historians used to be absorbed by the question of whether or not hospitals had doctors on their staffs. Florence took the prize for precocity; England trailed in last, with the Savoy Hospital. Contrast, for instance, the hospital of Santa Maria Nuova in Florence with that of St Giles, Norwich (the "Great Hospital," as it became known after the Reformation). Santa Maria Nuova had its retained corps of physicians who admitted only patients with acute but not life-threatening conditions and discharged them rapidly.[32] St Giles helped the chronically sick and elderly to live out their days in minimum pain. It had no doctors until after the Reformation.[33] The contrast could hardly be starker. The future of hospitals seems to lie on one side, in Tuscany. Their past lies on the other, in East Anglia. Medicalization of this kind – medicalization in the literal sense of the arrival of *medici* – is easily seen as the one development that really mattered. It

---

29 Cited from Rawcliffe, "Hospital Nurses," 57.

30 Ibid., 62.

31 Mikkele, *Hygiene*, p. 17.

32 Katherine Park and John Henderson, "'The First Hospital among Christians': The Ospedale di Santa Maria Nuova in Early Sixteenth-century Florence," *Medical History*, 35 (1991), 164–88; Henderson, "Splendide case di cura: spedali, medicina ed assistenza a Firenze nel trecento", in *Ospedali e città: L'Italia del Centro-Nord, XIII–XVI*, ed. A.J. Grieco and L. Sandri (Florence, 1997), pp. 15–50; Henderson, "'Antechambers of Death'? Poverty and Sickness in the Hospitals of Renaissance Florence," in *Forme di povertà e innovazioni istituzionali in Italia dal Medioevo ad oggi*, ed. V. Zamagna (Bologna, 2000), 111–29.

33 Carole Rawcliffe, *Medicine for the Soul: The Life, Death and Resurrection of an English Medieval Hospital* (Stroud, 1999).

V

becomes the *Leitmotif* of an implicit teleological narrative, from caring to curing, from the medieval to the modern.

The work of Carole Rawcliffe and John Henderson (among others), on English and Florentine hospitals respectively, undermines this contrast and subverts this teleology. Later medieval hospitals in both cities, as they have shown, were above all quasi-monastic religious institutions, with liturgy at their heart. Patients in both Norwich and Florence lay within sight of the sacrament, either because the ward opened out into a chapel or because there was an altar within the ward. In both places, daily life was punctuated by the monastic hours more than by the ward round.[34] The cure of the soul, through the medicine of the sacraments, was more important than the relief of bodily infirmity, not least because, as the fathers of the Fourth Lateran Council had reminded the faithful (Canon 22), the soul's health was an essential precondition for the recovery of the body. Exposure to the host, even without reception; regular confession, without which one sin might remain to contaminate the whole hospital; the proximity of relics in the hospital chapel; contemplation of devotional imagery – all these are likely features of the overriding purpose of hospital life. They erode the stark contrast between England and Italy, rendering the presence or absence of physicians less decisive for our estimation of the hospital's therapeutic capacity.[35]

Against those who maintain that doctors make all the difference, it could be said that the true medicine of hospitals is religion. Hospitals, in their ideal form, exemplified that subordination of the care of the body to the care of the soul, and of the earthly physician to *Christus medicus*, which the Church attempted to diffuse through society at large. Yet the analysis need not stop there. *Medicina sacramentalis*, the medicine of the soul, is acknowledged by its latest historians as potentially affecting the body as well: exposure to the host was supposed, for example, to alleviate bodily infirmities.[36] In his *Instructions for Parish Priests* (*c.* 1400), John Myrc claimed that anyone who saw a priest bearing the host would be safe for the rest of the day from death and blindness.[37] It was, presumably, on the basis of similar beliefs that, *c.* 1500, a local priest left money for masses to be sung every week in the hospital of

---

34 John Henderson, "Healing the Body and Saving the Soul: Hospitals in Renaissance Florence," *Renaissance Studies* 15 (2001), 188–216.

35 Carole Rawcliffe, "Medicine for the Soul: The Medieval English Hospital and the Quest for Spiritual Health," in *Religion, Health and Suffering*, ed. John R. Hinnells and Roy Porter (London, 1999), 316–38.

36 Rawcliffe, *Medicine for the Soul*, p. 103. Compare Oliver Sacks, *The Man who Mistook his Wife for a Hat* (London, 1985), p. 36, for the relief from the effects of extreme amnesia (Korsakov's syndrome) brought to a patient by taking communion.

37 Edward Peacock, ed., Early English Text Society (London, 1868), p. 10. On such "virtues" of the Mass, see further Adolph Franz, *Die Messe im deutschen Mittelalter: Beiträge zur Geschichte der Liturgie und des religiösen Volkslebens* (Freiburg im Breisgau, 1902, repr. Darmstadt, 1963), pp. 36–72.

the Holy Cross, Orléans, "for the sustenance of the *bodies* and souls of the poor."[38] Still, despite such examples, secularist historians may be tempted, first, to conceive of soul medicine as really only a spiritual remedy, and second, *a fortiori*, to conceive of that same medicine as medicine only by analogy – as not quite the real thing.

These misconceptions obscure medieval understanding of the phenomena in question, an understanding predicated upon the non-naturals. The contrary argument can be put in dialectical form. Thesis: hospitals are medical only if they have attendant doctors. Antithesis: the primary medicine of all hospitals is religion. Synthesis: the religion of hospitals is a type of medicine. Spiritual medicine is genuinely medicinal, not just in theological but also in medical terms. It is another kind of medicine without doctors. Anything that promotes medicine for the soul – sacraments, devotional images and the like – can be seen as altering the accidents of the soul. Medieval doctors knew this. In a *consilium*, Bartholomaeus da Montagnana urges the study of moral or theological narratives, along with the singing of psalms, as among the exercises "that bring delight" and therefore health.[39] In the sixteenth century, Alvise Luisini claimed that physicians could detect physical improvements in patients who had confessed one day previously. The ensuing freedom from anxiety led directly to better health, including the remission of fever.[40]

This is not only a "professional" medical insight. To the examples of public understanding of the non-naturals adduced above (Chaucer, Scrope et al.) can now be added that of the fathers of the Fourth Lateran Council. In what might seem to be their most emphatically theological mode, they also, in Canon 22, embrace basic medical psychosomatics. That is, they recognize the disease of fear:

> This among other things has occasioned this decree [that "physicians of the body" must persuade their patients to summon "physicians of the soul" before they treat them], namely that some people on their sickbed, when they are advised by physicians to arrange for the health of their souls, *fall into despair and so the more readily incur the danger of death.*[41]

If summoning a physician of the soul to the bedside became routine at the outset of treatment, instead of a later sign that the case was considered terminal, then fewer patients would succumb to the disease of fear and make their physical conditions more perilous.[42]

---

38 Annie Saunier, *"Le pauvre malade" dans le cadre hospitalier médiéval: France du Nord vers 1300–1500* (Paris, 1993), p. 104; italics added.

39 Olson, pp. 61–2.

40 Richard Palmer, "The Church, Leprosy and Plague in Medieval and Early Modern Europe," *Studies in Church History*, 19 (1982), 86, citing [Alvise] Luisini, *Tractatus de confessione a die decubitus instituenda* (Venice, 1563), 74–5.

41 Norman Tanner, ed. and trans., *Decrees of the Ecumenical Councils*, 2 vols (London and Washington, DC, 1990), 1:245–6; italics added.

42 For the resistance of some physicians to any summoning of priests, see Michael McVaugh, "Bedside Manners in the Middle Ages," *Bulletin of the History of Medicine*, 71 (1997), 217.

For illustration of the psychosomatic potential of the sacraments, even in a terminal case, we can return for a moment to the last, measured, hours of Hubert Walter as represented by Ralph of Coggeshall. Gilbert the physician advised his patient to confess. "On doing so, the fire of the archbishop's remorse and charity rose up and caused the moisture in his brain to dissolve, bringing forth from him a torrent of tears and great relief."[43] After receiving the last rites Hubert was again much relieved.[44]

Hospital Inmates

Of course, this evidence does not relate specifically to hospitals. But there is no reason why hospital patients should have responded any differently to the sacraments. According to the statutes of one thirteenth-century English hospital, for example, the steward of the sick was the "distributor" of relics, presumably because he paraded them around the ward to "irradiate" the patients.[45] The surrounding religious images that, along with the administration of the sacraments, constituted the hospital as a religious house could also have encouraged a salutary cheerfulness. Consider the most medicalized of Renaissance hospitals, Santa Maria Nuova. From about 1420 onward, a half-length statue of Christ showing his wounds stood in the lunette above the doorway to the hospital cemetery, and a terra cotta Coronation of the Virgin adorned the tympanum of the entrance to the church of S. Egidio, the hospital chapel. Both were images of healing and redemption, potential promoters of a salutary optimism. The Virgin, present not only here but, later on, inside the chapel in the famous Portinari altarpiece and in a fresco cycle, was, in her compassion, a role model of the hospital nurse, and her coronation signified triumph over death. Christ, meanwhile, "came as a doctor not just to visit us but to cure us."[46] His corporeal sufferings, so emphasized in the statue, were a "bitter medicine" which he took on our behalf to heal us of the "sickness of sin." Such is the Augustinian interpretation of *Christus medicus* provided by the early fifteenth-century Dominican friar Domenico Cavalca. It comes in a treatise sometimes entitled *Medicina del cuore*, as in a manuscript of 1410 that originated in a convent contiguous with Santa Maria Nuova. The title nicely captures the interpenetration of medicine and theology in the statue's message.[47]

It is obviously not only the religious aspects of the hospital that can be conceived in this medical fashion. Anything that promoted optimism among the patients is susceptible of the same kind of interpretation. The contributions of diet, rest, and

---

43 The paraphrase of Getz's *Medicine in the English Middle Ages*, p. 3.

44 Ralph of Coggeshall, *Chronicon Anglicanum*, p. 158.

45 Sethina Watson, "*Fundatio, ordinatio* and *statuta*: The Statutes and Constitutional Documents of English Hospitals to 1300" (DPhil. Thesis, University of Oxford, 2003), p. 258.

46 Henderson, "Healing the Body," 196–9, with n. 21.

47 Ibid.

good nursing have already been mentioned. A royal visit might work equally well. When, in 1405, Christine de Pisan urged the merits of charitable work and extolled the benefits of such a visit, she too was a "non-naturalist." The good princess, she wrote, should tour the hospital in all her grandeur and with a magnificent retinue because this honoring of the poor inmates would raise their spirits.[48] Sound medical theory chimed with common sense. In the non-natural scheme of things, the most therapeutic emotion was a moderate cheerfulness.

The dialectical synthesis extends, therefore, beyond religion, and embraces any aspect of the hospital, whether involving persons or things; whether working directly on the body, or indirectly on it through the accidents of the soul. That is why the hospital is, at least potentially, a *total non-natural environment*. It is vital to stress the "potentially" in that formulation. This is an ideal type, perhaps a Platonic hospital. It scarcely needs stating that not every real hospital functioned in this way. Not all potentially therapeutic aspects of any one establishment were equally efficacious.[49]

Nor can it be argued that the creation of such an environment inevitably formed part of a hospital founder's plan, unless that founder was an educated physician. Some benefactors may have had a lay awareness of the non-naturals; others will have cared little for them. This paper offers a conjecture, less about the *origins* of hospitals than about their *evolution* during the later Middle Ages, when, as Michael McVaugh has proposed, there was considerable popular appetite for medical theory.[50]

Just occasionally, some association of the non-naturals with a hospital can even be documented. John Mirfeld (d. 1407) lived for forty years in rooms near St Bartholomew's Hospital, London. While there, he composed a *Breviarium* of excerpts from medical texts for those without a suitable library.[51] It includes a discussion of the non-naturals as indispensable to basic hospital know-how. Toward the end of his life, Mirfeld prepared a comparable anthology of religious texts, the *Florarium*. In that later work, he reproduced the passages on regimen from the *Breviarium*.[52] As a model of self-discipline, regimen belonged first to medicine and then to religion. According to an inventory of 1448, another London hospital, St Mary Elsyng, Cripplegate (dedicated to the care of sick clergy), had a copy of the *Florarium* in its library.[53] This is unusual evidence. Mostly, the non-naturalness of the hospital

---

48 Christine de Pisan, *The Treasure of the City of Ladies*, trans. Sarah Lawson (London, 1985), p. 53.

49 It seems unlikely that, quite generally, medieval "hospitals, clinics, and health spas sounded with rhythm and melody," treating the soul with music therapy: Madeleine Pelner Cosman, "Machaut's Medical Musical World," *Annals of the New York Academy of Sciences* 314 (1978), 1–36, quotation from p. 1. This confuses ideal type with typical reality.

50 Michael McVaugh, *Medicine before the Plague: Practitioners and their Patients in the Crown of Aragon, 1285–1345* (Cambridge, 1993).

51 Getz, *Medicine in the English Middle Ages*, pp. 49–50.

52 Percival Horton-Smith Hartley and Harold R. Aldridge, *Johannes de Mirfeld of St Bartholomew's, Smithfield: His Life and Works* (Cambridge, 1936), p. 154.

53 J.P. Malcolm, ed., *Londinium Redivivum*, 4 vols (London, 1803–7), 1:29, cited by Carole Rawcliffe, "The Eighth Comfortable Work: Education and the Medieval English

V

can only be inferred. But if there is any general validity in what is here suggested, then many more medieval hospital patients were getting their medicine than might have been thought. Their non-naturals were being regulated, both spiritually and somatically. It was just that they were not necessarily getting that regulation, that medicine, through doctors. Even in Santa Maria Nuova, with its medical personnel, the medicine *without* doctors that was provided by religion and by the rest of the environment may have been as significant as the medicine *from* doctors.

Conclusion

There are many ways in which those propositions could be further illustrated. Carole Rawcliffe has, for example, emphasized the role of hospital gardens not just as sources of food and medicinal herbs, but as vehicles of aromatherapy and objects of aesthetic, and thus non-naturally beneficial, delight.[54] She has also proposed the later medieval English monastic infirmary, together with its "seyney house" in which monks were prophylactically bled, as one likely setting for the fullest realization of a regimen based on the non-naturals. Sick or elderly monks, or simply those for whom the liturgical round was proving oppressive, were granted a holiday from their duties, a nourishing diet, and ready access to the gladdening beauties of nature.[55] Elsewhere I have explored medical conceptions of the non-natural impact of the liturgy in hospital chapels.[56]

Slowly, the different aspects of this non-natural environment are being colored in. And doctors are scarcely to be seen.

Hospital," in *The Church and Learning in Late Medieval Society: Studies in Honour of Professor R. B. Dobson*, ed. Caroline Barron and Jenny Stratford (Donington, 2002), 390.

54 Rawcliffe, *Medicine for the Soul*, pp. 51–3; Rawcliffe, "Hospital Nurses," 58–9. See also William C. Cosgrove, "Medicine in the *Twelve Books on Rural Practices* of Petrus de Crescentiis," in *Manuscript Sources of Medieval Medicine*, ed. Margaret R. Schleissner (London, 1995), pp. 86–7.

55 Rawcliffe, "'On the Threshold of Eternity': Care of the Sick in East Anglian Monasteries," in *East Anglia's History: Studies in Honour of Norman Scarfe*, ed. Christopher Harper-Bill, Carole Rawcliffe and Richard G. Wilson (Woodbridge, 2002), 71–2; see further Mary Yearl, Chapter 11 in this volume.

56 Horden, "Religion as Medicine" (see note 2 above).

VI

Family History and Hospital History in the Middle Ages

> *'If I am sick, do they come and nurse me?*
> *... If I am out of work for weeks in bad*
> *times... does the rich man share his plenty*
> *with me, as he ought to do, if his religion*
> *was not a humbug? ... No, I tell you, it's*
> *the poor, and the poor only, as does such*
> *things for the poor.'*
> (Mrs Gaskell, Mary Barton, ch. 1)

1.1 How can the medievalist seize the realities of poverty and charity in the European city? Not, I shall argue, by weighing aggregates of supply and demand; rather, by searching out stories. Here are two introductory examples of the sort of story I have in mind.

1.2 One night in the winter of 1276, Jehanne de Sarris, wife and mother, who had migrated to the capital from a village in the diocese of Paris, lost the use of her legs.[1] Ramrod stiff, she remained housebound for a month, hoping every day for deliverance. She was poor; and since there was no one who could help her (not even her children), and since her maintenance was apparently beyond her husband's means, she was taken to the Hôtel Dieu. This was the largest general hospital of Paris, with room for several hundred poor, ill, or abandoned inmates.[2] There, sick and incapable, she stayed for over four months, until the feast of Sts Peter and Paul. The servitors in the hospital made crutches for her so that, gradually, she could move about and

VI

start to visit the hospital chapel. Once she was again mobile to this extent, she wanted to return to her husband and children and recover her independence. But she was unable to manage the journey and her husband had to carry her home. Thereafter, however, he again seemed unwilling to care for her. So in great pain she went on her crutches to her parish church to beg for alms. Then she heard that many miracles were taking place at the tomb of St Louis in St-Denis and that the sick were being cured there. The remainder of her story can be surmised. The dead king's intercession brought a happy issue out of all her afflictions.

1.3 Here is a second story.[3] The following year, 1277, a twenty-eight year old woman, Emmelot de Chaumont, came to St-Denis with two other women. Emmelot asked for lodging from Marguerite de Rocigni in the rue St-Jacques. Marguerite said she could not accommodate her, but she did pass her on to another woman in the same street, Emmeline la Charonne, who took in both Emmelot and her two companions. It was a Sunday, at vespers, when they entered their new lodging. The following day Emmelot stayed around the house and performed the chores which seem to have been her recompense for shelter: washing, making beds, fetching water, bringing in bread and fuel. Towards midnight on the following Tuesday, when she was in the bed she shared with one of her companions, Emmelot became ill. She too lost the use of her limbs, and indeed all feeling in them. She made a vow to St Louis and was taken to his shrine by a group of women: her 'landlady', one of her two companions, a neighbour, and one other. This was only the first of a number of visits, made with great difficulty, on crutches. Her cure came on the morning of Easter Sunday. Later she went on pilgrimage and then returned to lodge with Marguerite, the woman whom she had first approached for lodging in St-Denis. She became a chambermaid in a bourgeois establishment. But when she fell ill again she was taken, not to the shrine, but to the hospital of Saint-Denis. There she died.

1.4 Before I comment on these tales of families, neighbours, hospitals and shrines, let me explain how I came upon them, and why I think they illustrate the kind of evidence in which historians of the social policies of the medieval city should interest themselves.

2.1 Almost fifteen years ago, in the course of reviewing several then recent monographs on later medieval hospitals, I ruminated about the appropriate context within which to set the history of such institutions of poor relief.[4] I argued that the way to evaluate them was to dispense with the specious calculation of ratios: the ratio of the number of hospitals to total population (by which standard, in the later Middle Ages, Cambridge and Pistoia scored more highly than London and Florence), or the ratio of the number of beds to likely demand. Neither procedure is rewarding. We cannot establish the aggregate populations nor do we have any reliable estimates of the numbers of those who might be termed poor and needy (not least because we have no agreed definition of the latter). More importantly, for no medieval hospital, other than some monastic infirmaries,[5] can we be sure of the likely turnover of patients or of the numbers who occupied each bed. And the result of such exercises is predictable. Charitable institutions always come out of them badly. They always appear insufficient in size and number.

2.2 So I proposed, in that review-article, that we try to get away from the sharp dichotomy between major institutions and a generic backdrop of unsatisfied need. Our assessments of institutions must always be relative – relative, first, to a spectrum of other forms of public assistance, such as monastic distributions, confraternal charity, dowry funds, private almsgiving, the (sometimes) benevolent lordship of manor and *seigneurie*, and so forth. Relative also, and more significantly, to the actual demand for relief on the part of the poor and the variety of ways in which that demand might be met. Before we can see how much help the poor ideally required of institutions or individual benefactors, we have to make some attempt, however speculative, to assess how far, and by what means, they were able to help themselves. This cannot be done by citing profiles of living standards – wages and prices, diets and the like.[6] Nor can it be conveyed by what were, in 1988, the usual historiographical generalizations about solitary beggars or the predo-minance, among the remainder of the poor, of simple intra-familial care.[7] Some much more specific analysis is needed: an analysis, in relative terms, of each of the ways in which 'horizontal' relations within and between individuals, households, kin groups and neighbourhoods functioned as forms of welfare provision; and a further analysis of the ways in which these various resources could interact with the 'vertical' relations of patronage, lordship, almsgiving, or admission to a hospital.

2.3 This proposal – essentially for a view of poor relief that included the poor as active providers as well as passive recipients – was hardly new or controversial. Yet for the authors of the monographs on the Middle Ages that I was reviewing, it embodied an almost impossible brief. There was little that one could cite by way of pertinent example. The studies that were available concerned later periods. Most of them could not explore fully the highly localized, domestic context of self-help or the circumstances in which the need for charity arose.[8] The studies that moved furthest in the right direction concerned the workings of the Poor Law in early modern England.[9] Yet the force of this particular example – the possibility of extrapolating from it – seemed to be weakened by the presumption of its historians that 'the English are different, the English are best' because there was, supposedly, no equivalent form of regulated outdoor relief on the European mainland (Switzerland was highly exceptional in that regard). What my proposal might yield if implemented at monographic length, and for the Middle Ages, could only be imagined.

2.4 Imagine, I suggested, a book that combined a study of charitable foundations, like Miri Rubin's *Charity and Community in Medieval Cambridge* (1987), with one of social structure and the resources of poor citizens and transients, like Charles Phythian-Adams's *Desolation of a City: Coventry and the Urban Crisis of the Later Middle Ages* (Cambridge, 1979). Looking back into the fifteenth century from the vantage point of a 1523 census return, Phythian-Adams offered details about almost all the important demographic and familial factors determining the support that an individual might hope for when unable or unwilling to resort to an institution: the numbers never marrying, the typical age at first marriage (which affected parents' chances of being looked after in old age by their children), the rules of household formation and the proportion of nuclear to extended households (both of which influenced the availability of help from close relatives), the residential pattern (which affected the quality of neighbourliness), the sex ratio (which bore on the possibilities of remarriage for poor widows), and the employment opportunities for the young (service, apprenticeship) and older women (whether supplementing a husband's inadequate wage, supporting a sick spouse, or fending for themselves).[10]

2.5 Since 1988, of course, a number of studies have appeared that give us unexpectedly detailed group portraits of the recipients of charity in Renaissance to early modern times.[11] A smaller number have moved towards the fuller integration of family history (of the kind exemplified by Phythian-Adams) and the history of charity.[12] And a few have even explored the possibilities of pressing into service such evidence as charters and court rolls to gain some notion of the domestic resources of the medieval poor.[13] Even so, in his synopsis of *Poverty and Deviance in Early Modern Europe* (Cambridge, 1994), Robert Jütte could still note that 'only recently' had historians 'remarked upon the extent of self-help and mutual aid among the labouring poor' (p. 83).[14] My own recent involvement with the topic suggests, moreover, that, having ignored it so long, historians may now have turned to overestimating it. Partly on the basis of a collection of essays· that I co-edited with Richard Smith,[15] partly from a broad survey of the potential of ethnographic and ancient to medieval evidence,[16] four assertions have seemed warranted:

2.6 (a) There has been no 'golden age' of *intra-household* self-help among the poor in the European and Mediterranean worlds however far back we look: no period or area in which large supportive families have been efficiently responsible for the overwhelming bulk of welfare provision.

(b) Networks of connections *between* households, not necessarily involving kin, have probably been of immense importance to the needy, but such networks seem often to have been limited in strength and capacity. At this level of generality, it is argued, continuity in the history of households and networks is more evident than some fall from grace (the 'golden age' hypothesis).

(c) Historians of the sick poor should envisage a broad spectrum of resources beyond the household and its immediate connections – patrons, formalized community organizations, institutions and so on – as having been called upon for a very long time – indeed for millennia – to supplement informal assistance. To that extent, there is nothing new or modern about the 'mixed economy of care'.[17]

(d) Some of the major geographical distinctions in the history of European poor relief must also be called into question. The first is the presumed contrast between relief in early modern England – typically of the 'outdoor' kind, parish-based, comprehensive, and funded by a Poor Rate – and 'continental' European relief – supposedly haphazard and limited in its finances and scope, and based on the 'indoor' assistance provided in large hospitals. Underlying this contrast, it is held, and indeed perhaps one of its causes, is a second one (equally questionable). It is a contrast between demographic regimes and types of household organization. In early modern England, the argument goes, families were predominantly nuclear, their members were individualistic in outlook and the idea that they might look after their needy relatives was an alien one; responsibility for such people therefore fell upon the wider collectivity, beyond the household, and was met by public welfare measures such as the Poor Law. In contemporary southern Europe, on the other hand, families were allegedly larger, extended rather than nuclear; and they exhibited greater solidarity. Hence outdoor relief was rarer and other institutions less widespread and sophisticated.[18] Wrong on three counts. First, outdoor relief was far from being an English peculiarity. Second, households of the poor were generally small. Third, even where they were large, no simple correlation is discernible between size and willingness to care. Sandra Cavallo's work on early modern Turin, for example, shows that the families revealed in requests for admission to the Ospedale di Carità were, on the whole, no more ready to shoulder the burden of their dependants than were their English counterparts. It also shows that the welfare system of her area was far from exclusively indoor in its application. The contrast with England seems at least to have been exaggerated.[19]

Family History and Hospital History in the Middle Ages

3.1 That was the point I had reached when I read an article by Sharon Farmer which drew attention to the value of the Miracles of St Louis for an understanding of self-help and the resort to charity among the poor of thirteenth-century Paris and its satellite, St-Denis.[20] Farmer has been the first to notice the immense value, for the social historian, of the stories contained in this miracle book. They were faithfully summarized by Guillaume de Saint-Pathus in around 1303 from the records of the painstaking enquiry into the king's sanctity conducted between 1282 and 1283.[21] And their incidental detail – of names, dates, streets, kin relationships, living conditions – has the ring of verisimilitude. Farmer shows, moreover, how these stories can in many respects be corroborated by what else we know of the economy, the demography, and the institutional charity of contemporary Paris – charity from hospitals, religious houses, gilds, employers, and parishes. The whole context is skilfully drawn. One reads this article with a mixture of relief and annoyance: relief to find confirmation of pre-conceived ideas; annoyance that such capital evidence has been analysed so thoroughly as to leave little more to be said about it.

3.2 What I may hope to achieve in the present paper is therefore extremely modest. I can publicize Farmer's achievement and explore the miracles a little further, bringing in some stories concerning men to complement her focus on women's support networks. I can stress the perhaps surprising frequency with which charitable institutions are mentioned in the stories as an obvious resort for the sick and incapacitated, if only a temporary one.[22] I can bring out the corresponding fragility of the horizontal relationships described and the need for them to be supplemented by vertical ones, both informal and institutional. And I can adduce some further (less vivid) evidence of a similar kind from other places and periods.[23]

3.3 This programme needs a 'key note', and the one I should like to propose is that of the 'patient biography'. 'Patient' in the loose sense of the individual poor and needy person, often sick; 'biography' in terms of the sequence of welfare resources called upon. Ideally, too, there will be an implicit element of autobiography: we want to get as close as we can to the individual self-narration of the pauper, to the ways in which he or she conceived and connected the various forms of relief sought. The self-narration will of course be mediated – often heavily – by the verbal formulae of those recording (say) a court case or an inquisition. Sometimes it will be no more than a fiction, of which the value to us may be simply that the fiction must once have had sufficient general plausibility to engage its readers. Such an anecdotal approach would not satisfy a historian of recent centuries. But it may be preferable to the hazy aerial view of the subject with which medievalists have usually had to content themselves.

3.4 Before I proceed to further examples, a caveat. There is a danger in trying to envisage the whole spectrum of welfare agencies, from institutions at one end to solitary self-help at the other: the juxtaposition of so many forms of assistance can create the impression of a single well-tuned system. Now the haphazardness and lack of discrimination among later medieval forms of urban poor relief has certainly been exaggerated, and only recently have some of the continuities between these and sixteenth-century projects and institutions been fully appreciated.[24] None the less the various measures that analysis should now embrace were hardly able to keep a significant proportion of the population from extreme destitution. We cannot usually tell how big that proportion was, but we can at least sense its presence.

3.5 One corrective to any tendency to idealize the effects of welfare initiatives would be to seek out the complete failures. Rubin has valuably pointed to the need to look for evidence of those for whom charity and self-help proved ultimately inadequate – those found dead of hunger and exposure by the wayside.[25] These unfortunates have their patient biographies that deserve more extensive collection and analysis. So also do any who committed suicide as an escape from poverty.[26] Another corrective is to emphasize the self-interest and varying self-promotion of charitable donors, the lack of correlation between fashions in donation and the perceived needs of the poor.[27] If hospitals have empty beds, it is not necessarily because everyone in need is safely ensconced in some caring household, but because hospital patrons are highly selective and unresponsive to socio-economic shifts.[28] We should, then, think in terms not of a system but of a wide range of interacting 'sectors' – a jumbled, fumbling, sometimes uncaring 'mixed economy', but one which, if it should not be seen as a unity, ought certainly to be viewed in the round.

4.1 The first difficulty for the medievalist is of finding how informal support among the very poor might actually work, regardless of contact with institutions. There is a substantial sociological literature[29] and some historiographical classics.[30] But it seems to me that social anthropology offers the most evocative point of entry into this type of world – the modern equivalent to the 'autobiographies' that I would like to be able to hear in the medieval past. It is, particularly, the anthropology of the Americas that has produced some of the most sustained accounts of informal support networks among the poor.[31] Larissa Adler Lomnitz's *Networks and Marginality* (1977)[32] is a translation of a study originally published under a more revealing title meaning 'how did marginals survive?'. It reports on field work carried out between 1969 and 1971 in a shantytown of about 200 dwellings in Mexico City. The inhabitants are all first or second generation immigrants from the countryside, somewhat like the poor people who figure prominently in many of the Miracles of St Louis. They belong to the very bottom of the social scale. Many heads of household are unskilled labourers, the rest are in a variety of service occupations. None has much job security and underemployment is the norm. Indeed the average monthly earnings per residential unit are less than $100.

4.2 The first strikingly pertinent feature of the discussion concerns the complexity of living arrangements. Neither family nor household are easily conceptualized. 'A cluster of seemingly independent one-room dwellings may contain a single household. Conversely, a set of rooms with a single entrance may contain several households.'[33] Another pertinent theme to emerge from Lomnitz's study concerns the extent of cooperation and reciprocity between families and households. Of her informants she writes: 'they have literally nothing. Their only resources are of a social nature: kinship and friendship ties that generate social solidarity'. Ties between families are obviously at their closest in those 'extended' households, both under a single roof and on a single plot of land, that share cooking duties and living expenses. But even among those that do not share in this way, there is 'an intense reciprocal exchange including a variety of domestic functions'. And this occurs even though each co-resident or adjacent family leads a separate economic life. Of the independent nuclear families, meanwhile, the majority have relatives living in the same shantytown with whom they interact. No type of household is therefore typically isolated.[34]

4.3 Because of rigidly defined gender roles, the emotional content of marital relations is meagre. So men and women each tend to form their own circles. Men band into *cuate* (twin-brother) groups of five to ten in size. They get drunk, play games, or go to a bullfight together. But they also help each other in finding employment or building a home. It is the women who, as Farmer intuits, play the dominant role in cementing networks of reciprocity within and between families, networks that only a few relatively-affluent families can afford to ignore. These networks are not large, however. The majority of them link only two or three nuclear families. If their members all live under one roof or on a single plot of land, then network and household are, in a sense, coextensive. Relations of kinship dominate in the formation of networks. But some networks include close neighbours as well as kin; and a few, mostly on the smaller side, comprise neighbours only.

4.4 Three general aspects of the form of life that Lomnitz describes seem especially significant in the present context. First, the levels of economic security created are minimal: there is nothing cosy and readily sustaining about these networks. Second, networks can easily be diminished by friction or hostility between kin. Third, assistance is not always exchanged between those approximately equal in resources: asymmetric patron-client (vertical) relations may develop out of symmetric (horizontal) exchange networks. For instance, foremen become brokers between casual labourers of the shantytown and the employing builders or engineers.[35]

5.1 With this bleak modern example in mind, we can return to the historical evidence and press further back in time than the thirteenth century. The evidence must occasionally be rural: there is too little of it to preserve a strictly urban focus. It will be literary, anecdotal, and mostly drawn from hagiography; but other forms of narrative should not, of course, be excluded, especially those of pagan antiquity: 'To King Ptolemy greeting from Ctesicles. I am being wronged by Dionysius and my daughter Nike. For though I had nurtured her... when I was stricken with bodily infirmity and my eyesight became enfeebled she would not furnish me with the necessaries of life. And when I wished to obtain justice from her in Alexandria... she gave me a written oath by the king that she would pay me twenty drachmae every month... Now, however, corrupted by that bugger Dionysius, she is not keeping any of her engagements to me, in contempt of my old age and my present infirmity.'[36]

5.2 How should we interpret such complaints to high authority from Hellenistic Egypt? It might seem that they present an acutely biased view of informal, domiciliary care: much of the failure, none of the success. Yet even from the relatively abundant papyri of pre-Roman and Roman Egypt, we cannot be certain that the solidarity of the local kin group could usually be counted upon in such cases of need.[37] All we can say is that the evidence's occasional shafts of light do not illumine a happy scene. For example, some time around the end of the fourth century A.D. (to move forward into the Roman period) a city councillor fell in love with a public prostitute, but eventually, over dinner, he murdered her. The case came to trial before the governor. According to a transcript of the official record, the prostitute's mother, 'an old woman and a pauper, asks that [the councillor] be compelled for her support to provide some small consolation for her daughter's life. For she said, "this is why I gave my daughter to the pimp, so that I might have a means of support. Now that my daughter is dead I am deprived of my support..." '[38]

5.3 Seemingly no kin group to the rescue there. Nor do such groups figure prominently in that body of material that throws the broadest, if not always the most powerful, beam on social relations among the needy in late antiquity and the early Middle Ages – the biographies of saints.[39] Groups of friends and neighbours do occasionally appear as helpers, for example in the 'outdoor' care of the mentally ill or the possessed.[40] But they are not portrayed as large groups; nor (to my knowledge) is their charity ever extolled.[41]

5.4 Were even neighbours so dependable? A second-century A.D. poet imagines the following appeal from one peasant farmer to another – a rural scene, yes, but from the hand of an urban writer: 'A violent hailstorm has sheared off our standing grain, and there is nothing left to keep us from famine. Because we have no money we cannot buy imported wheat. But I hear that you have something left over from last year's good harvest. So please lend me twenty bushels, to give me the means to save my own life and that of my wife and children. And when a year of good harvest comes along, we will repay you... Please do let good neighbours go to ruin in times such as these.'[42] The answer to the plea for help is not given. The typical character of reciprocity among the poor, with its ethos of calculation and instrumentality, could not be better evoked, however. The resources in question are perceived as scarce; in ancient as in modern times, competition for them is a zero-sum game; neighbours are as likely to steal your possessions as to make good your losses;[43] horizontal networks of reciprocity seem delicate creations and always have to be supplemented 'vertically', by support from 'higher up'.[44]

5.5 Which is not to argue that horizontal ties functioned hardly at all. There is certainly evidence of the sorts of local interchange that we have been extracting from the record of much later centuries. Some of that evidence is again – inevitably – literary. In the early second century A.D. the orator Dio Chrysostom paints an elaborate and clever picture of rustic simplicity contrasted with urban decadence.[45] Unlike the farmer in the earlier literary vignette, the family depicted here have diversified their means of subsistence. They have plenty of wheat, barley and millet in store – though not beans, 'because they didn't grow this year'. Their other resources include a garden, two vines, the produce of hunting, and some livestock. But they also look to the benefits of having a functionally extended family. Their daughter has married a man of some substance in the local village. 'We don't want for anything', the woman of the house says, 'but they [her daughter and the husband] take a bit of game when we have it or fruit or vegetables – they don't have a garden. And last year we had some of their wheat, threshed seed, and gave them it back as soon as harvest was in.' The detail is imagined – no equivalent of an ethnographic record. But Dio's presentation, though stylized, does need to be plausible.

5.6 Moreover, aspects of it can be matched from non-literary sources. Gallant provides what is in effect an extended commentary on it with respect to earlier Greek material.[46] For the Roman period, we have in rabbinic sources hints of a similar level of exchange, even across religious boundaries.[47] In the small towns and the villages of Galilee during the second and third centuries, a Jewish woman might lend her blouse to a gentile friend or a Jewish man his ass or some farm equipment. Between, just as within, religious communities, there could be mutual aid in the work-place or in the sharing of a storehouse to deposit goods. Men living in the same alleyway or courtyard might pool their resources so as be able to buy in bulk; women living close together lent each other sieves or ovens.[48]

5.7 What we do not find men or women doing, in these or indeed in any equivalent sources, is cooperating with, or benefiting from, other members of a large supportive *household*. The co-resident groups encountered in the preceding *aperçus* have been nuclear or sub-nuclear. Neighbours sharing courtyards and rooftops emerge from such evidence with more credit than do kin. It is the same in rabbinic texts generally. The rabbis assume that people have only nuclear families to assist them – apart from occasional hired help. 'There is little evidence of any kind of the extended family sticking together in this period. One text alone suggests that a young couple might dwell in the same courtyard or house as the husband's parents, whereas there is a striking absence of halakha dealing with relations between a woman and her mother-in-law or with property relations between a man and his father.'[49] There are no early versions of the retirement contract, then. And, more generally, there are, it appears, few extended households.

5.8 Of course extension both vertically and laterally was a phase that numerous households would go through at some point in their developmental cycle. But any demographic 'snapshot' that we can envisage seems likely to reveal as great a preponderance of nuclear households among the poor as would later be characteristic of many parts of early modern Europe. 'All the instruments we have agree', Auden wrote in his elegy for Yeats. For our present purpose, those instruments include the very narrow circle of family members commemorated on the tombstones that survive in their thousands from the ancient and late antique worlds, and have been submitted to computerized analysis; the oblique references to household membership in hagiography and other literary genres; legal texts; the registers of dependent peasants on the great estates of the early medieval West; and the more limited evidence from that period of property transmission among peasants. By any measure, and with respect to any period, from the late Roman Republic to the tenth century A.D. and indeed further into the Middle Ages, in both southern Europe and Germanic lands, most poor households were small and many of these were simply conjugal.[50]

5.9 This does not mean that they were isolated. We may guess – though can never prove – that the household was no more the fundamental unit and source of welfare provision in this late-ancient to earlier-medieval period than it would be in Lomnitz's shantytown. Informal mutual support would, typically, be operating *between*, at least as much as *within*, dwellings. To say more about these systems than has already been said, and to show how they relate to patterns of residence, is extremely difficult. All that can be asserted for the moment – upon the basis of a considerable volume of source material – is that there is no sign, either around the ancient Mediterranean or in early medieval Europe, of the widespread existence

among the poor of households large and cohesive enough to be self-suffi-
cient.

5.10 The household or family history of the poor intersects, then, at
every turn with the world of 'vertical' relations, at least part of which com-
prises institutions of welfare and healing. There are isolated vignettes showing the scope and the limits of neighbourly and familial assistance in some Dark Age texts not hitherto exploited in this context, such as Anskar's
Miracles of St Willehad.[51] But, for the most ample illustration, we should
look to the corpus of hagiographies written by Gregory, bishop of Tours,
in the later sixth century.[52] In Gregory's miracle narratives pauper households appear predictably small, mostly conjugal. Neither the immediate
family nor the kin group is ever represented as supportive. Instead, there
is seemingly a ready resort to institutional or informal charity. For example: 'a woman named Foedamia was restricted by swelling due to paralysis and felt pain whenever she moved any part of her body. Her relatives
brought her and put her on display at the blessed church [of St Julian in
Brioude], so that she might earn her keep from almsgivers.' The martyr
Julian appeared to her and she was cured. Gregory fails to tell us how old
she was, but he does say that she had been paralysed for eighteen years.
So we should not accuse her relatives of too hastily ridding themselves of
the burden of an unproductive member, in need, presumably, of continual
nursing. But it is very striking how entirely matter of fact and non-judg-
mental Gregory is in his report of their decision to put the woman out to
beg.[53]

5.11 In another story, from the *Miracles of St Martin of Tours*, Gregory
does offer an excuse for a similar familial response to incapacity. A blind
child was 'given to beggars, so that he might wander about with them and
receive some alms; for his parents were very poor'.[54] Elsewhere, neighbourly support is represented as somewhat out of the ordinary. A slave
named Veranus, stricken with gout, lost the use of his feet. 'After Veranus
was afflicted for an entire year with such pains that even his neighbors located nearby carried him [*ut etiam vicina in proximo posita commoveret*],

suddenly his nerves stiffened and he was completely crippled'. That is why his master, 'grieved at the loss of a faithful slave' (or rather, one surmises, at the loss of his labour), had him brought to the shrine of St Martin.[55]

5.12 These stories focus on healing shrines, not on an institution of poor relief in the usual sense. Yet assistance to the poor was hardly alien to the purposes of those promoting a saint's cult. Gregory's narratives have the merit of showing us how an early medieval hagiographer depicted the patient biographies of those who found healing at his favoured shrines. There is, moreover, some reinforcement from another quarter for their implication that informal ties of family, kin or neighbours were not thought automatically able to sustain the poor, sick and disabled during the early Middle Ages. The reinforcement comes from Iceland.

5.13 Like all other Scandinavian countries apart from Finland, Iceland is conventionally included within the sphere of the north-western European household formation system, which always tended towards nuclearity.[56] Iceland is also the country for which the greatest degree of continuity in welfare arrangements, particularly care for the elderly, has been hazarded by historical demographers – a continuity from the early Middle Ages to the nineteenth century.[57] The national law book of Iceland is a vernacular compilation dating, in its surviving version, from the later twelfth century; but it embodies material from before the Christianization of the country over two centuries previously.[58] In it we read: 'A man must first maintain his mother. If he can manage more, then he must also maintain his father. If he can do better still, then he must maintain his children. If still better, then he must maintain his brothers and sisters. If better again, then he must maintain those people whose heir he is and those he has taken in against the promise of inheritance. If yet better, he must maintain the freed man to whom he gave liberty.'[59]

5.14 Anyone unable to support his parents as the law prescribed should approach the nearest kinsman with any resources to spare and should offer to work as his slave in order to pay off the loan of whatever was necessary to keep his parents alive. If some such family support proved impossible, then responsibility passed to the *hreppr*, a commune of twenty or so farms. It is all highly reminiscent of the Elizabethan Poor Law ('the father and grandfather, mother and grandmother, and children of every poor... person... shall at their own charges relieve and maintain every such poor person...'[60]). But the Icelandic law-makers seem to take an even less optimistic view of the potential of family support and of the range of kin from whom it might be expected. They do not expect much spontaneous generosity. They know that institutions will have to be relied upon. Nor is their gloomy outlook unique. It might be tempting to hypothesize that the need for such a law arose in Iceland from the breakdown of traditional means of supporting the needy caused by the trauma of migration from Norway in the ninth century.[61] But that is to ignore partial analogues in other Scandinavian codes, where it is insisted that kin rather than non-kin take in the poor and elderly – in return for a right to the inheritance.[62]

6.1 It is against this early medieval backdrop that we can return to the high and later Middle Ages. Again there are some fragmentary pieces of evidence that could be brought into the reckoning. In the twelfth-century Miracles of St William of Norwich we encounter, for instance, a representative of the labouring poor (as they would later be called) who accommodates a blind man in his home. There is also a priest who houses and clothes a severely paralysed woman, taking her from one healing shrine to another thrown face down over the back of a horse; and there are parents who bring their incapacitated child to a shrine in a wheelbarrow (*manuali vehiculo*).[63] In the Miracles of King Henry VI, reworked in the early sixteenth century, we see how a poor unskilled worker can descend into vagrancy and can mix, albeit unwittingly, with criminals; and we learn how neighbours gather round anxiously when they think a house is on fire (mistakenly as it happens: the glow is that of a vision of King Henry).[64] Such details show local self-help and mutual support in operation – but not very extensively. They are briefly introduced into the texts only to explain the dire circumstances in which resort to the saint came to seem the obvious solution.

6.2 Or resort to the hospital. The Miracles of St Louis, to my knowledge the fullest evocation from medieval hagiography of the interaction of pauper self-help and institutional charity, are especially suggestive in this respect. They include, on one hand, several minor success stories – stories of informal care among the poor in operation rather than breaking down. On the other hand, they also show the 'market penetration' of institutions.

6.3 To take some success stories first: Contesse lived in the same boarding house as Nicole on the Rue des Lavandières. Nicole had what appears to have been a severe stroke and was left paralysed and scarcely able to eat. But Contesse, who 'mout l'amoit', cared for her for more than two months, making her bed, helping her in and out of it, and bathing her. A neighbour then also lent her assistance. She owned a cart and between them the two women carried Nicole to the shrine of St Denis.[65]

6.4 Two other narratives: Richard, a draper, lived with his sister in St Denis. She looked after him and kept him from beggary for four years when he became so ill that he could not work.[66] Luce, who had emigrated to St Denis from Normandy, began to suffer from an acute eye disease sometime after she had given birth to a child. Within two years she became completely blind, and remained so for another eight years. During that time, however, she was able to produce, and nurse, no fewer than three further children. Her husband had no property and lived by his labour. And since Luce sold pickled fish once she regained her sight, we may presume that she had been working before the onset of disability. Yet Luce never had to beg. There was, surprisingly, a servant in the household, and Luce was also assisted by her nine-year old daughter. So the family was able to keep going without resort to charity, despite the number of children and the probable loss of the wife's earning power.[67]

6.5 In general, the Miracles of St Louis show us needy people – mostly but not entirely women – able to find lodging or help. But not necessarily in the long term. Many of the arrangements are makeshift. Employers are more often than not represented as jettisoning their servants when they become too ill to function. And it is worth remarking that, in the narratives, we do not find any cases of single women who find board with parents or siblings.[68] With a few exceptions, such as that of Luce, family economies are too fragile. Interactions among neighbours – within or between tenements – are far more prominent, and even they have their darker side: failure in reciprocity can lead to an accusation of sorcery.[69]

6.6 We can thus balance the success stories in the Miracles against the instances of breakdown in local informal care and the frequency with which institutional relief enters the picture (as in the story of Jehanne with which I opened).

6.7 When, for instance, Amile got up in the middle of the night (some time in 1271-2) to give a drink to one of her children she suddenly became paralysed. A lump appeared in her groin and grew eventually into a large open sore. After she had endured in this condition for three or four months her husband left her 'par ennui' and quitted Paris (perhaps in search of work). Hobbling on a crutch she had to beg for alms at her local church. It was her brother, not her husband, who took her to St Denis in the hope of cure.[70]

6.8 Elsewhere in the Miracles we meet a sixty-year old man whose body began to shake so much that he could not work normally and was reduced to begging and selling keys, and a blind man who, though helped by others (named in the text but not specified as relatives), still also had to beg.[71] In another narrative, Moriset could not keep his job as a doorkeeper when he became mildly ill; he went to lodge with his brother Colin. There, however, his afflictions became far more serious. Though he remained thus in his brother's house for about two months, his brother was poor and had his wife and five children to support. So Moriset decided to go to the hospital in Saumur, which was not far from where he thought his step-mother lived. On arrival in the hospital, however, he discovered that his relative was dead (although she had left a son living in the area). Worse, he soon developed such a huge and noisome aposteme on his backside that, eventually, the hospital was no longer willing to look after him. Thence he travelled, not to his half brother but as a solitary to various shrines, and finally to that of St Denis.[72]

6.9 The Miracles of St Louis are a particularly valuable set of narratives for two reasons. First, they give us a wider view of informal relief among the poor than the usual tales, which highlight moments of failure. Granted, they concentrate on the hardships created by illness rather than by sheer impoverishment, and they have little direct to say about illnesses other than paralysis. Like so much medieval evidence, too, they for the most part stare resolutely through the vast mass of the labouring poor. None the less they do show us families and individuals just managing to survive, as well as those at the end of their resources. They show or at least hint at the full range of vertical and institutional ties upon which those in need had to draw because their own horizontal means of support were inadequate. They do so in detail, giving personal names and dates, street names and places. So there is plenty of vividness. But the second reason why these miracles are, or should be, so precious to the social historian of the Middle Ages is that their details are ones upon which we can generally rely. This is not only because of the thoroughness of the ecclesiastical enquiry into Louis IX's posthumous miracles. It is much more because the detail is presented with almost no moralizing. The husband who abandoned his wife is not treated sympathetically. But otherwise the details in the narratives do not seem to have been subordinated to some ethical purpose. Unusually, no interest is shown in the sins that might have led to illness. An illness simply strikes, as part of the natural order of things. To be cured, one needs first to have confessed, of course. But even that message is not emphasized within the narratives. So we do not need to suspect that incidental detail – of the sort which is here of so much interest – has been selected or distorted to suit some theological theme – other than that of demonstrating the accessibility of St Louis as intercessor to even the poorest, and the concern of this heroic and active monarch with even the most paralysed of his erstwhile subjects.

7.1 What we need, of course, are many more vignettes like his miracle stories. A picture could then be built up that is sufficiently broad to yield statistically significant conclusions. The way forward has recently been shown by two monographs dealing with a subject that I have omitted so far because it is enough here simply to cite these works. That subject is the perils of childhood. Medieval hagiography is full of children. It is a matter of some surprise that historians of childhood have not, a handful of articles apart, exploited it more rigorously.[73] Now, however, we have a pair of exemplary studies: Didier Lett's *L'enfant des miracles: enfance et société au Moyen Âge (XIIe-XIIIe siècle)* (Paris, 1997), and Ronald C. Finucane's *The Rescue of the Innocents: Endangered Children in Medieval Miracles* (Houndmills and London, 1997). They are exemplary, first, because both seem, overall, to suggest that the circle of those emotionally or practically involved with needy children was quite narrow – apart from extreme occasions when the very young had strayed well outside the home and neighbours came to the rescue.[74] Second, they replay for us the debate amongst historians between advocates of the theological and of the sociological approaches to the interpretation of miracle narratives. Finucane is inclined to treat his corpus of some 600 incidents as the equivalent of modern governmental health and accident data.[75] By contrast, Lett for instance reminds us how much the incidental detail in narratives involving children may owe to the popularity, in the High Middle Ages, of the apocryphal 'infancy gospels'.[76]

7.2 A germane conclusion tentatively proffered by Finucane should be assessed in this light. The eight major miracle collections which he has analysed were selected so as to bring out any possible discrepancies between north-western and Mediterranean Europe.[77] One of these may, perhaps, be detected in the range of the adult participants in the various childhood dramas that the miracle tales recall.

More kin were involved in all categories (birth, accidents, illnesses) in southern Europe than in the north. Among the 156 child victims of accidents, only 28 cases were reported from southern Europe. This is a narrow basis for comparison, but it is striking that kin (apart from parents) were explicitly referred to in 9 of the 28 instances, i.e. in 32 percent of the southern cases. Northern Europe provided 128 examples of child accidents, but here non-parental kin were mentioned in only 15 cases, or 12 percent of the sample. 'Even though, in accidents, often a neighbor or stranger discovered the child's body rather than a kinsman, whenever kin were involved, they were more than twice as likely to show up in southern cases than in northern... Among the 334 illnesses, 62 reports (19 percent) included an explicit reference to kin beyond the nuclear family... Of 124 cases reported from the north, kin were mentioned in 6 instances (5 percent of cases); but in southern Europe, of 210 illnesses kin were present in 56 cases (27 percent)... It is just possible that these differences reflect a distinction between the conjugal northern, and extended southern, family models.'[78]

7.3 In terms of the effectiveness of households as welfare providers, that north-south distinction has already been called into question; but the evidence was early modern rather than medieval. Finucane's sample of hagiographical cases is far more substantial than anything I have been able to present above. It is, nonetheless, still too small to be conclusive.

8.1 The literary evidence adduced in this paper, coupled with a comparative analysis that brings in ethnography and detail from later periods, seems to me to offer something that, however provisional, really is counterintuitive – a conclusion which does *not* simply confirm what we had always suspected. It seems to show that the economy of welfare was always a mixed one in the Middle Ages; hospitals, paradoxically, have a larger place in it than might have been predicted from the simplistic calculation of ratios or from estimates of general standards of living. Families, households, neighbourhoods, have a less dominant role than might have been expected from the assertions that historians customarily make. Informal welfare is vital, certainly. Yet it is not as capacious as it has been projected because pauper households are too small and pauper networks too fragile to sustain very much in the way of extra burdens.

8.2 In the Preface to his *Historia Brittonum*, the Dark Age chronicler, Nennius, set out his methodology in the way that all good historians should: 'I have made a heap [*coacervavi*] of all that I have found'. Those who want to discover the workings of informal networks of mutual support amongst the medieval poor and the connections between such networks and charitable institutions are still at the stage of heap-making. Finucane's heap is larger than most. Farmer's is perhaps the most revealing. My own is, if nothing else, the most eclectic. There is a lot more work ahead for all of us.[79]

Notes

1 Guillaume de Saint-Pathus, *Les miracles de Saint Louis*, Editor P. B. Fay, no. XLII, Paris, 1931.
2 B. Geremek, *The Margins of Society in Late Medieval Paris*, Cambridge, 1987, pp. 170-1.
3 *Miracles de Saint Louis*, II.
4 P. Horden, *A Discipline of Relevance: The Historiography of the Later Medieval Hospital*, in "Social History of Medicine", 1, 1988, pp. 359-74.
5 See now B. Harvey, *Living and Dying in England 1100-1540: The Monastic Experience*, Oxford, 1993, ch. III. 4.
6 Which is not to belittle the importance of such works as C. Dyer, *Standards of Living in the Later Middle Ages*, Cambridge, 1989, ch. 8.
7 Cf. C. Dyer, review of M. Rubin, *Charity and Community in Medieval Cambridge*, in "Social History", 13, 1988, pp. 233-5.
8 Cf. John Henderson (Ed.), *Charity and the Poor in Medieval and Renaissance Europe*, special issue of "Continuity and Change", 3, 1988.
9 R. M. Smith (Ed.), *Land, Kinship and Life-Cycle*, Cambridge, 1984.
10 Horden, *A Discipline of Relevance*, p. 372.
11 E.g. J. Henderson, *Piety and Charity in Late Medieval Florence*, Oxford, 1994; J. Arrizabalaga, J. Henderson and R. French, *The Great Pox*, New Haven and London,

1997, ch. 7.

12 E.g., John Henderson and Richard Wall (Eds.), *Poor Women and Children in the European Past*, London, 1994; M. Daunton (Ed.), *Charity, Self-Interest and Welfare in the English Past*, London, 1996; S. Mendelson and R. Crawford, *Women in Early Modern England*, Oxford, 1998.

13 E.g. E. Clark, *Social Welfare and Mutual Aid in the Medieval Countryside*, in "Journal of British Studies", 33, 1994, pp. 381-406, as well as her contribution to Henderson and Wall; P. Skinner, *Gender and Poverty in the Medieval Community*, in *Medieval Women in their Communities*, Editor D. Watt, Cardiff, 1997, pp. 204-21.

14 Which does some injustice to O. Hufton, *The Poor of Eighteenth-Century France*, 1974, chs. 3-4.

15 With R. M. Smith, *The Locus of Care: Families, Communities, Institutions, and the Provision of Welfare since Antiquity*, London, 1998.

16 *Household Care and Informal Networks: Comparisons and Continuities from Antiquity to the Present*, in *The Locus of Care*, pp. 21-67.

17 Cf. J. Lewis, *Family Provision of Health and Welfare in the Mixed Economy of Care in the Late Nineteenth and Twentieth Centuries*, in "Social History of Medicine", 8, 1995, pp. 1-16.

18 J. Hajnal, *Two Kinds of Preindustrial Household Formation System*, in "Population and Development Review", 8, 1982, pp. 449-94; P. Laslett, *Family, Kinship and Collectivity as Systems of Support in Pre-Industrial Europe: a Consideration of the Nuclear Hardship Hypothesis*, in "Continuity and Change", 3, 1988, pp. 153-75.

19 S. Cavallo, *Family Obligations and Inequalities in Access to Care in Northern Italy, Seventeenth to Eighteenth Centuries*, in *The Locus of Care*, Editors P. Horden and R. M. Smith, 1998, pp. 90-110.

20 S. Farmer, *Down and Out and Female in Thirteenth-Century Paris*, in "American Historical Review", 103, 1998, pp. 345-72, to which I am immensely indebted.

21 Farmer, pp. 349-50.

22 Cf. Farmer, p. 360.

23 Drawing substantially, but no means entirely, on my contribution to *The Locus of Care*.

24 S. Cavallo, *Charity and Power in Early Modern Italy: Benefactors and their Motives in Turin*, Cambridge, 1995, pp. 23-8.

25 Rubin, *Charity and Community*, p. 267 with n. 178; Horden, *A Discipline of*

Relevance, pp. 371-2 with n. 41.

26 A. Murray, *Suicide in the Middle Ages*, vol. 1, Oxford, 1998, has no direct evidence on poverty (pp. 400-3). Perhaps it was not a significant factor.

27 Cavallo, *Charity and Power*, is exemplary on this topic. See also her *Charity as Boundary Making: Social Stratification, Gender and the Family in the Italian States (Seventeenth-Nineteenth Centuries)*, in *Charity, Philanthropy and Reform: From the 1690s to 1850*, Editors H. Cunningham and J. Innes, London, 1998, pp. 108-29.

28 Contrast J. W. Brodman, *Charity and Welfare: Hospitals and the Poor in Medieval Catalonia*, Philadelphia, 1998, p. 72.

29 M. Nolan, G. Grant and J. Keady, *Understanding Family Care: A Multidimensional Model of Caring and Coping*, Buckingham and Philadelphia, 1996, is a handy synthesis and literature survey.

30 E. Ross, *Survival Networks: Women's Neighbourhood Sharing* in *London before World War I*, in "History Workshop Journal", 15, 1983, pp. 4-27. Compare also L. Page Moch and R. G. Fuchs, *Getting Along: Poor Women's Networks in Nineteenth-Century Paris*, in "French Historical Studies", 18, 1993, pp. 34-49, cited by Farmer, p. 346 n. 6.

31 See also C. B. Stack, *All Our Kin: Strategies for Survival in a Black Community*, New York, 1974; though cf. I. Pardo, *Managing Existence in Naples*, Cambridge, 1996, p. 90ff. for a recent Italian example.

32 L. A. Lomnitz, *Networks and Marginality: Life in a Mexican Shantytown*, New York, 1977. I here reproduce a discussion from *The Locus of Care*, ch. 1.

33 Lomnitz, *Networks*, p. 89.

34 Quotations from Lomnitz, *Networks*, pp. 3, 101.

35 Lomnitz, *Networks*, p. 202.

36 Trans. A. K. Bowman, *Egypt after the Pharoahs 332 B.C.-A.D. 642*, 2nd edn, London, 1996, p. 58; cf. P. Garnsey and G. Woolf, *Patronage of the Rural Poor in the Roman World*, in *Patronage in Ancient Society*, Editor A. Wallace-Hadrill, London, 1989, pp. 155-6.

37 Garnsey and Woolf, *Patronage of the Rural Poor*, p. 155; although cf. R. S. Bagnall, *Egypt in Late Antiquity*, Princeton, 1993, p. 203, for some interaction among members of nuclear households.

38 *Aegyptische Urkunden aus den Koeniglichen Museen zu Berlin: Griechische Urkunden*, vol. 4.1 (Berlin, 1904), no. 1024.7 (pp. 19-20); trans. M. R. Lefkowitz and M. R. Fant, *Women's Life in Greece and Rome*, 2nd edn, London, 1992, p. 125;

Bagnall, *Egypt in Late Antiquity*, p. 197.

39 L. Theis, *Saints sans famille? Quelques remarques sur la famille dans le monde franc à travers les sources hagiographiques*, in "Revue historique", 225, 1976, pp. 3-21; J. L. Nelson, *Family, Gender and Sexuality in the Middle Ages*, in *Companion to Historiography*, Editor M. Bentley, London and New York, 1997, pp. 153-76.

40 P. Horden, *Responses to Possession and Insanity in the Earlier Byzantine World*, in "Social History of Medicine", 6, 1993, pp. 177-94.

41 Marc le Diacre: *Vie de Porphyre évêque de Gaza*, Editors H. Grégoire and M.-A. Kugener, Paris, 1930, ch. 97 (p. 74).

42 Alciphron, *Letters 2 (Letters to Farmers)*, 3, translator B. Shaw, in "Social History of Medicine" 2, 1989, p. 205.

43 T. W. Gallant, *Risk and Survival in Ancient Greece: Reconstructing the Rural Domestic Economy*, Oxford, 1991, pp. 144-5, 148, 158.

44 Gallant, *Risk and Survival*, p. 158, cf. p. 155.

45 *Euboicus* (= *Oratio* 7) 69, in *Dio Chrysostom: Orations VII, XII and XXXVI*, Editor D. A. Russell, Cambridge, 1992. Cf. P. Garnsey, *Famine and Food Supply in the Graeco-Roman World*, Cambridge, 1988, pp. 56-7.

46 Gallant, *Risk and Survival*, ch. 6.

47 M. Goodman, *State and Society in Roman Galilee, A.D. 132-212*, Totowa, NJ, 1983, p. 44.

48 M. Peskowitz, *Family/ies in Antiquity: Evidence from Tannaitic Literature and Roman Galilean Architecture*, in *The Jewish Family in Antiquity*, Editor S. J. D. Cohen, Atlanta, GA, 1993, p. 33.

49 Goodman, *State and Society*, p. 36.

50 For supporting references, ranging from late antiquity to well into the Middle Ages, see B. Shaw, *Latin Funerary Epigraphy and Family Life in the Later Roman Empire*, in "Historia", 33, 1984, pp. 457-97; Nelson, *Family, Gender and Sexuality in the Middle Ages*.

51 *Miracula S. Willehadi auctore S. Anskari episcopo Bremensi*, IX, XII, *Acta Sanctorum*, November, vol. 3, p. 349.

52 P. Horden, forthcoming, *The Sick Family in the Early Middle Ages*.

53 *De virtutibus Juliani*, IX, translator R. Van Dam, *Saints and their Miracles in Late Antique Gaul*, Princeton, 1993, p. 170.

54 *De virtutibus Martini*, III.16, translator Van Dam, pp. 266-7.

55 *De virtutibus Martini*, II.4, translator Van Dam, p. 231.

56 Hajnal, *Two Kinds*, p. 449; although on Finland see now B. Moring, *Marriage and*

Social Change in South-Western Finland, 1700-1870, in "Continuity and Change", 11, 1996, pp. 91-113.

57 G. A. Gunnlaugsson and L. Guttormsson, *Transitions into Old Age: Poverty and Retirement Possibilities in Late Eighteenth- and Nineteenth-Century Iceland*, in *Poor Women and Children in the European Past*, Editors P. Henderson and R. Wall, pp. 251-68. P. Laslett, *A Fresh Map of Life: The Emergence of the Third Age*, 2nd edn., London, 1993, pp. 158-9.

58 M. Stein-Wilkeshuis, *The Right to Social Welfare in Early Medieval Iceland*, in "Journal of Medieval History", 8, 1982, pp. 343-52.

59 *Grágás*, cap. 128, translated in P. Foote and D. M. Wilson, *The Viking Achievement*, London, 1970, p. 120. Cf. Stein-Wilkeshuis, *Right to Social Welfare*, pp. 345-6.

60 39-40 *Elizabeth I*, caps. 3-5.

61 Stein-Wilkeshuis, *Right to Social Welfare*, p. 351. Cf. J. L. Bycock, *Medieval Iceland: Society, Sagas, and Power, Berkeley and Los Angeles*, 1988, pp. 52-4, 57. On medieval Icelandic kinship structures, not redolent of breakdown to the non-specialist, see K. Hastrup, *Culture and History in Medieval Iceland*, Oxford, 1985, ch. 3.

62 Stein-Wilkeshuis, *Right to Social Welfare*, p. 346.

63 *The Life and Miracles of William of Norwich by Thomas of Monmouth*, Editors A. Jessop and M. R. James, Cambridge, 1986, pp. 168, 242, 245; cf. also pp. 148 (for year-long residence in a hospital), 159, 206, 223, 226, 228 (role of 'friends').

64 *The Miracles of King Henry VI*, Editors and Translators R. A. Knox and S. Leslie, London, 1923, XL (89), CLXVI (213); cf XXXVII (81) for resort to hospital.

65 *Miracles of St Louis, XXXIX*, with Farmer, p. 345; quotation from 120.

66 *Miracles of St Louis, XXIV* (p. 81).

67 Farmer, pp. 357-8,

68 Farmer, p. 363.

69 Farmer, pp. 364-5.

70 *Miracles of St Louis, LII* (p.159 ff.).

71 *Miracles of St Louis*, VIII-IX (pp. 27, 30).

72 *Miracles of St Louis*, XIV.

73 E.g. B. A. Hanawalt, *Narratives of a Nurturing Culture: Parents and Neighbors in Medieval England*, in Hanawalt, *'Of Good and Ill Repute': Gender and Social Control in Medieval England*, New York and Oxford, 1998, ch. 10.

74 Finucane, pp. 30, 57, 70-1, 84-5, and, for 'first finders' of accident victims, pp. 147-8; Lett, ch. 13.

75 E.g. Finucane, p. 141.

76 Lett, p. 91 ff.

77 Finucane, pp. 3-6.

78 Finucane, p. 166.

79 I am greatly indebted to John Henderson, Carole Rawcliffe and Ian Wood for advice and references.

Post Scriptum: since the above paper was written, in 2000, Sharon Farmer has published an extended analysis of the Miracles of St Louis in *Surviving Poverty in Medieval Paris: Gender, Ideology, and the Daily Lives of the Poor*, Ithaca and London, 2002. I regret not have been able to take account of this important monograph.

VII

A DISCIPLINE OF RELEVANCE: THE HISTORIOGRAPHY OF THE LATER MEDIEVAL HOSPITAL

A discipline of relevance: knowing what to include, what connections to make. That is how F. R. Leavis repeatedly characterized literary criticism. It is also how the historiography of medieval hospitals can suitably be conceived. In this above all journals, there need be no embarrassment in protesting against the 'tunnel vision' of narrowly institutional hospital histories, content to string together star names and momentous dates.[1] The subject clearly requires more than the equivalent of an elementary knowledge of literary plot.[2] Agreement on that, however, still leaves the big question open. How should the history of pre-modern hospitals be written? The now habitual response is that it should be analytical; that it should invoke the widest cultural and economic contexts—in short, that hospital history is inescapably social history. This response is uplifting but hardly precise.[3] Perhaps the appropriate contexts have not yet all been identified, let alone properly explored.

The present essay is no 'literature survey'.[4] I can merely sample the voluminous recent work dealing with hospitals in western Europe during the later

[1] J. R. Guy, 'Of the Writing of Hospital Histories there is No End', *Bulletin of the History of Medicine*, lix (1985), 415–20.

[2] Hospital histories that exhibit little more are still, however, being published. See J. Henderson's review in *Bulletin of the History of Medicine*, lxii (1988), 122–3.

[3] I owe the distinction between descriptive and analytical approaches to various pieces by John Henderson that he kindly allowed me to read in typescript. See also 'Editorial Introduction', *Social History of Medicine*, i (1988), v.

[4] Each of the works to be discussed below has a wide range of references. See also the bibliographies in C. Lis and H. Soly, *Poverty and Capitalism in Pre-Industrial Europe* (Sussex, 1979); in M. Mollat, *The Poor in the Middle Ages: An Essay in Social History* (New Haven and London, 1986), translation of *Les Pauvres au Moyen Age* (Paris, 1978); in various papers in *Continuity and Change*, iii (Aug. 1988), a special issue edited by J. Henderson on 'Charity and the Poor in Medieval and Renaissance Europe'; and in L. Granshaw and R. Porter (eds.), *The History of Hospitals* (forthcoming). See also A. Vauchez, 'Assistance et Charité en Occident, XIIIe–XVe siècles', in V. Barbagli Bagnoli (ed.), *Domanda e Consumi: Livelli e Strutture (nei Secoli (XIII–XVIII)* (Prato and Florence, 1978), pp. 151–62. J. Imbert (ed.), *Histoire des Hôpitaux en France* (Toulouse, 1982) is a valuable collection but has a very meagre bibliography. I regret not yet having seen two recent books by B. Geremek: *Mendicanti e Miserabili nell'Europa Moderna (1350–1600)* (Rome, 1985), and *La Pietà e la Forca: Storia della Miseria e della Carità in Europa* (Rome, Bari, 1986). I also regret lacking space for Spanish examples. See A. Rubio Vela, *Pobreza, Enfermedad y Assistencia Hospitalaria en la Valencia del Siglo XIV* (Valencia, 1984), and L. Matz, *Poverty and Welfare in Hapsburg Spain: The Example of Toledo* (Cambridge, 1983), now to be read in conjunction with D. Goodman, *Power and Penury: Government, Technology and Science in Philip II's Spain* (Cambridge, 1988).

Middle Ages. My primary focus will be Miri Rubin's book, *Charity and Community in Medieval Cambridge.*[5] I shall rehearse some of its findings concerning hospitals and compare them with those of new (or newly published) work on three European cities. Then, returning to the Cambridge evidence, I hope to suggest aspects of the subject in which a compelling discipline of relevance has yet to be attained. In particular, I shall emphasize the importance of understanding the role of the very smallest hospitals, too often confined to the background of modern accounts, and of viewing hospitals of all sizes from the vantage point of family history.

I

As Rubin's scholarly and comprehensive monograph demonstrates, the one significant hospital—also the best documented—in Cambridge and its environs was the Hospital of St John, later to become St John's College in the University. Its origins and early development cannot be fully established. But it appears to have been founded at the beginning of the thirteenth century on an area of wasteland near the town centre. In collaboration with the borough community, a burgess erected a small house for the poor and sick. He later asked the bishop of Ely for permission to add an oratory and cemetery. The establishment thus enjoyed all the immunities and privileges of a church; and the bishop, possibly not without opposition, became its patron (Rubin, pp. 99–111).

There is no evidence of any medical involvement with the hospital beyond the attestation of a charter of donation to it (dating from before 1230) by a *Robertus medicus* and the recorded payment of wages by the hospital to a barber (-surgeon?) in 1485 (p. 152). The sick and poor inmates may not have required 'professional' scrutiny, however. The hospital's rule—by no means an eccentric one—forbad the admission of pregnant women, lepers, the wounded, cripples, and the insane. The rationale can be surmised. Pregnant women seeking a hospital bed were likely to have conceived out of wedlock, and in any case could not with propriety be accommodated in a male community; lepers were catered for elsewhere; the wounded might have been involved in a brawl and hence were dangerous to know; and, like cripples and the mentally ill, they probably could not look after themselves (pp. 157–9).

The hospital avoided admitting those that would inevitably place too great a strain on its resources. Nor did it open its doors wide. An apostolic twelve is a reasonable estimate of the number of sick and poor with which it generally coped. The process by which these were selected is unknown. But the quasi-monastic life-style imposed on them after admission can be reconstructed quite easily. It followed the same essentially Augustinian rule kept by the lay and clerical brothers (perhaps ten in all) and the hospital's master, who, along with some half-dozen servitors, completed the establishment (pp. 159–76).

Altogether, then, hardly more than thirty men lived or worked in the

---

[5] Cambridge, Cambridge University Press, 1987. Pp. xiv + 365. ISBN 0-521-32392-4.

hospital, and the poor were in the minority. When the hospital was refounded as an academic college in the early 1500s, the poor had, apparently, long ceased to merit any space in it at all. The apostolic twelve had yielded to a variable gathering of corrodians (who purchased accommodation and sustenance in the hospital for the remainder of their lives in return for a handsome benefaction or promised legacy), poor scholars, paying guests, and, periodically, members of the bishop's consistory court (pp. 110–11, 171–3, and 183).

Not all Cambridge hospitals changed in this way. For instance, the alms-houses founded in the second half of the fifteenth century seem to have endured well. And a leper hospital dating from about 1361 was still functioning as such in Tudor times—although, in nice conformity with Foucault's account, it may also have admitted the mad.[6] But most local charitable concerns did not survive as such. The earliest foundation—possibly a royal one—the leper hospital at Stourbridge on the outskirts of Cambridge, had by the mid-thirteenth century become simply a free chapel in the patronage of the bishops of Ely. Other communities were dissolved around the time of the Black Death (pp. 129–47).

A broadly similar picture emerges from another recent monograph, devoted to a town much larger than Cambridge but still not one of the major centres, nor one that has held much attraction for hospital historians: Liège.[7] Pierre de Spiegeler's systematic and sensible (if unambitious) collection of the evidence supplies the first of my three other examples of recent historiography.[8] It reveals an apparent lack of medical concern with hospital patients comparable to that in Cambridge (barbers were employed in two institutions, but for the hirsute only: de Spiegeler, pp. 207–8). The book's catalogue of the eighteen hospitals functioning in Liège at one time or another between the late twelfth and late fifteenth centuries suggests a pattern of foundation and transformation reminiscent of Rubin's survey. In Liège, as in Cambridge, corrodians seem to have preponderated toward the close of the Middle Ages. The number of beds remaining for the city's poor and sick was clearly small. Yet it was still further diminished by the allocation of an increasing amount of space to transients and pilgrims, something that the town's economic and cultic significance can hardly

---

[6] M. Foucault, *Folie et Déraison: Histoire de la Folie à l'Age Classique* (Paris, 1961). The best discussion of this work is by H. C. E. Midelfort, 'Madness and Civilization in Early Modern Europe: A Reappraisal of Michel Foucault', in B. C. Malament (ed.), *After the Reformation: Essays in Honor of J. H. Hexter* (Pennsylvania, 1981), pp. 247–65. The whole question of how the insane were treated in later medieval and early modern Europe needs to be reopened in a way wholly independent from that of Foucault, especially now that the Islamic 'background' of hospitals for the insane and the treatments available in them has been investigated by M. W. Dols. See his *Majnun: the Madman in Islamic Society* (forthcoming). Rubin's brief discussion, pp. 157–8, does not mention or use R. Neugebauer's work on the jurisdiction of the Crown over the mentally disturbed. See his 'Treatment of the Mentally Ill in Medieval and Early Modern England: A Reappraisal', *Journal of the History of the Behavioural Sciences*, xiv (1978), 158–69, and 'Medieval and Early Modern Theories of Mental Illness', *Archives of General Psychiatry*, xxxvi (1979), 477–83. See also n. 13 below. I hope to return to the matter elsewhere.

[7] Though several contributions to the journal *Annales de la Société Belge d'Histoire des Hôpitaux* should certainly not be undervalued.

[8] P. de Spiegeler, *Les Hôpitaux et l'Assistance à Liège (X^e-XVe Siècles): Aspects Institutionnels et Sociaux*, Bibliothèque de la Faculté de Philosophie et Lettres de l'Université de Liège, fascicule CCXLIX (Paris, 1987).

be said to have justified. Meanwhile, pregnant women, foundlings, orphans, and suchlike continued to be without institutions of their own (pp. 151-5 and 212).

How very different from my two remaining examples, Florence and Paris, according to the most recent reports that we have on each. Florentine hospitals of the later Middle Ages have been expertly surveyed by John Henderson.[9] The survey is modestly described as a preliminary one. That is because the outstandingly rich archives of these establishments have yet to be properly exploited. None the less, it is already possible to build up a remarkably clear picture. There are two major features of Florence which set the agenda for Henderson's enquiry. The first is that the city was one of the largest in Europe, with a population of the order of 100,000 on the eve of the Black Death.[10] This presumably generated a correspondingly large number of potential hospital inmates. The second feature is that Florentine hospitals were regarded as exceptional and worthy of imitation by contemporaries. It is therefore tempting to assess these hospitals in terms of broad demographic trends, and also to try to establish what exactly contemporaries found so distinctive about them.

A graph of the overall development of the fifty-eight hospitals known from the period 1000-1500 (derived from dates of foundation or earliest mention) shows a different pattern from that of Cambridge or Liège (Graph 1). It begins early by Cambridge standards (though not those of Liège). It is relatively uneventful during the later twelfth and earlier thirteenth centuries, when we might have expected a wave of new foundations. But it rises quite sharply during the later thirteenth and much of the fourteenth centuries—when Cambridge hospitals were disappearing and those in Liège were mostly being transformed.[11] As might have been predicted, the fifteenth century is quieter (though hardly bereft of foundations) until there is what seems like a wave of new ones toward 1500 (an illusion created by the availability of tax returns for 1495?). The graph of foundations thus seems to accord quite well with the graph of population as it rises to a peak before the Black Death and declines over a long period thereafter, mainly because of recurrent epidemics.

The history of these hospitals subsequent to their foundation is, especially in its earlier phase, a familiar one of corruption or apparent decline.[12] At any one time, though, between thirty and thirty-five hospitals would have been

---

[9] J. Henderson, 'The Hospitals of Late-Medieval and Renaissance Florence: A Preliminary Survey', forthcoming in Granshaw and Porter (eds.). Dr Henderson very kindly sent me a copy of the typescript, which I shall cite by footnote rather than page number to facilitate eventual reference to the published version.

[10] D. Herlihy and C. Klapisch-Zuber, Les Toscans et Leurs Familles: Une Etude du Catasto Florentin de 1427 (Paris, 1978), pp. 165-77.

[11] At n. 14, Henderson proposes that the Florentine pattern does not differ markedly from that of other cities. It may conform broadly to the pattern of the Avignon region, for which see J. Chiffoleau, La Comptablité de l'Au-delà: les Hommes, la Mort et la Religion dans la Région d'Avignon à la Fin du Moyen Age (Rome, 1980), pp. 314-21. But compare J. Caille, Hôpitaux et Charité Publique à Narbonne au Moyen Age de la Fin du Xᵉ à la Fin du XVᵉ Siècle (Toulouse, 1978), part i.

[12] The survey in R. Davidsohn, Storia di Firenze, trans. G. B. Klein (Florence, 1972), vii. 87 ff. has not been replaced.

active. Many were restricted in their clientèle. Indeed, a significant proportion of those new later thirteenth-century hospitals were not dedicated to the poor in general, despite their rapidly increasing numbers. Rather, they were exclusively for the benefit of the artisan confraternities that founded them (nn. 26 and 27). The rest—hospitals for the poor and sick at large, and also, perhaps earlier than we might have expected, for the mad—were generally on the small side.[13] Even the hospital of S. Maria Nuova, which was to become one of the most important in Florence, had only twelve beds for the poor at its foundation in 1288. It enlarged its scope, at least in part, by functioning as a centre from which sums of money were distributed to the needy in their own homes (n. 30).

So to the Black Death and its repercussions. Rubin sees the various epidemics as reducing both the demand for charity amongst the poor and the availability of funds to supply it (Rubin, pp. 49–53 and 291). Like de Spiegeler, she registers a decline in the frequency with which hospitals enjoyed testamentary benefactions, and she links that to what we might call the rise of the corrodarians (de Spiegeler, pp. 175 and 186; Rubin, p. 262). Henderson (n. 10) remarks no such evolution—and thinks that more wealth, not less, would have been available for charity after the Black Death. Hospitals in Florence did not benefit from testators to anything like the extent that the great alms-giving confraternity of Orsanmichele did. But, Henderson implies, the major hospitals responded to sharp demographic change in the fourteenth century by increases in both size and degree of specialization, not by contraction.[14] Hundreds of children were housed in three main fifteenth-century orphanages. Poor women, especially widows, gained from a variety of charitable services, including the sizeable Orbatello hospital, founded in 1372. The poor enjoyed medical treatment in other hospitals on a wholly new scale and level of efficiency.[15] These were the institutions that attracted the praise of contemporaries and produced a discernible sequence of imitations. The advantage of the Florentine archives, however, is not only that they enable us to glimpse these great institutions as it were from the inside. It is that they are sufficiently detailed to remind us that S. Maria Nuova flourished at the same time as, for example, S. Maria del Carmine, a hospice with its seven widowed inmates, at least two of whom were moribund (Henderson, n. 48).

Of Parisian hospitals less can confidently be said. The archives have suffered

[13] At n. 44, Henderson quotes an early fourteenth-century sermon that, without comment, includes the insane among the various categories of patient to be found in Florentine hospitals. The sermon raises the possibility that there was a long tradition of hospitalizing the insane in parts of Europe of which we can now be only dimly aware. Compare Midelfort, 'Madness and Civilization', p. 253. See also N-E. Vanzan Marchini, *L'Ospedal dei Veneziani: Storia-Patrimonio-Progretto* (Venice, 1986).

[14] Compare Chiffoleau, *Comptabilité*, p. 320, for continued testamentary favour of Avignon hospitals.

[15] K. Park, 'Hospitals and Medical Welfare in Renaissance Florence', paper advertised as forthcoming by Henderson at n. 36. See for the moment K. Park, *Doctors and Medicine in Early Renaissance Florence* (Princeton, 1985), p. 106, and R. J. Trexler, 'Hospital Patients in Florence: San Paolo, 1567–68', *Bulletin of the History of Medicine*, xlviii (1974), 41–59.

greatly, and there is no recent synoptic yet detailed study of them comparable to those of Rubin, de Spiegeler or Henderson.[16] But Bronisław Geremek does devote a portion of his *The Margins of Society in Late Medieval Paris* to them (pp. 169–79), and brings to light some pieces of evidence of more than local interest.[17] In this perhaps most densely populated of European cities (200,000 in the thirteenth century?[18]) Geremek first briefly identifies a wave of early foundations ending in the thirteenth century. Later initiatives were nearly all very modest in scale. But, as in Florence, a few hospitals were clearly much larger than the rest and inevitably dominate the scene. There was the Hôtel-Dieu, with which doctors had been associated since the early thirteenth century, and which catered for poor cripples, all those who were seriously ill, abandoned or homeless children, and pregnant women. In the fifteenth century it was generally looking after 400–500 people at a time, although, exceptionally, that number could almost double—or fall to as little as 100. Pilgrims and poor travellers were diverted to two fourteenth-century foundations.

As in Florence, there were some more specialized establishments—for women, former prostitutes, orphans destined for apprenticeship, and outcast or unfit members of various guilds. But these seem to have originated well before the Black Death, not to have changed very much after it, and therefore to have had nothing particular to do with the new economic conditions of the later fourteenth century.[19] Two other institutions deserve mention. With one, the leper house of Saint-Lazare, it is sufficient to note that in the earlier fourteenth century it had a staff of ten brothers and two sisters, but only five male and six female lepers for them to look after.[20] The other hospital was that of Quinze-Vingts, founded by Louis IX for 300 blind people. It was reserved for those born in Paris, and their admission (along with that of the occasional guide or wife) was subject to the agreement of the royal almoner. The hospital had not, however, been designed to keep its inmates off the streets. They groped their way round Paris in small groups, begging wherever they could. Their numbers declined during and after the Hundred Years War, but there

[16] See also Imbert, op. cit., pp. 79 and 132. Modern French work has been focused elsewhere: Caille, *Hôpitaux à Narbonne*; N. Gonthier, *Lyons et ses Pauvres au Moyen-Age (1350–1500)* (Lyon, 1978).

[17] Cambridge, 1987. Originally published in Polish in 1971 and translated into French in 1976; surely destined for new currency in its English version. The footnotes are out of date in places but the detail and the analysis remain compelling.

[18] Geremek, op. cit., p. 7. *Histoire de la Population Française*, under the direction of J. Dupâquier (Paris, 1988), i. 306.

[19] Caille, op. cit., part 2, suggests, plausibly, that ostensible specialization may not, in any case, have meant the exclusion of other categories of the poor.

[20] Like the response to insanity, the treatment of lepers in the later Middle Ages—the other arm of the 'Foucault hypothesis'—is sorely in need of reassessment. Was the incidence of leprosy declining throughout Europe (with a few very northern exceptions)? Were there not enough lepers to fill the leprosaria or were people becoming less afraid of infection? (One might expect that increasing rarity bred more intense fear of the disease and greater desire to shut away the few lepers remaining.) K. Manchester, 'Tuberculosis and Leprosy in Antiquity: An Interpretation', *Medical History*, xxviii (1984), 162–73, is better on pathology than on history. R. I. Moore, *The Formation of a Persecuting Society* (Oxford, 1987), is the most stimulating recent discussion of changing attitudes to the disease from the twelfth century onward.

were still a hundred resident in the hospital at the beginning of the sixteenth century.

Continuity seems, indeed, to be the general theme of hospital history in Paris. Many of the changes that have been noticed in Cambridge, Liège, and Florence are not to be found there. Like de Spiegeler and, to some extent, Rubin, Geremek makes use of wills to show which charities were singled out for bequests. His sample is somewhat limited. But it is still big enough to suggest that Parisian hospitals did not fall from testamentary favour toward the end of the Middle Ages. The suggestion is encouraged by the early fifteenth-century accounts of the two permanent collecting boxes deployed by the Hôtel-Dieu, one inside, the other outside, the building. Whatever their statistical value, these accounts constitute Geremek's most attractive piece of evidence. The box inside the hospital naturally attracted fewer and smaller donations since only those visiting the sick poor went past it. In 1416 it received one gold piece but over 500 deniers or half deniers. The box outside the hospital, in contrast, held over twelve times as much. Eleven per cent of that was gold coin and more than 87 per cent silver (pp. 182–90).

II

A discipline of relevance must be one in which appropriate comparisons are drawn. It is tempting to see regional studies or details of particular hospitals as indicative of a much larger field and to look for reassuring parallels elsewhere, no matter how partial. (Rubin's footnotes, a bibliographical *tour de force*, are exemplary in this respect. Their frequent adversion to hospitals of many different periods and places creates the general impression that Cambridge is a part of the main, even if the precise point of individual references is often unclear.) It may be, however, that greater 'discipline' yields a more instructive context. Places of different size and political or economic significance, as widely scattered as possible, need to be juxtaposed. For even a secondhand and superficial comparison of four hospital centres reveals a variety of chronologies, building types, and larger evolutionary patterns that at once casts doubt on broad descriptions or explanations of change.

We have not, after all, seen a predictable institutional response to the Black Death. We have not found any widely discernible graph of foundation and decline. Further, we have had little occasion to refer to those great themes of increasing lay control, centralization, and confinement that may well be appropriate to the early modern period, but should not too eagerly be invoked when dealing with the preceding centuries. The major social and demographic changes of the fourteenth century doubtless gave rise to new attitudes for example, with labour scarce, beggars and vagrants, the under- and the unemployed were not highly regarded. But was this wholly new? Philanthropy in the early and central Middle Ages had been far from indiscriminate. And even when those sterner attitudes did emerge, beggars were by no means all cut off from the charity of their social superiors. The later medieval hospital is thus not a unitary or clearly bounded phenomenon. Nor is it a subject of which we may yet claim to have got the measure.[21] The few really large institutions that have left detailed archives, and that seem so modern in their medical and administrative sophistication, inevitably capture historians' attention. But these cannot by themselves provide an adequate basis for grand theory. A discipline of relevance turns aside, if only briefly, to the less ambitious foundations— those that make the outstanding problems of interpretation and context harder to evade.

If we are to understand the later medieval hospital—and, indeed, the hospital in earlier centuries too—it is with St John's, not S. Maria Nuova, that we must first come to terms. At this level, comparisons and parallels should certainly be sought. All over Europe, it seems, there were similarly modest establishments: the actual, as distinct from the historiographical, stuff of the charitable past. How should we respond to them? The most extreme response would be to decide that they were not 'true' hospitals at all. Since they offered 'care' rather than 'cure', they now have little place in the social history of medicine.[22] (It could be added that, since most of them offered support to only a small number of paupers, they are hardly more important for the history of poor relief either.) A second response, implicitly that of Rubin, would be to concede that they were founded as hospitals but that many of them rapidly declined into something else. Decline, perversion, loss of vocation: these are, indeed, the obvious terms for any concluding analysis.[23] Their undisciplined use is, however, to be resisted.

First, let us dispense with the dubious antithesis of care and cure, which should not automatically be equated with the presence or absence of hospital doctors.[24] This is not the place to rehearse the range of medical regimes available

[21] See B. Pullan, 'Support and Redeem: Charity and Poor Relief in Italian Cities from the Fourteenth to the Seventeenth Centuries', *Continuity and Change*, iii (1988), 177–208, for the latest analysis, showing the differences between 'the old' and 'the new philanthropy', but also emphasizing the survival of 'the old philanthropy' into the early modern period. Compare Geremek, 'Renfermement des Pauvres en Italie (XIV–XVIIᵉ Siècle): Remarques Préliminaires', in *Mélanges en l'Honneur de Fernand Braudel: Histoire Economique du Monde Méditerranéen 1450–1650* (Toulouse, 1973), ii. 205–17. The whole tradition of respecting the shame-faced poor (for whom see n. 28 below)—a tradition going back to the patristic period—can be interpreted as one of hostility to beggars. See also the various evidence cited by Mollat, *Poor in the Middle Ages*, pp. 16, 29, 45, 71–2, 85, etc., for the earlier Middle Ages. It seems to me that many later medievalists have idealized charity in the period preceding their own, placing far too much emphasis on Mendicant attitudes.

[22] See T. Miller, 'The Knights of St John and the Hospitals of the Latin West', *Speculum*, liii (1978), 709–33, for an extreme view. Compare Henderson, 'Hospitals of Florence', at n. 94, and Pullan, 'Support and Redeem', p. 188.

[23] C. Rawcliffe, 'The Hospitals of Later Medieval London', *Medical History*, xxviii (1984), 1–21, at pp. 17–18.

[24] P. Horden, 'The Byzantine Welfare State: Image and Reality', *Society for the Social History of Medicine Bulletin*, xxxvii (1985), 7–10; M. Pelling, 'Healing the Sick Poor: Social Policy and Disability in Norwich 1550–1640', *Medical History*, xxix (1985), 115–37, especially section II, for the more subtly differentiated spectrum of restorative regimes on offer. I have not seen R. L. Numbers and D. W. Amundsen (eds.), *Caring and Curing: Health and Medicine in the Western Religious Traditions* (London and New York, 1986).

during the period, compare their clinical techniques, and pronounce on their relative effectiveness. Nor is it the place to discuss the therapeutic value of religious consolation for those who believed that the remission of illness could originate only in the remission of sins. It will have to be enough to propose the general appropriateness of the nursing, food, and shelter provided in hospitals like St John's to the needs of their carefully selected inmates, whether poor, leprous, or otherwise diseased. (We could also remark that hospitals as medically well equipped as S. Maria Nuova or S. Paolo could rapidly discharge a large number of apparently cured patients because the majority of these had suffered from acute ailments: fevers very often, or skin diseases such as scabies. The Florentine hospitals tailored their admissions to their resources quite as much as St John's did. Their therapeutic successes should be judged accordingly (Henderson, nn. 45 and 101).)

Secondly, let us dispense with the calculation of ratios. Hospital historians offer these supposed means of comparison and tests of adequacy in various forms. The ratio of number of hospitals to total population may be given—by which standard Cambridge and Pistoia rank somewhat higher than Florence and London (Henderson at n. 15). That of number of beds to total population has also been calculated for several areas—an unrewarding procedure, since the demographic aggregates with which medievalists must operate depend more on bold estimates than on evidence, and both the 'turnover' of patients and the number of them in each bed, though essential to the calculation, can seldom be conjectured. The results of such efforts are, moreover, predictable. Hospitals always come out of them badly.[25]

A more subtle analysis is needed, both of what hospitals such as those in Cambridge had to offer and of their immediate contacts with the wider urban community. Thanks to Rubin, the Hospital of St John provides the clearest example of the various directions that such an analysis can take. First, though obvious, it has to be emphasized that, like any hospital with a chapel, St John's was above all a religious house. Liturgy, not therapeutics, was the centre of its life. Whatever changes it underwent during the later Middle Ages were minor in comparison with that enduring feature, and we should not expect, or subconsciously wish, it to have been otherwise. Hospital history in this period, whatever lay influences came to bear on it, was ecclesiastical quite as much as social history.[26] The intercessory prayers of the inmates, poor or not, aided living benefactors and associates and speeded through purgatory the souls of departed ones (Rubin, pp. 184–92). And that, we might allow, is a form of social welfare. Wealth given (or sold) to the hospital in the expectation of this metaphysical return should not be seen as originating in self-regard rather than genuine compassion for the poor. To operate with that antithesis is to impose

---

[25] Except to E. J. Kealey, *Medieval Medicus: A Social History of Anglo-Norman Medicine* (Baltimore, 1981). Compare Geremek, op. cit., p. 175, de Spiegeler op. cit., pp. 191–2.

[26] And can be written as such. See, for example, J. Avril, 'Le Statut des Maisons-Dieu dans l'Organisation Ecclésiastique Médiévale', in *Santé, Médecine et Assistance au Moyen Age, Actes du 110ᵉ Congrès National des Sociétés Savantes, Montpellier 1985* (Paris, 1987), pp. 285–97.

an anachronistic definition of altruism on the Middle Ages (compare Rubin p. 3 n). Welfare provision was not something separable from its religious expression.

Rubin places great emphasis on the fact that the categories of welfare recipient at St John's changed during the later Middle Ages. The change can perhaps be seen as more apparent than real. St John's began by admitting paupers and turned to admitting poor scholars and corrodians. How much difference to the overall character of its community did that actually make? Throughout, St John's continued to act as a refuge and source of employment—a hospital of a kind—for its relatively poor brothers and servitors.[27] Whatever their projected length of stay, the few poor and sick who could originally be accepted were presumably chosen with great care from a much larger 'pool'. If, as theology urged, they were Christ's truest representatives, they were presumably respectable, and perhaps not of the very poorest: 'of good governance and . . . fallen in poverty'[28]—the shame-faced poor, as they would be called in Tudor times, who could hardly be expected to beg and were doubtless a model of comportment.[29] It is a defensible generalization—applicable to the whole of the Middle Ages—that nearly all hospitals were more like almshouses than doss-houses.

St John's inmates had to be able to look after themselves. They were expected to participate as fully as possible in the religious life of the community. They had to be worthy objects of their superiors' benevolence and also suitable intercessors. Perhaps very little, beyond education, distinguished them from the poor scholars who came to take their place. Yet the historiography of charity still tends to keep the welfare of scholars in a separate—and relatively neglected—category from that of the poor, as if scholars did not have to endure genuine poverty.[30] Rubin devotes a substantial section of her book to university and collegiate charities for scholars. It is distanced from her account of life in St John's by almost 100 pages. And the analogy between a college and a hospital—both of them charities, chantries, and welfare agencies—seems not to interest her. She is far more concerned with the intrusion of corrodians. But perhaps these, too, were sometimes quite close in character and circumstance to the poor whose beds they usurped. And even if they were indeed better off, they might still augment rather than diminish the hospital's potential for poor

[27] Henderson, op. cit., after n. 93; B. Pullan, 'Institutional Charity and Employment in Early Modern Europe: The Service of Hospitals and Conservatories in Italy and France in the Sixteenth and Seventeenth Centuries', paper read at Istituto Internazionale di Storia Economica Francesco Datini, XIV Settimana di Studio: 'L'Emergenza Storica nelle Attività Terziarie (Sec. XII/XVIII), Prato, 1982.

[28] As in an Essex almshouse founded in the 1480s. See M. K. McIntosh, *Autonomy and Community: The Royal Manor of Havering, 1200–1500* (Cambridge, 1986), pp. 239–40.

[29] On the shame-faced poor see G. Ricci, 'Naissance du Pauvre Honteux: entre l'Histoire des Idées et l'Histoire Sociale', *Annales*, xxxviii (1983), 158–77; A. Spicciani, 'The "Poveri Vergognosi" in Fifteenth-Century Florence: The First Thirty Years' Activity of the Buonomini di S. Martino', in T. Riis (ed.), *Aspects of Poverty in Early Modern Europe* (Stuttgart, 1981), pp. 119–82.

[30] See J. M. Reitzel, 'The Medieval Houses of Bons-Enfants', *Viator*, xi (1980), 179–207; Geremek, op. cit., chap. 5.

relief by attracting donations.[31] Florentine hospitals admitted corrodians or pensioners: their presence in, or association with, an establishment is not necessarily a symptom of corruption or decline.[32] It might, indeed, be interpreted as a tribute to the quality of the accommodation offered to the few exemplary paupers already there.

A small medieval hospital had many possible functions, all of them interrelated. Rubin connects the apparent mutation of St John's with changing conceptions of charity (pp. 111 and 295). It might be preferable to see the hospital as embodying at one time or another different aspects of a single concept—a concept that had a much broader scope than Rubin's long exposition (chap. 3) of the theology, canon law, and preaching of charity suggests. Her concern is essentially with alms-giving: 'descending' charity as we might call it. But charity was surely intended to operate in other directions. There was (one hopes) fraternal charity within the hospital amongst brethren and inmates, charity between the house and its benefactors, charity between the poor and the rich for whom they interceded. 'Caritas quippe est amor Dei atque proximi': love of God and neighbour.[33] It has its 'ascending' and 'horizontal' kinds, too.

The charitable functions of St John's were not, of course, confined to its premises. Its very existence advertised to the community the ideals in which it had originated, and which its liturgical round and its provision for inmates continued to embody. It was built in the area of Cambridge's Jewry, no doubt deliberately as 'a symbol and monument of Christian welfare'—an assertion, in effect, of Christian superiority in that regard.[34] It is no coincidence that one of the 'external services' that St John's came to offer was money-lending. A benefactor would make assets over to it *in perpetuum* in return for a substantial sum that would 'acquit me of the Jewry' (Rubin, pp. 218–19). Other ways in which the hospital could be a source of welfare in the wider community stemmed from its pastoral responsibility for those parishes that were appropriated to it (augmenting its revenues with their tithes) and in its paternal responsibility for tenants on its estates (p. 193). Under the latter heading, for example, a poor widow was given a tenement for life and two bushels of corn annually. This largesse was not (or not only) a reflection of the fact that her late husband had been one of the hospital's benefactors: other tenants enjoyed concessions such as reduced rent (pp. 230–1). Also, it seems that paupers could be buried in the hospital's cemetery even if they had not previously been inmates (p. 181).

III

A minor charitable establishment thus insinuates itself into local society in more ways than mere bed-counting can reveal. Describing those ways is one

---

[31] *Calendar of Patent Rolls, Richard II vol. 4, 1388–92* (London, 1902), p. 484 (16 Oct. 1391), cited by Rawcliffe, 'Hospitals of Later Medieval London', p. 4; de Spiegeler, op. cit., pp. 152–5.

[32] I. Chabot, 'Widowhood and Poverty in Late Medieval Florence', *Continuity and Change*, iii (1988), 291–311, at p. 300.

[33] F. Courtney, *Cardinal Robert Pullen: An English Theologian of the Twelfth Century* (Rome, 1954), p. 197, cited from Rubin, p. 58.

[34] C. N. L. Brooke, 'The Churches of Medieval Cambridge', in D. Beales and G. Best (eds.), *History, Society and the Churches: Essays in Honour of Owen Chadwick* (Cambridge, 1985), p. 60.

means of estimating its local importance. But the search for the right context clearly cannot end there. If charity is construed in the broadest sense, and taken (as it is by Rubin) to be among the principal bonds of society, then the essential context for St John's will be an account of Cambridge's entire social structure (something that Rubin's title might be thought to promise, even though she clearly did not intend to deliver it).

Of more immediate concern here is the question of how the hospital can be assessed as a source of charity in the more usual, 'descending', sense of the word. A comparative approach is again called for—not now between hospitals but between hospitals and other sources of medical help and poor relief. A convincing assessment of the hospital's therapeutic value to the community should be a relative one. It should go beyond description of facilities (or lack of them) and ask what alternatives existed in the area, both for those whom the hospital turned away (such as pregnant mothers) and for the sick poor whom it admitted. That would, naturally, require investigation of a considerable variety of evidence—concerning miraculous healing as well as both 'folk' and 'learned' medicine, midwifery, and nursing.[35] Incompleteness and imprecision will always attend such an enterprise, but that is no excuse for evading it. The supposed 'medicalization' of hospitals in the later Middle Ages is a process about the course and consequences of which conclusions should not be drawn without reference to this larger curative context—especially since medicalization only concerned a tiny proportion of all hospitals.

A similarly wide-ranging enquiry is also the only way in which the hospital's importance for the relief of the poor can convincingly be established. The four studies under review earlier show that part of the job has been done. For Liège, De Spiegeler has brief sections on the minor role of monastic distributions, on capitular *mandata* (daily foot washing and bread doles for several weeks a year), and on the city's 'poor table' or almonry (pp. 89–96). For Paris, Geremek describes the role of confraternities as sources of relief for their own members and, occasionally, for the needy at large—by admitting well-dressed paupers to their banquets or by scattering left-overs. He also gives details of distributions to beggars at the gates of colleges, churches, and hospitals (pp. 179–89). Rubin (chap. 7) provides further evidence for comparison under several of these headings (St John's, we might note, seems not to have been a favoured centre for distributing the bequests of others: pp. 247–8). And she adds three further ones: alms-giving at funerals and obits (anniversaries); the neighbourly relief

[35] Rubin, pp., 148–52 with references, to which add J. K. Mustain, 'A Rural Medical Practitioner in Fifteenth-Century England', *Bulletin of the History of Medicine*, xlvi (1972), 469–76. For Italy, see Park, *Doctors and Medicine*, and I. Naso, *Medici e Strutture Sanitarie nella Società Tardo-Medievale: le Piemonte dei Secoli XIV e XV* (Milan, 1982), an excellent conspectus of both 'professional' and 'alternative' medicine—as is, for France, D. Jacquart, *Le Milieu Médical en France du XIIe au XVe siècle* (Geneva, 1982). See also papers in *Santé, Médecine et Assistance au Moyen Age* for midwifery and quackery in France and Catalonia.

promoted by episcopal indulgences for families that had suffered loss by robbery or fire and for individuals with a severe physical handicap; and the redistribution of tithes and bequests by the parish priest or his vicar, who were also, of course, expected to offer hospitality and to visit the sick.

For Florence, Henderson shows how research on the major hospitals is inseparable from research on a number of other institutions of comparable size: the enormously wealthy Confraternity of Orsanmichele, for instance, which, unlike most confraternities in Paris or Cambridge, made a very substantial contribution to poor relief;[36] or the *Monte delle Doti*, the Dowry Fund, which complemented the work of the various hospitals for women.[37] Other work on Renaissance Italy enables us to extend this catalogue to the *Monti di Pietà*, pawnshops that offered cheap credit to the poor and, like the loans offered by St John's, kept the needy from the clutches of the Jews.[38] And other work on later medieval England—fragmentary, incomplete, in urgent need of development and synthesis—suggests that we add the manor as a source of welfare provision.[39]

Hospitals clearly should not be studied in isolation from these various other institutions, which together probably did far more to alleviate distress. Embracing them within the discipline of hospital history, and so arriving at some relative estimate of the hospital's place in the institutional history of healing and poor relief, does not, however, quite bring us to the end of what is potentially relevant. Institutions are not enough. There remains a world beyond them. Part of that world is, of course, the domain of individual, private alms-giving, well known in outline but usually impossible to quantify.[40] But there is more—an area of activity that historians of charity have occasionally conjectured but are only now beginning to investigate.

Some English evidence shows what is at issue. One of the most arresting details in Rubin's book is tucked away in a footnote. It concerns cases of death

[36] On which see Henderson, 'Piety and Charity in Late Medieval Florence: Religious Confraternities from the Middle of the Thirteenth to the late Fifteenth Century' (unpublished Ph.D. thesis, University of London, 1983).

[37] J. Kirschner and A. Molho, 'The Dowry Fund and the Marriage Market in Early Quattrocento Florence', *Journal of Modern History*, 1 (1978), 403–38, the most accessible of their several articles on the topic.

[38] Pullan, 'Support and Redeem', pp. 191–3.

[39] M. K. McIntosh, 'Local Responses to the Poor in Late Medieval and Tudor England', *Continuity and Change*, iii (1988), 209–45, with full bibliography; R. M. Smith, 'The Manorial Court and the Elderly Customary Tenant in Later Medieval England', forthcoming in Z. Razi and R. M. Smith (eds.), *The Manor Court and Medieval English Society: Studies of the Evidence*. The continental seigneurie does not seem to have been studied from this point of view.

[40] Rubin, op. cit., pp. 298–9; Geremek, op. cit., p. 190; Mollat, *Poor in The Middle Ages*, pp. 266–7. For a recent example of the quantification possible with the almsgiving of a powerful individual see P. Contamine, 'La Pieté Quotidienne dans la Haute Noblesse à la Fin du Moyen Age: l'Exemple de Charles d'Orléans (1463–1465)', in H. Dubois, J-C. Hocquet, and A. Vauchez (eds.), *Horizons Marins, Itinéraires Spirituels (Ve-XVIIIe Siècles)* (Paris, 1987), i. pp. 35–42.

from hunger and exposure reported at the Cambridge assizes of 1260.[41] What had been lacking to such unfortunates, who presumably died unattended? Not only admission to a hospital, entitlement to a dole, help from a manor court, a confraternity, a priest, or a private almsgiver. Their chief deprivation has rather to be construed as lack of access to a range of informal systems of health care and material support that centred variously on family and household, kin group and neighbourhood. To recall Rubin's title, when such people died unattended, it was not only charity that had failed but the sentiment of community as well. An integrated history of welfare provision in the later Middle Ages, giving more or less equal space to both institutional and informal systems of relief, has not yet been written. But it could be. Imagine a book that combined Rubin's chapters on charitable foundations with those on social structure in Charles Phythian-Adams's study of Coventry.[42]

In the latter, we find details about almost all the important demographic and sociological factors that determined where the poor might look for support if they were unwilling or unable to turn to an institution: the number of those who never married; the characteristic age at first marriage, which affected parents' chances of being looked after in old age by their offspring, who might already have died or who might be overburdened by children of their own; the rules of household formation and the proportion of nuclear to extended families, both of which affected the availability of help from close relatives; the residential pattern, which affected the availability of members of the wider kin group and of unrelated but well-disposed neighbours; the sex ratio, which had a strong bearing on the possibility of remarriage for poor widows; and the employment opportunities for two vulnerable groups, the young and unmarried, who might become servants in other households, and older women, who might have to supplement a husband's inadequate wage or, as widows, fend for themselves.[43]

In dissecting Coventry society Phythian-Adams had the distinct advantage of being able to utilize a recently discovered census return of 1523, and he could extrapolate backwards from then into the previous century. Such an

---

[41] Rubin, p. 267 n. 178, cites W. M. Palmer (ed.), *The Assizes Held at Cambridge, AD 1260* (Linton, 1930), pp. 2 and 19. Much more remains to be done here. The frequency of such cases in periods when there was no serious food shortage, the manner of death, and what contemporaries perceived to be lacking to those involved, would repay investigation. R. M. Smith kindly draws my attention to the value of the coroners' rolls. See, for example, R. F. Hunnisett (ed.), *Sussex Coroners' Inquests 1485–1558*, Sussex Record Society, 74 (Lewes, 1985), p. 7, no. 27; (ed.), *Bedfordshire Coroners' Rolls*, Publications of the Bedfordshire Historical Record Society, 41 (Streatley, 1961), p. 74, no. 165; p. 89, no. 208. Compare P. Laslett, *The World We Have Lost—Further Explored*, 3rd edn. (London, 1983), p. 133. Such evidence casts doubt on the existence of the tightly knit rural community that historians have frequently claimed to detect in the Middle Ages.

[42] *Desolation of a City: Coventry and the Urban Crisis of the Late Middle Ages* (Cambridge, 1979), chaps. 6, 10, 13, 14, 20, and 22.

[43] Female labour opportunities (somewhat neglected by Rubin) are now at last being seriously investigated in this period. See, for example, P. J. P. Goldberg, 'Women in Fifteenth-Century Town Life', in J. A. F. Thomson (ed.), *Towns and Townspeople in the Fifteenth Century* (Gloucester, 1988), pp. 107–28, with full bibliography, and Chabot, 'Widowhood and Poverty'.

analysis would be impossible for a historian of medieval Cambridge, and difficult for most other places.[44] But there are historical studies of later periods and anthropological monographs in which to find analogies.[45] Sources like the Florentine *catasto* of 1427 have yet to yield more than a fraction of the information that they contain on topics of this kind.[46] And, from what relatively little work has already been done, some related general conclusions are emerging that can form the starting-point for more systematic research: about the numerical predominance—or, at least, significance—of the nuclear family in most of western Europe, possibly since Roman times; about the concomitant weakness of the kin group as a source of welfare provision; about the consequent indispensability of some source of extra-familial assistance; and about the ways in which particular demographic and charitable regimes may determine one another.[47] Some provocative thoughts by Peter Laslett on this whole field of

[44] Compare Rubin, op. cit. pp. 41, 135, and 267–8. Geremek throughout exhibits horizontal ties amongst his 'marginals'—thieves, prostitutes, beggars, jongleurs, clerks, *et al.*—that belie his frequent and heavy emphasis on the rootlessness of such people.

[45] For the early modern period, even in England with its abundance of demographic data, work that links poor relief to the domestic context of poverty is only just beginning. It is indicative of the state of the field that virtually the only studies in it on which P. Slack can draw for his excellent *Poverty and Policy in Tudor and Stuart England* (London and New York, 1988) are those in R. M. Smith (ed.), *Land, Kinship and Life-Cycle* (Cambridge, 1984). See Henderson, 'Introduction', *Continuity and Change*, iii (1988), 145–51, and id., 'The Parish and the Poor in Florence at the Time of the Black Death: the Case of S. Frediano', ibid., pp. 247–72, at pp. 263–4, for the provision at neighbourhood level of free or subsidized accommodation. Compare R. M. Schwarz, *Policing the Poor in Eighteenth-Century France* (Chapel Hill and London, 1988), pp. 93–119; D. Garrioch, *Neighbourhood and Community in Paris, 1740–1790* (Cambridge, 1986), pp. 19–26, 64–5, 93–4—admirably detailed and, for a medievalist, suggestive; S. Woolf, *The Poor in Western Europe in the Eighteenth and Nineteenth Centuries* (London and New York, 1986), chaps. 1, 7 and 8. Anthropology: most useful are L. A. Lomnitz, *Networks and Marginality: Life in a Mexican Shantytown* (New York, San Francisco, and London, 1977), and D. S. Pitkin, *The House that Giacomo Built: History of an Italian Family, 1898–1978* (Cambridge, 1985), a moving account of the functioning of a poor extended family, now to be read in conjunction with D. I. Kertzer, *Family Life in Central Italy, 1880–1910* (New Brunswick, New Jersey, 1984).

[46] See the quotations in the footnotes to Chabot, 'Widowhood and Poverty'.

[47] The subject is large and I plan to return to it elsewhere (see n. 48 below). It will be enough here to cite a handful of studies that exemplify the current direction of research. On family and household the beginning and end of the Middle Ages are very much better served than the centuries in between. (Something more rigorous than D. Herlihy, *Medieval Households* (Cambridge, Mass., 1985) is needed.) See, therefore, R. P. Saller and B. D. Shaw, 'Tombstones and Roman Family Relations in the Principate: Civilians, Soldiers and Slaves', *Journal of Roman Studies*, lxxiv (1984), 124–56; P. Guichard, 'De l'Antiquité au Moyen Age: Famille Large et Famille Etroite', *Cahiers d'Histoire*, xxiv (1979), 45–60; R. R. Ring, 'Early Medieval Peasant Households in Central Italy', *Journal of Family History*, iv (1979), 2–25; G. Duby, *The Early Growth of the European Economy* (London, 1974), p. 34; R. M. Smith, 'The People of Tuscany and their Families in the Fifteenth Century: Medieval or Mediterranean?', *Journal of Family History*, vi (1981), 107–28; J. Hajnal, 'Two Kinds of Preindustrial Household Formation System', *Population and Development Review*, viii (1982), 449–94; M. Mitterauer and R. Sieder, *The European Family* (Cambridge, 1982), chap. 2. On the much-neglected topic of the balance in welfare provision between kin, neighbours, and the wider social world, see again next note; also P. Garnsey, *Famine and Food Supply in the Graeco-Roman World: Responses to Risk and Crisis* (Cambridge, 1987), pp. 55–63; works cited by Henderson, 'The Parish and the Poor in Florence', p. 267, n. 2; R. M. Smith, 'Kin and Neighbours in a Thirteenth-Century Suffolk Community', *Journal of Family History*, iv (1979), 219–56; id, 'Welfare and the Management of Demographic Uncertainty', in M. Keynes, D. A. Coleman, and N. H. Dimsdale (eds.), *The Political Economy of Health and Welfare* (London, 1988), pp. 108–35.

welfare at both familial and extra-familial or institutional level have long been available, and have recently been presented in revised and expanded form.[48] It should not have been left to a historian of Africa to demonstrate the fruitfulness of the union of disciplines that Laslett presupposes.[49]

In this essay I have been concerned virtually exclusively with the 'supply' side of hospital history: the sorts of institution available, the services that they offered, and their necessary context in the history of other charitable institutions and of informal networks of mutual aid. I have said little about the 'demand' side as it appeared to contemporaries—the causes and extent of poverty in this period, the links between poverty and disease, and so forth—although here too there are some received ideas that a discipline of relevance might eventually come to modify. That is mainly for lack of space. But it is also because our estimates of demand depend crucially on our estimates of the informal level of supply. We must have some idea of the extent to which the poor were able to help one another before we can decide how much help they ideally needed from institutions. The urgent task is therefore the integration of hospital history and family history. A discipline of relevance: knowing where to go next.

---

[48] P. Laslett, 'The Family and the Collectivity', *Sociology and Social Research,* lxiii (1979), 432–42; id., 'Family, Kinship and Collectivity as Systems of Support in Pre-Industrial Europe: A Consideration of the "Nuclear Hardship" Hypothesis', *Continuity and Change,* iii (1988), 153–75. Partly in response to Laslett, I have suggested the establishment of an agreed typology of the possible categories and directions of welfare requirements and provisions so that the whole subject can be set on a more secure conceptual base: 'Nuclear Hardship, Conventional Hardship: Toward a Framework for the Comparison of Welfare Systems', paper read to the Oxford University seminar 'Issues in the History of Poverty' in June 1988, of which a version is forthcoming.

[49] J. Iliffe, *The African Poor: A History* (Cambridge, 1987), p. 8: 'The intimate connection between poverty and family structure has been neglected by historians of Europe and may be Africa's chief contribution to the comparative history of the poor.'

VIII

PAIN IN HIPPOCRATIC
MEDICINE

'About suffering they were never wrong,/The Old Masters,'
W.H. Auden wrote in 'Musée des Beaux Arts'; 'how well they
understood/Its human position . . .'[1]

It is not difficult to produce quotable 'old masters' from either
classical or late antiquity on this subject of sick and suffering
humanity – Aeschylus, in the *Agamemnon*, on 'wisdom through
suffering', the encapsulation of a whole philosophy with pain at its
focus;[2] Aristotle: 'pain perturbs and destroys the nature of the
sufferer but pleasure does nothing of the sort';[3] Epicurus: 'pain
does not last continuously in the flesh: when acute it is there for a
short time . . . and chronic illnesses contain an excess of pleasure in
the flesh over pain';[4] Seneca: 'pain is slight if not reinforced by
opinion';[5] Jesus, as quoted in the *Epistle of Barnabas*: 'those who
wish to see me and attain to my kingdom must lay hold of me
through pain and suffering';[6] the pagan Caecilius in Minucius
Felix's *Octavius*, strikingly characterizing Christians in somatic
rather than doctrinal terms, as 'parched with fever, racked with
pain';[7] Jerome: 'am I in good health? I thank my Creator. Am I sick?
In this case, too, I praise God's will.'[8] Very particular pains, not just
pain and illness in general, may be similarly 'theory-laden'.
Contradicting any notion of the Virgin's Immaculate Conception,
there is a tenth-century (or earlier) 'Praise of the Archangel
Michael' written in Coptic: a lengthy prayer for healing in which
the individual labour pains of the Virgin are not only invoked but
even named.[9]

All these quotations derive from 'old masters' who give pain and
suffering a 'human position' rich in ethical implication, often in the
form of theodicy. In this paper, however, I am concerned with old
masters of medicine, chiefly the writers of the *Corpus Hippocraticum*

(CH) but also, more briefly, Rufus of Ephesus and Galen. And these masters are different from those represented above – far more so, I suggest, than we might expect from the obvious contrast of literary genre between, for instance, high tragedy and medical treatise. The difference can be characterized under three headings.

First, *philosophy*. Hippocratic authors and physicians do not articulate any philosophically elevated theory of pain – any conception of its place in the human scheme of things. Undoubtedly they evolve physiological *explanations* of pain; but they go no further than that. Pain, for them, is no 'lived metaphysics'.[10] It is simply 'a message composed, sent, and delivered by illness'.[11] That is, the Hippocratics step aside from the religious and ethical frameworks within which pain can acquire meaning. They offer, for example, no more than occasional recognition of the possibility that an illness is of supernatural origin.[12] Nor did the passing centuries soften this outlook. At the other end of the classical period, a comparable detachment is to be found in the work of the early Byzantine medical encyclopaedists, writing in an overwhelmingly Christian environment. Perhaps in part reflecting religious change, these encyclopaedists guardedly include a few more magical remedies than their Hippocratic-Galenic authorities did; but they are otherwise difficult to distinguish from them in tone and broad intellectual outlook.[13] Their conservatism shows the narrow limits of learned medicine's accommodation to Christian theodicy in late antiquity.

Philosophies of a less elevated kind were registered no more fully. In the conclusion to his admirable account of 'Hippocratism' in antiquity, Owsei Temkin writes that Hippocratic medicine offered a counterbalance to the claims of the spirit. Especially in late antiquity, he argues, medicine sided with the majority of the people – with the rationally disciplined claims of the flesh, rather than with the extreme ideals of chastity and asceticism that, according to some modern scholarship, are such a prominent feature of the culture of the later Roman world.[14] Temkin's argument is plausible enough. But it should be noted in the present context that, at least in the major texts through which it has come down to us, ancient medicine did not explicitly discuss the high level of background pain with which most 'rationally disciplined' people were presumably resigned to living until only decades ago. Stepping aside from metaphysics, ancient medical writers were apparently no more responsive to the presumed world-view of common men and

PAIN IN HIPPOCRATIC MEDICINE

women – for whom pain was simply painful, and unwelcome, but very often unavoidable. Whatever actual doctors' practice, Hippocratic medicine does *not* see some pain as inevitable, as intrinsic to 'the human condition'.

The second of the three headings is *distinctiveness*, or rather the lack of it. The writers of CH do not, I suggest, see pain as a distinct or even an especially important subject. It blends easily into the rest of medicine. To my knowledge, no ancient doctor wrote a treatise on pain *tout court*. The eminent Muslim physician Razi preserves fragments of what he refers to as a work on pains in various parts of the body by that major first-century figure, Rufus of Ephesus. Razi is, however, likely to have been mistaken as to the literary integrity of the fragments' original.[15] Rufus, like other ancient medical authors, doubtless discussed pain *en passant* in a variety of works. For undoubtedly pain could have enormous diagnostic-prognostic significance. Indeed, *pace* Foucault, no ancient doctor of any calibre would have been so epistemically challenged as to fail to ask 'where does it hurt?'.[16] But that was only one among a number of appropriate questions, equivalent in prognostic potential: it was not necessarily the primary question. And it did not necessarily deserve a treatise to itself.

The third heading is *vocabulary*. Whatever clinically transpired between doctor and patient was (I propose) seen as too diffuse, too 'sub-theoretical', to be recorded in subtly-differentiated terminology. For the literate physicians or medical authors of the CH, pain seemed, perhaps, a subject on which there were narrow limits to what could – and therefore need – be written. There was no call for sophisticated taxonomies.

I have introduced the last of my three headings only briefly because I now want to explore it in some detail. I take it first because it is fundamental to the other two. Looking at the ways in which Hippocratic doctors wrote – or failed to write – about pain will, I believe, simultaneously show its lack of metaphysical significance for them (the initial heading) and will also begin to open up, for subsequent consideration, the second topic, distinctiveness.

The corpus of over sixty treatises associated with the name of Hippocrates was composed at sundry times over the course of a century or more, beginning *c.* 450 BC. It is the product of a diversity of authors, perhaps including Hippocrates himself, and its contents reveal a variety of genres and intellectual allegiances.[17] The Corpus does none the less exhibit a certain coherence: its authors partake of shared assumptions and beliefs. Therefore it can, for present purposes, be considered as a whole: a dossier of ancient medical thought second only to the output of Galen in size and compendiousness.[18] Given this abundance of material, we should hardly be surprised to find scholars asserting that in CH 'the semantic field of pain is extremely important' and, indeed, 'rich' – as rich as the semantic field of disease.[19]

Is that really so? With all respect to specialists in this material, I want to argue that CH's language of pain is somewhat undifferentiated, even impoverished. Far from offering its readers a rich terminology, it deals for the most part in synonyms; moreover, these synonyms are attended by only a small repertoire of adjectives and adverbs. Pain is not an especially vivid subject in CH. To support this proposition, some statistics will be helpful, though alas they will be no more exciting than the vocabulary that they represent – statistics of the kind that the splendid Concordance to CH now available makes it almost perilously easy to generate.[20]

Undoubtedly the number of references to pain in CH is considerable, larger perhaps than the number of occurrences of *nosos*, the basic word for disease or illness, and its family.[21] Four principal terms are involved. Of the immediate ('nuclear') family of *algos* and *algema* over 400 uses have been counted; members of the *ponos* family appear almost 700 times; *pathos* is favoured on some 150 occasions; there are precisely 772 uses of *odyne*.[22] We can leave aside the rare *lype* (a mere 59 entries), the single instance of the Homeric *pema*, and the obviously specialized *odis*, meaning labour pain (12 references). We should also discount the uses of *ponos* for exercise and *pathos* for emotion and so on. Still, the total number of occurrences of some kind of word signifying pain must still approach 2,000. The Hippocratic writers certainly did not keep silent on the subject. One could be forgiven for supposing that it was important to them.

Now that we have the statistics, they should be put to analytical use. Before we confront the obvious question of definition, it is worth pausing to consider whether the vocabulary shows any great historical development. For instance, *algema*-based words appear more frequently in *Epidemics V* and *VII*, sometimes dated to *c*. 350 BC, than they do in Books *I* and *III*, perhaps written some seventy years earlier.[23] But since the dating of individual Hippocratic works is fraught with controversy, it is impossible to hazard any large conclusions about when a particular term found or lost favour – and still less about why it did so.

PAIN IN HIPPOCRATIC MEDICINE

In her ambitious *History of Pain*, the late Roselyne Rey tries a different tack. She asks which words occur how often in which treatises, and tries to infer something about the respective preferences of those two great medical schools, Cnidus and Cos, between which scholars have often attempted to divide the authorship of the Hippocratic treatises. *Odyne*, the most popular word for pain overall, appears with the greatest frequency in the supposedly Cnidian writings, *Diseases II*, *Epidemics VII* (traditionally seen as the runt of the litter), *Internal Affections*, and the gynaecological works. 'At most,' Rey writes, 'one could conclude that the so-called Cnidian treatises concentrate more on pain and that, when they do so, it is the word *odyne* that is used to convey it'.[24]

There is indeed a contrast to be drawn between the 'Cnidian' texts, with their preference for *odyne*, and the *Coan Prenotions* or Prognoses. In the latter work *algema* predominates among pain terms (being used 70 times), *ponos* is the second most-favoured (63 uses), and *odyne* is chosen on only 18 occasions. As with the chronology of the different books of *Epidemics*, however, no great hypothesis can be erected on such a basis. Rey, for instance, conjectures that *odyne* is characteristic of the supposedly more primitive Cnidians, and that they place more emphasis on pain, and on its usefulness in localizing disorders, than do their 'rationalist' Coan rivals. But it is time Hippocratic scholarship removed the dichotomy between 'primitive/archaic' and 'rational' from its conceptual armoury;[25] such thinking, one might almost say, is a vestige of a now archaic mode of thought – the mode of Victorian evolutionism. Moreover, as Lonie and others have demonstrated, none of the distinctions between the two schools that some scholars propose has ever been adequately justified; they rest more on contrasts of topic and literary form than on any differences of mentality or underlying theory.[26] I conclude, then, that the vocabulary of pain did not develop in any now obvious ways as the constituent texts of CH were slowly and spasmodically set down. Their authors' attitudes to, and vocabularies of, pain cannot be distinguished by either historical period or institutional origin.

A fashionable question to raise next would be that of whether pain is 'gendered' in CH. In modern times women are perhaps more likely to report experiencing a variety of recurrent pains than are men, although they are also more aggressive in combating pain.[27] In that, they distinguish themselves from the women patients referred to in the Hippocratic *Diseases of Women*:[28] these render themselves incurable through ignorance of the source of their condition and through being too ashamed to talk to the doctor until there is little that can be done. According to the Hippocratic writers, female pathology is determined predominantly by the reproductive system (the Hippocratic woman is essentially, as has often been noted, a tube with an orifice at either end).[29] Therefore, if women menstruate regularly, they will not suffer serious illnesses as often as men do; and that compensates to some extent for their lesser but perhaps more frequent ailments arising from innate bodily weakness.[30] Are Hippocratic female patients depicted as being more often in pain than male ones? I undertook some sample counts of the number of pain references in the case histories in *Epidemics*, and it may well be that pain is on average referred to as a symptom with greater frequency in female cases than in male. But there is no characteristic vocabulary of female pain. Nor, apart from the delusions of certain suicidal virgins (on which more below), do women's afflictions seem to be rendered particularly expressively. And that is true of both the *Epidemics* and the gynaecological works – a point which may have some indirect bearing on the continuing debate among specialists about whether women's voices are 'audible' in the *gynaikeia*.[31]

So the semantic field of pain in CH cannot be divided up by period, medical school, or gender. The major question of course remains: are there detectable differences of overtone between the various pain words? Roselyne Rey and Helen King have both argued that there are. They concede that the *algema* family need not be discussed: *algema* is indisputably an all-purpose word for pain. But they do contend that the contexts in which *ponos* and *odyne* are used allow us to distinguish the two words' respective resonances. In King's scheme, '*to an extent* [my italics], in the medical texts *ponos* is often used for long-lasting pain, dull pain; *odyne* for sharp pain, pain which pierces the body'.[32] Rey proposes in similar fashion that the verb *poneo* 'is used without any qualification to describe a general state of suffering or illness, and that when the localisation of pain is referred to, it is almost always approximate, involving the use of prepositions such as *peri* or *es*, i.e. "in the area of" or "about"'. *Odyne*, she writes, is by contrast 'almost always used in a precise sense – either by qualifying, or by giving some clue as to the whereabouts of, the pain'.[33] My own sampling of the texts, via the Concordance, provides only limited support for such conclusions. Both terms, not just *odyne*, can be used of pain in a particular part;

PAIN IN HIPPOCRATIC MEDICINE

and the way *odyne* is localized seems hardly more precise than the manner in which *ponos* is deployed (*contra* Rey). If there is *odyne* in the hip, or throughout the belly, there may equally be *ponos* in the head or the hypochondrium. If *ponos* is for the most part chronic, dull pain (King), why do we find it qualified by *ischyros* (strong) or *sphodros* (violent) or *oxys* (sharp)? If *odyne* is sharp or piercing pain by definition (King again), it is perhaps odd that it should sometimes be qualified by an adjective such as *sperchnos* (rapid). For neither *odyne* nor *ponos*, it might be added, is the range of typical adjectives strikingly evocative: 'terrible' and 'sharp' are common; exotic analogies are hard to find. The Hippocratic authors provide little guidance as to what thinking (if any) lies behind their choice of pain words.

Rather than 'surf' the Concordance, playing with aggregates across the entire corpus, we might seek enlightenment from individual works. In absolute terms, the word *odyne* occurs more often in *Diseases II* than in any other treatise. And far from exhibiting any clear, single, meaning, it seems to be used as the all-purpose noun for pain. It is pain which can indeed be sharp, which suddenly seizes the patient's head, is violent, or presses.[34] In a rare metaphoric flight it is associated with the sensation of pricking needles or styluses.[35] It can be intense or excessive (*periodynie*). But, equally, it can also be light.[36] It can be localized with relative precision in the front of the head or, more loosely, in the side.[37] On other occasions, it clearly signifies lasting and more diffuse pain, linked to chills and fever, dizziness and heaviness. It can radiate, move gradually, or withdraw beneath the shoulder-blades.[38] This is humpty-dumpty writing: *odyne* apparently refers to whatever type of pain the author chooses. Everything depends on the context, which, as can be seen, displays some variety in this work.

More telling still, there are several passages in CH where major pain terms appear to be used synonymously. Two verbally similar *Aphorisms*, on pain in the diaphragm and the liver respectively, show *ponos* and *odyne* as equivalent;[39] while elsewhere *algema* is replaced now with *odyne* and now with *ponos* – though not in such a way as to suggest that *algema* is a general term embracing two distinct semantic sub-fields.[40] The phrase 'ponos de kai [and] odyne', which for instance occurs in *Places in Man*, does not suggest that, for the author of that particular work, there was much to choose between them.[41] Nor does the rapid shift from *algema* to *odyne* to *ponos* in a passage in the treatise on *Regimen in Acute*

301

Diseases betray a greater fastidiousness.[42] Indeed, in this undifferentiated lexical landscape only one manifestly specialized term can be discerned, and that is *odis* – occasionally used in CH, mainly in the gynaecological treatises, for the pain of childbirth – but never to the exclusion of *odyne* and *ponos*.[43]

What we today think of as the psychogenic pains of mental illness fail to elicit any richer descriptions. There is no mind-body problem for Hippocratic medicine; the problem arises only for its modern interpreters, handicapped by a conceptual dualism not evident in their sources. The Hippocratics' theory of mental illness was essentially physicalist, and therefore mental disorder did not seem to present any particular problem of description, aetiology or treatment.[44] As G. E. R. Lloyd has written, 'the doctors were concerned to collect cases of cold toes along with those of fear and despondency: all formed part of a total homogeneous epidemiological culture'.[45] The Hippocratics made no concessions to the Platonic view that certain kinds of madness, under divine patronage, were blessings rather than afflictions.[46] Emotions that were presumably in some way painful – the 'psychological' ingredients in somatic disorder that would later, in Galenic medical theory, be numbered among the 'non-naturals' – are therefore simply listed. Seldom do the Hippocratics give us any sustained evocation, any first-person account of 'how it felt'.

One striking exception is the often-quoted passage in a short gynaecological treatise describing the delirium of young virgins of marriageable age, virgins made ill by the retention of menstrual blood. Fears and terrors are said to be aroused in them; they become murderously inclined; delusions bid them leap into wells or hang themselves; they are more than half in love with death.[47] In Hippocratic eyes, however, such powerful emotions are still largely epiphenomenal to somatic disorders; they are not therefore generally described as in themselves painful. In one of the case histories of insanity in *Epidemics III* a woman is said to experience intense and continuous pains, but these are entirely somatic, mentioned separately from her 'psychological' symptoms.[48] In another work, it is *insensitivity* to pain in those with a physical illness that is taken as a sign that the mind also is afflicted.[49] Pain and psychological trauma are kept in separate diagnostic compartments.

The topic of insanity is a suitable point at which to relax the discussion's restriction to medical texts and bring into play the wider

PAIN IN HIPPOCRATIC MEDICINE

context of ancient Greek literature. Medical historians have often turned to literature for enlightenment as to the overtones that medical terms may possess. Helen King for example draws on the possible meanings of *ponos* in a range of texts from Hesiod to Plutarch to elicit a further medical definition: 'pain with a goal, a means to an end . . . very unlikely to be relieved in any way . . . divinely-ordained as part of the human condition'.[50] I have, by contrast, already argued that there is no evidence in CH of discriminable categories of pain of any type, let alone one so redolent of a whole philosophical anthropology. In some literary texts *ponos* undoubtedly refers to unevadable toils and pain; it is also used of the 'work' (for women) of sexual relations.[51] But not all the possible overtones of a word are necessarily present in any single use of it. And no ethical dimension to *ponos* is hinted at in the various references already surveyed. It might even have been the case that Hippocratic authors were intent on establishing their own particular, neutral, usages, purifying (in medicine at least) the dialect of the tribe.

Instead of pressing literature into the service of explaining medicine, I would prefer to emphasize the differences between the two. For beyond the medical corpus there does lie a rich semantic world of pain – a world in which more than two or three basic terms are in question, context supplies a way of gauging delicate alterations of register, physiology is inseparable from ethics, and somatic and psychological pain and distress lie on a continuum rather than either side of a conceptual chasm. There is no space here for detail. Mere allusions will have to suffice: to the representations of pain or wounding in Homer – those involving, say, Aphrodite and Agamemnon in the *Iliad* or the Cyclops in the *Odyssey*;[52] to Philoctetes' suppurating foot, its pain devouring his mind like a plague;[53] to the dementia of Io in *Prometheus Bound*; or, in a perhaps less familiar and later example, to Medea's torments of love in Apollonius's *Argonautica*:

> From her eyes flowed tears of pity, and within her the pain [*odyne*] wore her away, smouldering through her flesh, around her fine nerves and deep into the very base of the neck where the ache and hurt [*achos*] drive deepest, whenever the tireless Loves shoot their torments into the heart.[54]

How inordinately different from the Hippocratic tone of voice . . .[55] I have been suggesting that the Hippocratic vocabulary of pain is not rich or evocative – that it is replete with synonyms and predictable adjectives; also that it does not extend to psychological suffering. I now return to my second heading, distinctiveness. For the Hippocratic authors, pain is as it were all of a piece, important in the clinical encounter but perhaps in a uniformly banal and sub-theoretical way. It poses no insuperable problems, nor even ones that are very special. It is so intimately bound up with the rest of medicine as to exert no great independent leverage on the perceptions and mind of the theorist.

Granted, to feel pain in general is, for the Hippocratics, part of the human condition. We feel pain because, as *The Nature of Man* has it, we are not a unity[56]. If we were made up entirely of one element, pain would be impossible, for a unity would not exhibit change and corruption, excess and deficiency; and these, as we read in *Places in Man*, are the causes of pain.[57] But if pain arises inevitably in such disunited creatures, it does not follow that, when it does so, it must be endured. Medicine, we are told, is completely discovered; it has no frontiers left to cross.[58] Its goal is health, which is the absence of pain; and pain can be dealt with. *The Art* 3: 'I would define medicine as the complete removal of the pains (or troubles) [*tous kamatous*] of the sick.' *The Sacred Disease* 18: 'there is nothing in any disease which . . . is insusceptible to treatment'.[59] Of course, against those texts, one could cite *Prognostic* 1: 'it is impossible to cure all patients',[60] or the continuation of the passage from *The Art* just quoted: '. . . the complete removal of the pains of the sick, the alleviation of the more violent diseases [note that this still creates the impression that all minor pains can all be dealt with], and the refusal to undertake to cure cases in which the disease has already won the mastery, knowing that everything is not possible to medicine'.[61]

The resolution of the conflicting testimonies, as Heinrich von Staden proposes, is to conclude that, in Hippocratic eyes, no case is in principle hopeless, no pain *in principle* beyond removal or alleviation.[62] Hippocratic doctors did not uniformly refuse to treat those beyond help. Their underlying thought (according to von Staden's persuasive reconstruction) was that only in particular instances was a condition to be deemed untreatable. The condition – together with its attendant pains – could arise from heredity, or from some flaw in Nature; it might have been left untreated too long, or might lie beyond the skill of the individual doctor or the current resources of medicine. In that case, and if the pains were so nearly unbearable that the patient requested euthanasia, then the physician would not hesitate to assist.[63] But pains, even very severe ones, were not considered intrinsically beyond the reach of medical science.

All pain is in principle treatable because so are all diseases. Part of the reason why the Hippocratic authors are not much interested in the subtleties of pain, or very interesting when they do write about it, is that those statements about pain and disease are nearly tautologous. Having discoursed about disease, its symptoms and treatment, the Hippocratic authors have nothing of consequence to add. In *Ancient Medicine* 3, the reason medicine was founded is given as 'ridding man of the diet that caused pain, sickness and death'.[64] There, pain is a preliminary to disease or in effect a minor ailment, at the other end of the spectrum from the most serious ailment of death. In *Breaths* 1, the greatest evils are *lype, ponos* [two words for pain], and death. In *Places in Man* 42, 'pains are cured by opposites and there is something specific for each disease'.[65] Both texts show the approximate equivalence of pain and disease.

I must certainly avoid creating the impression that analgesia was never considered an end in itself. Precisely because of that intertwining of pain and disease, there was, I believe, no serious anxiety expressed by the Hippocratics (such as was later voiced by Caelius Aurelianus)[66] that concern with analgesia might distract from the main purpose of addressing the disease. A large repertoire of anodynes was available, for both local and general use: regimen, bathing, purgatives, fomentations, cataplasms, sneezing, and simply letting nature do the work. More remarkably, cauterizing was occasionally in order as an analgesic, for gout among other things – and it was also held by some that 'pain calms pain', can itself be an analgesic, and that if two pains occur simultaneously but in different places, the worse one cancels the other out.[67] The striking feature of this repertoire is that the treatments for pain are virtually coterminous with those for disease. Analgesics no more belong in a separate domain than do the sensations of pain against which they are directed.

Pain was thus of some concern to the Hippocratic physician, but as a subject it blended very well into the general medical context. Of course, what the patient said and showed about his or her pains might be crucial to prognosis. 'The spread of pains to the head without a sign, in the presence of fever, is fatal.' And again: 'pains which depart without obvious cause are fatal'.[68] In less extreme cases, pain might be particularly helpful in beginning to localize a disease or physical symptom, or in suggesting the direction of treatment, for instance by its position above or below the diaphragm.[69] 'When you question the patient and examine each thing carefully, do so first with regard to the state of his head, whether it is free of pain and has no heaviness in it; then the hypochondrium and the sides, whether they are free of pain . . .' and so on.[70] And yet – it is striking that in other extensive descriptions of clinical examination and diagnosis (i.e. descriptions longer than a few lines), such as that at the beginning of the treatise on *Prognosis* or in *Epidemics*, i. 3. 10, there is no mention of pain.[71] Was it taken for granted, or was it deliberately omitted? Perhaps at this learned level the Hippocratic physician was too anxious to assert his own 'professional' standing to grant the patient that limited degree of authority implicit in the description or demonstration of pain.[72] Or perhaps clinical conversation about pain was, as I have already proposed, thought too individual and subjective a matter to be added to the stock of theoretical wisdom: as remote from the rigidities of the treatise as (apparently) is a session with a psychoanalyst from a textbook on Freud.

The final question to raise – briefly – is that of how far, on this score, the Hippocratics can stand for the whole of ancient Greek medicine. The thrust of the answer depends hugely on the choice of texts to be adduced. In Aretaeus of Cappadocia's writing *On the Causes and Indications of Acute and Chronic Diseases*, we find for example some finely tuned representations of various types of headache.[73] On the other hand, in an anonymous work also dealing with acute and chronic diseases, and also of the first century AD, we encounter such bland statements as 'warmth applied by contact is fine for any pain'.[74] And we realize that we should not be seduced into associating the entire gamut of medical writing with the achievements of a few distinguished names. The legacy of Rufus of Ephesus, a greater and more famous clinician of the first century than Aretaeus, provides further warnings against expecting learned medicine under the Roman Empire to produce newly refined approaches to the problem of pain. As remarked here at the outset, Rufus may not actually have written a treatise on pain. The subject is none the less prominent in some of his case histories preserved in Arabic. For example:

> The pain did not subside but extended to the side of [a melancholic's] face . . . when I feared that it might pass to his eye and brain and that it might kill him, I asked him to have his blood

> let . . . Then, I cauterized his ribs where there was pain. The
> pain subsided completely . . .[75]

At first blush, pain seems important, a subject for treatment in its
own right. Then, however, it becomes apparent that Rufus is
virtually equating pain with disease, as the Hippocratics had often
done. The relative vividness of the passage does not proclaim a
novel or more sensitive theory. And in another work Rufus himself
tells us why that should be so. *Questions of the Physician* runs in
some detail through the ideal clinical interrogation of the patient –
enquiries concerning diet, defecation, previous experience with
doctors, and so forth.

> We must also ask what pains [*algemata*] the ailment is causing.
> It is true that one can judge in other ways when a person is in
> pain – by his groans and exclamations, by his uneasy
> movements, his embarrassment, the posture of his body . . . it
> is possible to recognize pains [*ponoi*] in a patient apart from his
> complaints.[76]

To ask where it hurt was not therefore absolutely essential, even
though Rufus did not consider that the question should be lightly
omitted from the clinical encounter. On the other hand, in *Questions
of the Physician* he immediately went on to caution against the
histrionics of the effeminate, whose representations of pain (*odyne*
this time) were as bad as those of tragic actors. And, most significantly for the present argument, enquiries about pain fall well
below the top of his list. Some six other topics are treated first in
Questions.

Perhaps for similar reasons, Galen, to close with the greatest
Hippocratic of them all, also had *relatively* little to say of a theoretical nature about pain. Of course, in some cases, Galen could prognosticate *solely* on the basis of questioning the patient, provided he
or she were intelligent and articulate. Moreover, to underpin that
virtuosity he elevated investigation of pain into a prime means of
locating the affected part. On the basis of his masterly synthesis of
Hippocrates and Aristotle with dashes of Platonism, and his
advances in anatomy and physiology, Galen elaborated a theory of
the production of pain to a degree of sophistication inevitably
lacking in the Hippocratic corpus. He enriched the descriptions
and extended the similes. He began classifying the different kinds
of pain (including sympathetic or referred pain) according to their

character and their potential for revealing not only the location of the diseased organ but also a general humoral imbalance.[77] As always, Galen is his own most best advocate:

> These organs [liver and kidneys] develop a feeling of heaviness, as if some kind of an unnatural tumor had taken hold of them. In the membrane surrounding each of the viscera mentioned above a nerve is inserted which is endowed with sensibility; when distended by the swelling of the organ it indicates to us the diagnostic classification according to the type of pain. Therefore Hippocrates was the first to write: 'pain in the kidneys feels heavy'.[78]

Hippocrates was the first to write it; Galen the first to explain it. Yet what is striking is that, despite all this, and despite the number of brief discussions of pain in his massive corpus, he seems to have devoted to the topic only one book of the one late treatise just quoted, *On the Affected Parts*. There is no reference to the significance of pain in his extended self-advertisement *On Prognosis*.[79] In comparison with the massive literary attention he paid to pulse and the almost over-refined descriptive vocabulary that he developed for that subject,[80] it is not very much. The best modern commentators on his clinical-diagnostic method find correspondingly little to say about patients' reports of pain or their involuntary signs of distress.[81]

That is surely because Galen rapidly came up against what he took to be the limits of the subject. Where his own recollected experience of pain was inadequate, he would have to rely, as he put it, either on those who did not understand their experiences or on those who understood but could not formulate their suffering in words, 'since it requires a considerable effort or cannot even be communicated verbally'.[82] Malingering, too, presented problems.[83] Hence, despite the distinctions advocated in *On the Affected Parts*, he generally seems to have used *algema*, *odyne*, and *ponos* interchangeably, just as the Hippocratics had done.[84] Pain was easier to deal with from a neurological than from a clinical point of view. The task of interpreting its verbal and behavioural representations was, on the whole, best left at the bedside and kept out of the treatises.

Did the general reluctance of ancient physicians to develop a sophisticated account of the experience of pain stem from inherent limits set to learned endeavour by the topic's irreducible subjectivity? Or was pain more deliberately marginalized? Galen would

PAIN IN HIPPOCRATIC MEDICINE

have responded to the enquiry by referring to subjectivity. He might have agreed with Virginia Woolf, had he lived to read her, on this if nothing else: that 'the merest schoolgirl when she falls in love has Shakespeare, Donne and Keats to speak her mind for her, but let a sufferer try to describe a pain in his head to a doctor and language at once runs dry'.[85] Galen would also have found congenial the twentieth-century surgeon René Leriche: 'in the suffering patient the pain is like a storm which hardly admits of assessment once it is over . . . and there you are, powerless to understand.'[86]

None the less, we must be wary of accepting either the Hippocratics' or Galen's attitude to pain as simply dictated by the inherent nature of the problem. Their attitude should, additionally, be given a cultural setting. But where? One approach, of which a great deal has lately been made, would place Galen in a context that he would not have appreciated: the emergence of Christianity. The period of the late Roman Republic and the earlier empire (the first two centuries) has been interpreted by historians of Foucauldian persuasion as witnessing a 'turn toward the body'. They have discerned an increasing literary emphasis on the representation of physical suffering – an emphasis which foreshadowed, and indeed facilitated, the cultural reception of Christianity's suffering martyrs and saints. Galen assumes a prominent role in such accounts, his fame and success suggesting a medicalization of Roman imperial society, even a medicalization of the notion of the self.[87] There is much evidence to favour such an interpretation. It is surely not coincidental – that is, not just a reflection of the greater abundance of the written evidence – that the type of quotation with which I began is easier to find in the age of Galen than in that of Hippocrates. Yet the history of pain in medicine suggests at least as much continuity as development in the centuries separating the two presiding genii of the subject. Pain does *not* come to dominate Roman medical 'discourse' in the manner predicted by the Foucauldians.

A rather different backdrop may be more appropriate. It has sometimes seemed tempting to divide the history of pain, if only implicitly, into three phases.[88] The third and most recent one began as recently as the 1960s and 1970s. It has witnessed the establishment of pain clinics for chronic sufferers, the founding of the journal *Pain*, a celebrated pain questionnaire, the burgeoning of an anthropological literature which attends to the culturally determined ways in which the afflicted fashion significant narratives around their pains,[89] and a steady increase in the number of doctors who do *not* separate mental suffering from somatic pain or confine treatment to the latter. Before all this, in Phase Two, came the advances in neuro-anatomy of the nineteenth and earlier twentieth centuries and the 'laboratory revolution' in medicine. It is this period, we have in effect been told, which first banished pain to the margins of medical interest and encouraged the view that non-somatic pain was unreal.[90] Phase One, which stretches back to antiquity, is therefore, on this account, pre-lapsarian: a phase in which power lay with the patient, and in which the holistic approach of humoral medicine ensured a much greater degree of attention to patients' suffering and its relief. Phase Three can thus be presented as to some extent a return to Eden – not (admittedly) to a paradise in which there is no pain, but at least to one in which pain is again accorded due status.

Galen and the Hippocratic authors, as I have been construing them, refute the ideas underlying all such nostalgic historical schemata. In their seeming indifference to the pains of mental illness, in their reluctance to give pain too prominent a place in diagnostic enquiry, in their unwillingness to elaborate a vocabulary of pain, above all in their refusal to philosophize about it, they can (in retrospect) be seen as performing two salutary tasks. First, they hinder our general attribution to Phase One of too great an interest in the causation or relief of pain.[91] But second, paradoxically, they also in a sense align themselves with the age of the laboratory, more readily seen as their cultural and intellectual antithesis. And this alignment seems appropriate: in each of the two ages, that of the Hippocratics and that of the laboratory, learned medical aspirations were, though expressed very differently, perhaps quite similar – aspirations towards scientific rationality and the prestige that went with it, aspirations towards authority over the patient, and thus over everything that he or she said as well as did. About suffering they were never wrong, the Old Masters?[92]

NOTES

1. Edward Mendelson (ed.), *The English Auden* (London: Faber and Faber, 1977), 237.
2. *Agamemnon*, line 177, with Eduard Fraenkel, *Aeschylus: Agamemnon*, 2 vols (Oxford: Clarendon Press), ii. 106.
3. *Nicomachean Ethics*, iii. 12.

PAIN IN HIPPOCRATIC MEDICINE

4. Epicurus, *Key Doctrines*, 4, trans. A.A. Long and D.N. Sedley, *The Hellenistic Philosophers*, 2 vols (Cambridge: Cambridge University Press, 1987), i. 115.

5. *Moral Letters*, lxxviii. 13, with P.H. Schrijvers, 'Pijn, waar is je overwinning? Over de 78e Brief van Seneca', in H.F.J. Horstmanshoff (ed.), *Pijn en Balsem, Troost en Smart: Pijnbeleving, en Pijnbestrijding in de Oudheid* (Rotterdam: Erasmus Publishing, 1994), 185–95.

6. Vii. 11. Cf. *Acts*, xiv. 22.

7. *Octavius*, 12, trans. Judith Perkins, *The Suffering Self: Pain and Narrative Representation in the Early Christian Era* (London/New York: Routledge, 1995), 38–9.

8. *Letters*, xxxix. 2. Cf. Darrel W. Amundsen, *Medicine, Society, and Faith in the Ancient and Medieval Worlds* (Baltimore/London: Johns Hopkins University Press, 1996), ch. 5.

9. Marvin Meyer and Richard Smith (eds), *Ancient Christian Magic: Coptic Texts of Ritual Power* (New York: HarperCollins, 1994), no. 135, p. 335.

10. Cf. David Melling, this volume; John Bowker, *Problems of Suffering in Religions of the World* (Cambridge: Cambridge University Press, 1970).

11. David B. Morris, *The Culture of Pain* (Berkeley/Los Angeles: University of California Press, 1991), 74.

12. James Longrigg, *Greek Rational Medicine: Philosophy and Medicine from Alcmaeon to the Alexandrians* (London/New York: Routledge, 1993), 26 n.l with refs.; G.E.R. Lloyd, *Magic, Reason and Experience: Studies in the Origins and Development of Greek Science* (Cambridge: Cambridge University Press, 1979), ch. 1.

13. Vivian Nutton, 'From Galen to Alexander: Aspects of Medicine and Medical Practice in Late Antiquity', *Dumbarton Oaks Papers*, xxxviii (1984), 8–9.

14. Owsei Temkin, *Hippocrates in a World of Pagans and Christians* (Baltimore/London: Johns Hopkins University Press, 1991), 256; Peter Brown, *The Body and Society: Men, Women and Sexual Renunciation in Early Christianity* (New York: Columbia University Press, 1988); Simon Goldhill, *Foucault's Virginity: Ancient Erotic Fiction and the History of Sexuality* (Cambridge: Cambridge University Press, 1995); Perkins, *The Suffering Self*.

15. Charles Daremberg and Charles Emile Ruelle (eds), *Oeuvres de Rufus d'Ephèse* (Paris: Imprimerie Nationale, 1879), nos 256–324; J. Ilberg, 'Rufus von Ephesos: ein griechischer Arzt in trajanischer Zeit', *Abhandlungen der philologisch-historischen Klasse der Sächischen Akademie der Wissenschaften*, xli. 1 (1931), 38–42. I am grateful to Vivian Nutton for advice.

16. Michel Foucault, *The Birth of the Clinic* (Tavistock: London, 1973), xviii.

17. No aspect of the *Corpus Hippocraticum* is free from continuing debate. I do no more than attempt to summarize the conventional scholarly wisdom. The most accessible means of entry into CH is through Paul Potter, *Short Handbook of Hippocratic Medicine* (Quebec: Editions du Sphinx, 1988), and G.E.R. Lloyd (ed.), *Hippocratic Writings* (Harmondsworth: Penguin, 1978).

18. The standard edition, Carl Gottlob Kühn, *Claudii Galeni: Opera Omnia*, 22 vols (Leipzig: Cnobloch, 1821–33), is only the upper part of an

iceberg. In what follows all references to CH will be by volume and page number in the standard edition of E. Littré (hereafter L), *Oeuvres complètes d'Hippocrate*, 10 vols (Paris: J.-B. Baillière, 1839–61).

19. Simon Byl, 'Le traitement de la douleur dans le *Corpus* hippocratique', in J.A. López Férez (ed.), *Tratados Hipocráticos* (Madrid: Universidad Nacional de Educacion a Distancia, 1992), 203, a study to which I am greatly indebted.

20. Gilles Maloney and Winnie Fromm (eds), *Concordantia in Corpus Hippocraticum*, 5 vols (Hildesheim/Zurich/New York: Olms-Weidmann, 1986).

21. Byl, 'Traitement', 203, has larger aggregates.

22. Cf. Roselyne Rey, *The History of Pain* (Cambridge, MA/London: Harvard University Press, 1995), 18.

23. On the dating, L. Conrad *et al.*, *The Western Medical Tradition* (Cambridge: Cambridge University Press, 1995), 22.

24. Rey, *History*, 19.

25. Contrast Lloyd, *Magic*, subtly distinguishing tradition and naturalism in Hippocratic ideology, with Longrigg, *Greek Rational Medicine*.

26. I.M. Lonie, 'Cos versus Cnidus and the Historians', *History of Science*, xvi (1978), 42–75, 77–92.

27. A.M. Unruh, 'Gender Variations in Clinical Pain Experience', *Pain*, lxv. 2–3 (1996), 123–67.

28. I. 62, L viii.126.

29. Useful conspectuses: Lesley Dean-Jones, *Women's Bodies in Classical Greek Science* (Oxford: Clarendon Press, 1994); Ann Ellis Hanson, 'The Medical Writer's Woman', in David M. Halperin *et al.* (eds), *Before Sexuality: The Construction of Erotic Experience in the Ancient Greek World* (Princeton, NJ: Princeton University Press, 1990), 309–38.

30. Dean-Jones, *Women's Bodies*, ch. 2, esp. 119, 125.

31. Helen King, 'Self-help, Self-knowledge: in Search of the Patient in Hippocratic Gynaecology', in Richard Hawley and Barbara Levick (eds), *Women in Antiquity: New Assessments* (London/New York: Routledge, 1995), 135–48.

32. Helen King, 'The Early Anodynes: Pain in the Ancient World', in Ronald D. Mann (ed.), *The History of the Management of Pain* (Carnforth, Lancashire/Park Ridge, NJ: Parthenon Publishing Group, 1988), 58.

33. Rey, *History*, 19.

34. 60 (L vii. 93), 6 (14) with 21 (36); 14 (27); 60 (93).

35. 66 (L vii. 101), 73 (111).

36. 14 (L vii. 25), 15 (167).

37. 8 (L vii. 16), 27 (44), 55 (87).

38. 4 (L vii. 12), 16 (30); 20 (33), 23 (38).

39. Vi. 40, vii. 52 (L iv. 572, 592); Byl, 'Traitement', 203.

40. Byl, 'Traitement', 203–4.

41. 7 (L vi. 290).

42. 7 (L ii. 268–72), *pace* King, 'Early Anodynes', 60, which seems to me overingenious. I am very grateful to Helen King for allowing me to read, in advance of its publication, a paper that elaborates some of the

PAIN IN HIPPOCRATIC MEDICINE

material there: 'Chronic Pain and the Creation of Narrative', forthcoming in Jim Porter (ed.), *Constructions of the Classical Body*.

43. Cf. again King, 'Early Anodynes', 60. In the early second century AD, Soranus still used both *odyne* and *ponos*; cf. his *Gynaecoloy*, ii. 6–8.

44. P.N. Singer, 'Some Hippocratic Mind-Body Problems', in López Férez (ed.), *Tratados Hipocráticos*, 131–43.

45. G.E.R. Lloyd, *The Revolutions of Wisdom: Studies in the Claims and Practices of Ancient Greek Science* (Berkeley/Los Angeles/London: University of California Press, 1987), 23.

46. E.R. Dodds, *The Greeks and the Irrational* (Berkeley/Los Angeles/London: University of California Press, 1951), ch. 3.

47. L viii. 468. Helen King, 'Bound to Bleed', in Averil Cameron and Amélie Kuhrt (eds), *Images of Women in Antiquity*, rev. ed. (London: Routledge, 1993), 109–27.

48. Xvii. 11 (L iii. 134).

49. *Aphorisms*, ii. 6 (L iv. 470).

50. King, 'Early Anodynes', 59–60, seeming to me to confuse (a) pain which cannot on a particular occasion be relieved, (b) pain which can *never* be relieved, (c) pain which *should* not be relieved.

51. Anne Carson, 'Putting Her in Her Place: Woman, Dirt, and Desire', in Halperin *et al.* (eds), *Before Sexuality*, 149.

52. *Iliad*, v. 336f., xi. 251f.; *Odyssey*, ix. 387f. F. Mawet, *Recherches sur les oppositions fonctionelles dans le vocabulaire homérique de la douleur* (Gembloux: Académie Royale de Belgique, 1979).

53. Sophocles, *Philoctetes*, lines 705–6. Philip van der Eijk, 'Pijn en Doodsstrijd in de Griekse Tragedie: Sophocles' *Philoctetes*', in Horstmanshoff (ed.), *Pijn en Balsem*, 71–83. For wider context and many further references: Bennett Simon, *Mind and Madness in Ancient Greece* (Ithaca/London: Cornell University Press, 1978); Ruth Padel, *In and Out of the Mind: Greek Images of the Tragic Self* (Princeton, NJ: Princeton University Press, 1992); Padel, *Whom Gods Destroy: Elements of Greek and Tragic Madness* (Princeton NJ: Princeton University Press, 1995).

54. Iii. 761–5, trans. Richard Hunter, *Jason and the Golden Fleece*, World's Classics (Oxford/New York: Oxford University Press), 84 (modified slightly). Mawet, 'Evolution d'une structure sémantique: le vocabulaire de la douleur – Apollonios de Rhodes et Homère', *L'Antiquité Classique*, 1 (1981), 499–516; Richard Hunter, *The 'Argonautica' of Apollonius* (Cambridge: Cambridge University Press, 1993), ch. 3, § 3.

55. *Pace* Padel, *In and Out of the Mind*, 50: 'doctors are as fascinated by pain and its causes as are epic and tragedy'.

56. 2 (Lvi. 34).

57. 42 (L vi. 334–6).

58. *Places in Man*, 46 (L vi. 342).

59. L vi. 394, trans. Lloyd, *Hippocratic Writings*, 251.

60. L ii. 110, trans. Lloyd, *Hippocratic Writings*, 170.

61. Adapted from Lloyd, *Hippocratic Writings*, 140.

62. Heinrich von Staden, 'Incurability and Hopelessness: the *Hippocratic Corpus*', in Paul Potter *et al.* (eds), *La maladie et les maladies dans la Collection hippocratique* (Quebec: Editions du Sphinx, 1990), 75–112.

63. Amundsen, *Medicine, Society, and Faith*, chs 2, 4; Ludwig Edelstein, *Ancient Medicine* (Baltimore/London: Johns Hopkins University Press, 1967), 11 f.
64. L i. 578.
65. L vi. 90, vi. 334.
66. Caelius Aurelianus, *On Acute and Chronic Diseases*, I.E. Drabkin (ed.) (Chicago: University of Chicago Press, 1950), Chronic Diseases, ii. 79 (p. 616).
67. *Aphorisms*, ii. 46 (L iv. 482). Byl, 'Traitement'; King 'Early Anodynes'.
68. *Coan Prenotions*, 366, 364 (L v. 660–2).
69. *Aphorisms*, iv. 31, 32 (L iv. 512).
70. *Regimen in Acute Diseases, Appendix*, 9 (L ii. 436f.), trans. Paul Potter, *Hippocrates*, vi, Loeb Classical Library (Cambridge MA/London: Harvard University Press and Heinemann, 1988), 285.
71. L ii. 110f., 668f.
72. The competitively rhetorical aspect of Hippocratic writing is well brought out by Lloyd, *Magic*.
73. *Chronic Diseases*, i. 2, Carolus Hyde (ed.), *Corpus Medicorum Graecorum* [hereafter CMG] (Berlin: Academy of Sciences, 1958), 36–7. Cf. Caelius Aurelianus, *Chronic Diseases*, i. 4 (pp. 610f., Drabkin).
74. Ivan Garofallo (ed.), Brian Fuchs (trans.), *Anonymi Medici de Morbis Acutis et Chronicis* (Leiden/New York/Cologne: Brill, 1997), vi. 10 (p. 44).
75. The standard edition of Rufus's *Krankenjournale* is by Manfred Ullmann (Wiesbaden: Harrasowitz, 1978). I quote a translation by Michael W. Dols from an Oxford Arabic MS: Dols, *Majnun: The Madman in Medieval Islamic Society* (Oxford: Clarendon Press, 1992), 479.
76. Hans Gärtner (ed.), *Rufus von Ephesos: Die Fragen des Arztes an den Kranken*, CMG Supplement 4 (Berlin: Academy of Sciences, 1962), 8 (p. 38).
77. Rosa Maria Moreño Rodriguez and Luis García Ballester, 'El dolor en la teoría y práctica médicas de Galeno', *Dynamis*, ii (1982), 3–24.
78. *On the Affected Parts*, ii. 4, trans. Rudolf E. Siegel (Basel: S. Karger, 1976), 47 (ed. Kühn, viii. 78–9), with *Epidemics VI*, i. 5 (L v. 268).
79. Vivian Nutton (ed.), *Galen: On Prognosis*, CMG, v. 8. 1 (Berlin: Academy of Sciences, 1979).
80. C.R.S. Harris, *The Heart and the Vascular System in Ancient Greek Medicine* (Oxford: Clarendon Press, 1973), ch. 7.
81. Vivian Nutton, 'Galen at the Bedside: the Methods of a Medical Detective', in W.F. Bynum and Roy Porter (eds), *Medicine and the Five Senses* (Cambridge: Cambridge University Press, 1993), 7–16; Luis García Ballester, 'Galen as a Medical Practitioner: Problems in Diagnosis', in Vivian Nutton (ed.), *Galen: Problems and Prospects* (London: Wellcome Institute for the History of Medicine, 1981), 13–46, esp. 26–30.
82. *On the Affected Parts*, ii. 7 (p. 51, Siegel; viii. 89, Kühn).
83. Galen's brief discussion of it is edited by Karl Deichgräber and Fridolf Kudlien in CMG, v. 10. 2. 4 (Berlin: Academy of Sciences, 1960), 113f.
84. Richard J. Durling, *A Dictionary of Medical Terms in Galen* (Leiden/New York/Cologne: E.J. Brill, 1993).

85. Woolf, 'On being Ill', *Essays*, Andrew McNeillie (ed.), iv (London: Hogarth Press, 1994), 318.
86. Quoted by Morris, *Culture of Pain*, 28.
87. Cf. Perkins, *The Suffering Self*, ch. 6.
88. The implication of Morris, *Culture of Pain*, which provides abundant supporting references.
89. Cf. Byron J. Good, *Medicine, Rationality, and Experience* (Cambridge: Cambridge University Press, 1994), chs 5–6.
90. Cf. Eric J. Cassell, *The Nature of Suffering and the Goals of Medicine* (Oxford/New York: Oxford University Press, 1991); Andrew Cunningham and Perry Williams (eds), *The Laboratory Revolution in Medicine* (Cambridge: Cambridge University Press, 1992).
91. Rey, *History of Pain*, chs 1–3, esp. pp. 26–7; Barbara Duden, *The Woman beneath the Skin: A Doctor's Patients in Eighteenth-Century Germany* (Cambridge, MA/London: Harvard University Press, 1991), 87–91; Porter, this volume.
92. I am grateful for references and advice to several 'modern masters' of the subjects touched on here: Edward Hussey, Jane Lightfoot, Vivian Nutton, and particularly Helen King, who has kindly tolerated my incursion into her field and my friendly disagreement with some of the conclusions of her stimulating work.

IX

Travel Sickness: Medicine and Mobility in the Mediterranean from Antiquity to the Renaissance

1. INTRODUCTION

He was evidently old when he passed away, for his unsurpassed accuracy in material detail indicates an advanced age. That he travelled to many parts of the world can be inferred from his wide knowledge of places. We must also suppose a great abundance of wealth to have been at his disposal, for long journeys call for much expenditure, especially in those times when it was not the case that all seas could be safely sailed or that people could easily visit each other.

Thus the late antique *Life* of Homer by one Proclus (possibly not the famous Platonist).[1] He implicitly contrasts the limited mobility of the Homeric age with the greater ease of maritime communications characteristic of Roman imperial times. He offers us a perception of increasing Mediterranean mobility.

This paper too is about perceptions. In *The Corrupting Sea* Nicholas Purcell and I offered a partial definition of the integrity and distinctiveness of the Mediterranean in terms of the region's fluid communications and the concomitant mobility of its peoples.[2] My aim now is not to defend our definition; it is to revisit it from an unusual angle—that of medicine. What were the connections between personal mobility and health in the ancient and medieval Mediterranean? How is mobility represented in the medical texts?

---

[1] Ch. 8, trans. M. L. West, who kindly directed me to this passage in his Loeb edition of the *Homeric Hymns, Homeric Apocrypha, Lives of Homer* (Cambridge, Mass. and London, 2003).

[2] *CS*, especially chs. II, V, IX.

First, some very wide context within which to locate my particular subject. Mobility and therapy interconnect in a variety of ways in pre-modern times. Doctors itinerate, and not just quacks but Galen and his like.[3] Living holy men and saints perform healing wonders *en route*—and hagiography provides some of our most detailed evidence of medieval Mediterranean mobility and its infrastructure.[4] Dead saints also heal 'on the hoof'—sometimes literally, as their relics are ceremoniously 'translated'.[5] Nor should we forget trade or transfers involving drugs,[6] medical texts, and healing artefacts such as magic bowls.[7] Patients, finally, move in search of therapy—like Aelius Aristides—to healer, to shrine.[8] They also travel to hospitals. They flee epidemics. And their travels bring on new pathologies: travel sickness.[9]

All that is obvious enough. Less well known are the two aspects of the topic on which I want to focus here. 1. Regimen *for* travel: medical advice on how to preserve health while mobile or how to restore it through self-help while away from one's usual healer. 2. Travel *as* regimen, or as therapy. These both counterbalance the familiar theme of the tribulations of Mediterranean movement—for example, the penitential

---

[3] Hence the need to pin some of them down in cities by offering retainers: V. Nutton, 'Continuity or Rediscovery? The City Physician in Classical Antiquity and Mediaeval Italy', in A.W. Russell (ed.), *The Town and State Physician in Europe from the Middle Ages to the Enlightenment* (Wolfenbüttel, 1981), 9–46.

[4] E. Malamut, *Sur la route des saints byzantins* (Paris, 1993).

[5] M. Heinzelmann, *Translationsberichte und andere Quellen des Reliquienkultes* (Turnhout, 1979); P. Geary, *Furta Sacra* second edn. (Princeton, 1990).

[6] V. Nutton, 'The Drug Trade in Antiquity', *Journal of the Royal Society of Medicine* 78 (1985), 138–46.

[7] F. Maddison and E. Savage-Smith, *Science, Tools and Magic*, i. *Body and Spirit, Mapping the Universe*, The Nasser D. Khalili Collection of Islamic Art 12 (London, 1997), 72–100.

[8] C. A. Behr, *Aelius Aristides and the Sacred Tales* (Amsterdam, 1968); R. Schlesier, 'Menschen und Götter unterwegs: Ritual und Reise in der griechischen Antike', in T. Hölscher (ed.), *Gegenwelten zu den Kulturen Griechenlands und Roms in der Antike* (Munich and Leipzig, 2000), 129–57. For medieval pilgrims see R. C. Finucane, *Miracles and Pilgrims: Popular Beliefs in Medieval England* (London, 1977), ch. 9.

[9] R. Wrigley and G. Revill (eds.), *Pathologies of Travel* (Amsterdam and Atlanta, 2000).

suffering required of the pilgrim or the shipwreck risked by the voyager.[10] They offer a more positive view of personal mobility. They also bring together two poor relations. Migration is the most neglected aspect of pre-modern demography.[11] Regimen—preventive medicine, diet—is the most neglected aspect of pre-modern medicine, mainly, I conjecture, because medical historians are still subconsciously in thrall to the therapeutic, interventionist, bias of modern biomedicine.[12]

2. MOBILITY AND FIXITY

Before I consider those two themes separately, let me next try to generalize about the perceptions of Mediterranean movement that the medical texts offer. I must warn in advance that no big demographic conclusions will emerge. It is not inevitable that mobility should engender a commensurate literature of advice. That is, the medical literature cannot, through any changes in emphasis or quantity, give us a reliable index of changing Mediterranean mobility. Still less is this evidence sufficiently detailed or geographically widespread to permit Mediterranean and non-Mediterranean comparisons—comparisons that might suggest where mobility was greater. What the medical material can do, however, is show how at least some contemporary authors perceived, classified, and evaluated mobility.

In the late fifth to early fourth century BC the author of the Hippocratic *Regimen* (*Peri diaites*) claims (ch. 68) to be writing for the majority of men: those who use ordinary, accessible, food and drink, who exert themselves as much as is essential, who undertake land journeys and sea voyages to collect their

---

[10] D. J. Birch, *Pilgrimage to Rome in the Middle Ages* (Woodbridge, Suffolk, 1998), 3–4, on the 'white martyrdom' of pilgrimage, contrasted, but not too strongly, with the 'red martyrdom' of death. See further C. Stancliffe, 'Red, White and Blue Martyrdom', in D. Whitelock, R. McKitterick, and D. Dumville (eds.), *Ireland in Early Medieval Europe* (Cambridge, 1982), 21–46. For the overrated dangers of Mediterranean sea voyages see *CS*, chs. V.3, X.4, with bibliography.

[11] *CS*, Bibliographical Essay to ch. IX.6.

[12] P. Horden, 'Religion as Medicine: Music in Medieval Hospitals', in P. Biller and J. Ziegler (eds.), *Religion and Medicine in the Middle Ages* (Woodbridge, Suffolk, and Rochester, NY, 2001), 135–53.

livelihood.[13] The claim is perhaps disingenuous. But the image of the small producer who of necessity sometimes has to travel long distances to gather sustenance, and who benefits from the maritime 'connectivity' of the Mediterranean, seems like a condensation of *The Corrupting Sea*.[14] It is exactly the form and degree of mobility that Purcell and I postulated. It contradicts the retrospective account of Mediterranean communications implied by that extract from the *Life of Homer* with which I began. In the early first century AD, Celsus (*De medicina* 1.1) offered a more aristocratic version. The healthy man, his own master, needs no medical attendants to stay healthy. Variety spices his life. He is now in the country, now in the town, and more often 'in agro'; he should sail, hunt, rest sometimes, but more frequently take exercise. He avoids common foods, goes to the baths but avoids athletics, and eats as much as he wants twice a day. In the Hippocratic-Galenic tradition, on which Celsus to some extent draws, the balance between mobility (usually meaning exercise) and rest is central. It is one of the 'non-natural' determinants of health hinted at in the Hippocratic corpus, mentioned unsystematically by Galen, and canonized by medieval Islamic medical writers.[15] Mobility is also figuratively present, in a variety of ways. For example, nautical metaphors abound in Plutarch's short treatise offering 'instructions for health' (*Hygieina paraggelmata*). In the tenth-century Muslim physician Razi, the illness itself is imaged as a journey. 'The patient's strength is like a traveller's provisions. Disease

[13] *Oeuvres complètes d'Hippocrate*, ed. and trans. E. Littré, 10 vols. (Paris, 1839–61), vi. 594. For guidance as to other editions see P. Potter, *Short Handbook of Hippocratic Medicine* (Quebec, 1988). Galen will be cited by reference to the standard (but incomplete) edition of C. G. Kühn (hereafter K), *Claudii Galeni: Opera Omnia*, 22 vols. (Leipzig, 1821–33), and to better editions where they exist.

[14] *CS*, chs. III, VI.

[15] L. García-Ballester, 'On the Origin of the "Six Non-Natural Things" in Galen', in G. Harig and J. Harig-Kollesch (eds.), *Galen und das Hellenistische Erbe*, *Sudhoffs Archiv* Beiheft 32 (Wiesbaden, 1993), 105–15; G. Olson, *Literature as Recreation in the Later Middle Ages* (Ithaca, NY and London, 1982), 40–4, esp. 41 n. 3 for earlier bibliography; H. Mikkeli, *Hygiene in the Early Modern Medical Tradition* (Helsinki, 1999), 9–10 (esp. 10 n. 4 for bibliography), 14–23.

is the highway, and the culmination of the disease his destination'.[16]

Beyond these generalities two contradictory tendencies are evident in the medical literature. On one hand, everyone is mobile. That is, the possibility of considerable movement is mentioned at the outset and presupposed in all the medical advice that follows. In the fourth century AD, the imperial physician Oribasius prefaced the advice on food that begins his massive *Medical Collections* (1.1) with the reminder that, 'on arrival in a foreign country one is obliged to eat something unusual', and one should test the food in advance (as well, other ancient authors recommended, as eating lots of garlic).[17] Movement is also presupposed in the institutional and social obverse of this regimen for the well to do. The late antique hospital, which was developing in Byzantium around the time Oribasius was writing, is a *xenodocheion*. It offers rest, nursing, and, sometimes, medicine—to *xenoi*, strangers: to the rootless poor, those who move to survive because they have no personal support networks.[18] At the extreme, the regimen of the mobile and that of the rooted are represented as almost identical. After all, as far as much dietary advice is concerned, where you are makes little difference. As Anthimus wrote in *De obseruatione ciborum* to Theuderic, a sixth-century king of the Franks: 'let us suppose that someone asks how anyone can take this sort of care [over food] when engaged in military manoeuvres or a long journey. I would say that if a fire can be lit... what has been suggested ought to be possible.'[19] The early medieval European compil-

---

[16] A. Z. Iskandar, *A Catalogue of Arabic Manuscripts on Medicine and Science in the Wellcome Historical Medical Library* (London, 1967), 4.

[17] Trans. M. Grant, *Dieting for an Emperor* (Leiden, 1997), 26–7, and see also 100.

[18] For the hospital see now P. Brown, *Poverty and Leadership in the Later Roman Empire* (Hanover and London, 2002), 33–44; P. Horden, 'The Earliest Hospitals in Byzantium, Western Europe and Islam', *Journal of Interdisciplinary History*, forthcoming. On networks of support, P. Horden, 'Household Care and Informal Networks: Comparisons and Continuities from Antiquity to the Present', in P. Horden and R. Smith (eds.), *The Locus of Care: Families, Communities, Institutions and the Provision of Welfare since Antiquity* (London and New York, 1998), 21–67.

[19] Anthimus, *De obseruatione ciborum, On the Observance of Foods*, ed. and trans. M. Grant (Totnes, 1996), 48–9.

ation of general medicine known as the *Medicina Plinii* was packaged as advice for travellers who would otherwise be at the mercy of ignorant and expensive quacks.[20] There, it is the perceived need of self-help that slants the text towards mobility. But the ninth-century medical handbook of Ibn al-Jazzar entitled, impartially, *Provisions for the Traveller and Nourishment for the Sedentary*, was addressed to physicians.[21] It was for use in regular consultation, even though its title suggested to Manfred Ullmann that its overt appeal was to 'Jedermann'.[22] In the eleventh century it was translated into Greek by one Constantine of Reggio, as the *Ephodia tou apodemountos*, and, by 1098, into Latin by 'the' Constantine—Constantine the African—as the *Viaticum peregrinantis*.[23] Both these translations obscured its titular appeal to the sedentary, however. It passed into the European medical curriculum of Bologna, Montpellier, and elsewhere as part of the *Articella*.[24] That guidance for travellers could subsume all the basics of medical learning thus in a sense became very widely accepted. What could the implication of the title *Viaticum* have been? That we are all in a literal sense travellers, all mobile at one stage or another? Or that, in some higher sense, we are all on the journey, the pilgrimage, of life?

[20] Prologue, *Plinii Secundi Iunioris qui feruntur de medicina libri tres*, ed. A. Önnerfors, *Corpus Medicorum Latinorum* 3 (Berlin, 1964), 4.

[21] *Ibn al-Jazzar on Sexual Diseases and their Treatment: A Critical Edition of 'Zad al-musafir wa-qut al-hadir, Provisions for the Traveller and Nourishment for the Sedentary, Book 6*, ed. and trans. G. Bos (London and New York, 1997), 8; M. G. Dugat, 'Études sur le traité de médecine d'Abou Djàfar Ah'mad', *Journal Asiatique*, 5th ser., 1 (1853), 287–353. Here and in what follows Arabic is represented in 'open transliteration'.

[22] M. Ullmann, 'Neues zu den diätetischen Schriften des Rufus von Ephesos', *Medizinhistorisches Journal* 9 (1974), 23–40, at 38.

[23] M. F. Wack, *Lovesickness in the Middle Ages: The 'Viaticum' and its Commentaries* (Philadelphia, 1990), ch. 2, for bibliography; C. Burnett and D. Jacquart (eds.), *Constantine the African and 'Ali ibn l-'Abbas al Magusi: The 'Pantegni' and Related Works*, Studies in Ancient Medicine 10 (Leiden, 1996).

[24] On the *articella*, see C. O'Boyle, *The Art of Medicine: Medical Teaching at the University of Paris, 1250–1400* (Leiden, 1998). See also J. Arrizabalaga, 'The Death of a Medieval Text: The *Articella* and the Early Press,' in R. French, J. Arrizabalaga, A. Cunningham, and L. García-Ballester (eds.) *Medicine from the Black Death to the French Disease* (Aldershot, 1998), 185–6, for summary and full bibliography.

The latter reading, perhaps implicit in medieval medicine, was to be made explicit in a Renaissance regimen to which I shall return at the end.

Against all this, on the other hand, are ranged what might be called the medical forces of 'fixity': those who image a static world to us.[25] This is the second of the contradictory tendencies to which I referred. Take the two corpora that came to dominate the medical output of antiquity and that thus moulded the medical learning of both Europe and the Middle East until at least 1700 (if not much later in some places). These are the Hippocratic corpus and the massive output of Galen. In the most significant of the earlier Hippocratic texts such as *Airs, waters, places* or *Epidemics I* and *III*, it is the healer who is on the move. Patients—my earlier quotation from the Hippocratic *Regimen* notwithstanding—are envisaged as closely related to their environments, which change with the seasons but are geographically stable.[26] Patients take exercises, *ponoi*, but they do not 'travel'. When the Hippocratic texts describe the questions that the physician should put to the patient (for example at the beginning of the treatise on *Prognosis* or in *Epidemics* 1.3.10) they do not juxtapose 'where have you been?' with 'where does it hurt?'. (For something approaching an enquiry of that sort we have to wait until Roman times (*c*.100 AD and Rufus of Ephesus, who also composed a regimen for travellers.)[27]

Galen is much the same as his Hippocratic exemplars.[28] In *De sanitate tuenda*, books 2–3, he writes at some length about the different ages of life, about exercise (including the long-distance exercise of riding and hunting) and fatigue.[29] But apart from a few stray asides he has virtually nothing else explicitly

---

[25] N. Purcell, 'Fixity', in R. Schlesier and U. Zellmann (eds.), *Mobility and Travel in the Mediterranean from Antiquity to the Middle Ages* (Münster, 2004), 73–83.

[26] e.g. *Epidemics*, 1.1–5.

[27] *Rufus von Ephesos, Die Fragen des Arztes an den Kranken*, ed. H. Gärtner, *CMG*, Suppl. 4 (Berlin, 1962).

[28] V. Nutton, 'Galen and the Traveller's Fare', in J. Wilkins, D. Harris, and M. Dobson (eds.), *Food in Antiquity* (Exeter, 1995), 359–70, is far more about Galen's dietetics in general than its title suggests.

[29] R. M. Green, *A Translation of Galen's Hygiene* (Springfield, Ill., 1951); 6.1–452K, *CMG* 5.4.2. For analysis, see G. Wöhrle, *Studien zur Theorie der Antiken Gesundheitslehre, Hermes* Einzelschriften 56 (1990), ch. 7.

directed at those on the move. Presumably he did not want his patients to feel they could do without him. Galen's practice is dedicated to (at the least) the wealthy in their villas, whom he counsels to stay put, avoiding urban insalubrities.[30] Some of his clearest recommendations to a sufferer who has to travel come in his letter of 'Advice for an epileptic boy'. Its sheer specificity perhaps indicates how marginal the topic was to him.[31]

A final point under this heading of 'fixity'. Galen's silence on the matter of travel extends to women, and is exemplary of the whole field of medicine for the mobile. Women should exercise, to the extent of going for a walk or riding in a carriage. But women do not travel. At least, they are not, I think, explicitly addressed, or represented, as travellers. Regimens for women and girls were composed by Rufus of Ephesus, yet, like almost all previous dietary advice directed at women, their purpose is to facilitate a reproductive marriage.[32]

3. TRAVEL AS THERAPY

I have arrived now at the first of my two principal themes, travel as therapy. Exercise (for both men and women) is pain, *ponos*. But travel is torture: Old French *travail* apparently descends, via the hypothetical verb *tripaliare*, from the medieval Latin *tripalium*, three-pronged instrument of torture on which the victim is stretched—an instrument attested in sixth-century Gaul.[33] Why should anyone welcome travel? Aelius Aristides underwent deliberate shipwreck at the prompting of a perverse deity.[34] His was an extreme case. Yet we still tend to think of ancient Mediterranean travel as fearful, whatever may be said about the ease of maritime communications in the region. It is

[30] *De curandi ratione per venae sectionem* 17, 11.299–300K.

[31] O. Temkin, *The Falling Sickness: A History of Epilepsy from the Greeks to the Beginnings of Modern Neurology*, 2nd edn. (Baltimore and London, 1971), 72–3, with Temkin's translation in *Bulletin of the Institute of the History of Medicine* 2 (1934), 179–89, from 11.357–8K.

[32] R. Flemming, *Medicine and the Making of Roman Women* (Oxford, 2000), 221–4, 316–17.

[33] W. von Wartburg, *Französisches Etymologisches Wörterbuch*, vol. 13.1 (Basle, 1966), s.v. **tripaliare*.

[34] *Oration* 48 (= *Sacred Tales* 2), 11–13, trans. C. A. Behr, *P. Aelius Aristides: The Complete Works* 2 (Leiden, 1981), 293–4.

clear, nonetheless, that travel for one's health is no invention of the age of 'grand tourism', or spas and sanatoria. Ebenezer Gilchrist's *The Use of Sea Voyages in Medicine* (London, 1756) may have been the first book of its kind in English. It could, however, have drawn on ancient example.

Not that ancient, though; a chronological change can be detected. This seems to be a Hellenistic and Roman rather than a classical Greek theme. (It may even, as Nicholas Purcell has suggested to me in conversation, have something to do with the Hellenistic vogue for pleasure boating.) Take Celsus (*De medicina* 3.22.8). In cases of true consumption, he says, if the patient is strong enough, then a long sea voyage, with a change of air, is called for—ideally the voyage from Italy to Alexandria. If the patient is not strong enough, he recommends *gestatio* (passive exercise while being transported), in a ship not going very far. If a sea voyage is impossible, the patient should be carried in a litter. (Compare Celsus 1.10 for the same 'fallback' in cases of pestilence.) Pliny asserts in the *Natural History* (31.62 ff.) that Egypt is not chosen for its own sake as the destination of therapeutic voyages but simply because of the time it takes to get there. Yet the young and 'consumptive' Seneca went to Egypt precisely to take the air in the Nile valley (*Letter* 78).[35] And Galen admits that many like him returned from Egypt seemingly cured, only to relapse later through self-indulgence.[36] Mountain air was also highly beneficial to consumptives, as Cassiodorus reminds us in the sixth century (*Variae* 11.10).

Sufferers from other diseases might also be helped by a long journey. Caelius Aurelianus, the fifth-century North African physician, recommends travel, preferably by sea, for more ailments than any other ancient authority—ailments including bladder problems, diseases of the colon, obesity, epilepsy, and elephantiasis. For headaches,

make use of natural waters, dry heat, and long sea voyages [*longa per maria navigatio*]. Voyages on rivers, bays, and lakes are considered

---

[35] M. Griffin, *Seneca* (Oxford, 1976), 43.

[36] *De simplicium medicamentorum temperamentis ac facultatibus* 9.1 (12.191K); L. Friedländer, *Roman Life and Manners under the Early Empire*, trans. A. B. Gough, 4 (London, 1913), 321.

unsuitable, since they cause the head to become moist and cold by reason of the exhalation from the earth; but sea voyages imperceptibly and gradually open the pores, give rise to a burning effect by reason of the saltiness of the sea, and, by working a change, repair the bodily condition.[37]

In the Methodist scheme of things, which Caelius represented, the relative constriction or dilation of the pores, rather than humoral balance, was the key to health. A long journey was a form of relaxation, but primarily in a physiological sense.

There are aspects of therapeutic travel that affront modern notions. For Pliny and others, the rolling and pitching of the boat, and the occasional bouts of seasickness that it brought on, were also beneficial for many ailments. Whether the patient was on horseback or in a carriage or on a boat, the rhythms of the journey were as much part of the cure as the air was. So also were the emotions induced. Among the 'non-natural' determinants of health in late antiquity were the 'passions of the soul', in effect positive emotions.[38] That is what, centuries later, permitted learned physicians to recommend 'wine, women, and song' as preventive measures against bubonic plague and syphilis.[39] In the context of the slightly different form of mobility that is the hunt, Galen explains: in hunting 'with dogs and all other kinds', exertion and pleasure combine. 'The motion of the soul involved is so powerful that many have been released from their disease by the pleasure alone.'[40]

I suggested that travel as regimen is noticeable in Hellenistic medicine but not earlier. Perhaps Hellenistic and Roman times together constitute its apogee. For I do not think we find nearly as much of it in the Middle Ages and later, although Burton would write in *The Anatomy of Melancholy* that 'peregrination

---

[37] *Chronic diseases* 1.44, ed. and trans. I. E. Drabkin, *Caelius Aurelianus On Acute and Chronic Diseases* (Chicago, 1950), 467.

[38] P. Gil-Sotres, 'Modelo teórico y observación clínica: las pasiones del alma en la psicología médica medieval', in *Comprendre et maîtriser la nature au Moyen Age: Mélanges d'histoire des sciences offerts à Guy Beaujouan* (Geneva, 1994), 181–204.

[39] P. Horden, 'Musical Solutions', in Horden (ed.), *Music as Medicine: The History of Music Therapy since Antiquity* (Aldershot, 2000), 24.

[40] *Exercise with the Small Ball* 1, trans. P. N. Singer, *Galen, Selected Works* (Oxford, 1997), 299 (5.900K = *Scripta Minora*, ed. J. Marquardt, I. Müller, and G. Helmreich, 1. 93–4).

charmes our senses with such unspeakable and sweet variety', and would of course urge it on melancholics; and Sydenham once reportedly cured a patient by sending him on a journey to see a non-existent physician in Aberdeen.[41] 'Dr Horse', as he became known, is the commonest recommendation. Sailing is rare; long sea voyages rarer still. In general, medieval doctors' regimens and *consilia* have little to offer on the theme of 'gestation' other than a few brief topoi.[42]

Between antiquity and the Middle Ages, the categories of personal mobility changed as well. That is a huge theme. Here, I simply want to stress the value of the medical evidence as an indicator of the sometimes alien ways in which the varieties of movement in space were conceptualized. Many of the texts I have been citing, and a number of others (for instance Book 2 of Galen's *De sanitate tuenda*), discuss different forms of exercise. And these discussions have obvious implications for the classification of more extensive movement. In the Hippocratic *Regimen* (chs. 2, 61) *ponoi* are either natural (*kata phusin*) or violent (*dia bies*). Perhaps to our surprise, natural exercises are those of sight, hearing, voice, and thought. Walking partakes of both the natural and the violent. We have seen different, but equally unfamiliar, taxonomies of movement in Celsus and Caelius. For those who could not afford to hunt, Galen recommended playing with a small ball, hardly the obvious alternative.[43] In the medieval learned tradition, physical

---

[41] *Anatomy of Melancholy*, pt. II, sect. ii, memb. 3, subs. 1, ed. T. C. Faulkner, N. K. Kiessling, and R. L. Blair 2 (Oxford, 1990), 65. K. Dewhurst, *Dr. Thomas Sydenham (1624–1689): His Life and Original Writings* (London, 1966), 53–4 (a story not told until the nineteenth century, and of other physicians, such as John Abernethy, as well; I am grateful to Alick Cameron and John Forrester for references).

[42] P. Gil-Sotres, 'The Regimens of Health', in M. D. Grmek (ed.), *Western Medical Thought from Antiquity to the Middle Ages* (Cambridge, Mass., and London, 1998), 291–318, at 307; D. P. Lockwood, *Ugo Benzi: Medieval Philosopher and Physician 1376–1439* (Chicago, 1951), 44–78, for a sample discussion of *consilia*.

[43] *Exercise with the Small Ball* 2, trans. Singer, 299 (5.900–1K = *Scripta Minora*, ed. J. Marquardt *et al.*, 1.94). For hunting see R. Lane Fox, 'Ancient Hunting: From Homer to Polybius,' in J. B. Salmon and G. Shipley (eds.), *Human Landscapes in Classical Antiquity: Environment and Culture* (London, 1996), 119–53, esp. 122, 147.

exercise is voluntary movement only; and 'voluntary' is defined in a way that separates the labouring from the leisured classes.

The work of carpenters, farmers, merchants, *et al.*, is not a physical exercise, since we do not observe voluntary movement, speaking properly, but rather forced movement. Moreover, merchants, bourgeois, and their like, walk a great deal, for long periods and over long distances; but here too we are not dealing with a genuine physical exercise. In order to have this one must walk at one's own initiative.

Thus Bernard of Gordon in the fourteenth century.[44] Exercise is for the few, not the many.

4. REGIMEN FOR TRAVELLERS

From travel *as* regimen, and the ways in which travel was understood, I turn to regimen *for* travellers, the second of my two themes. This is a topic on which, as I have indicated, the Hippocratics and Galen have very little to contribute. As the evidence comes down to us, the earliest we meet it is in the fourth century AD. I have referred to Oribasius' *Medical Collections*. The relevant material is not there (at least not in the 25 books that survive out of an original 70) but in one of the two Synopses of it that he later wrote. In the Synopsis addressed to his son Eustathius, he includes short regimens for travellers on foot (*pros tas poreias*) and for seafarers.[45] The context is this: preceding sections on exercise for out-of-sorts 'businessmen' (derived from Galen's *De sanitate tuenda*) and those with a corruption of food in the stomach; succeeding sections on drunkenness and sexual excess. In between the two regimens is some advice taken from Erasistratus (fragment 158)[46] on how to cope with a change of water. A train of thought is just detectable in Oribasius' layout and selection. From stomach problems he moves to 'the easiest way to depart on a journey on foot' (not, I submit, a 'walking-tour' as the passage's new editor-translator has it; that conjures up anachronistic

---

[44] *Regimen sanitatis*, MS. Cues 508, f. 52vb, trans. Gil-Sotres, 'Regimens of Health', 305.

[45] *Synopsis ad Eustathium* 5.31, 33, ed. I. Raeder, *CMG* 6.3 (Leipzig and Berlin, 1926), v. 166–8.

[46] In *Erasistrati fragmenta*, ed. I. Garofalo (Pisa, 1988).

images).[47] This 'easiest way' is 'with bowels emptied...in summer, with a soft band six or seven fingers wide and not more than five yards long wrapping up the loins as far as the flanks'. So now we know how to dress, or at least what underwear to don (to prevent chafing?). We are told about the use of a stick. We learn about what to drink, how to avoid being dried out by the sun, and so forth. As for sea voyages, the great thing is not to resist being sick—an empty stomach again being an advantage—and to counteract the stench of the bilge water.[48]

These are not Oribasius' own prescriptions. He takes them from writers of the fourth century BC who survive, for us, only in fragments (such as these extracts). They are among the numerous casualties of the Galenic near monopoly of subsequent medical learning and copying. Presumably Oribasius turned to these two writers because they were distinctive: because there was nothing like them in his principal source, Galen. The regimen for travellers comes from the works of Diocles of Carystus (fragment 184 van der Eijk), known to the Athenians of his time as 'the younger Hippocrates'.[49] The regimen for seafarers is from his rough contemporary Dieuches (fragment 19).[50] The latter, to judge by what remains of his writing, dealt mainly with food and drink, and also with the use of seawater as a purgative (fragment 18).[51]

Diocles reportedly wrote twenty or so books on a great variety of medical topics. Given his concern for the welfare of travellers, it is ironic that one of the most substantial fragments of his to come down to us (fragment 182) is a detailed daily regimen, from the moment of waking onwards, for the man who has no need to do anything more than sleep, eat, groom himself, walk, and visit the gymnasium. Beyond that, he does not go anywhere. Duties (if any there be) seem to occupy only a tiny

---

[47] P. J. van der Eijk, *Diocles of Carystus, A Collection of the Fragments and Translation with Commentary: Text and Translation* 1 (Leiden, 2000), no. 184, p. 323.

[48] Dieuches, ed. Raeder, *CMG* 6.3, 167–8.

[49] For context, apart from van der Eijk's admirable edition, see Wöhrle, *Studien zur Theorie*, ch. V.3.

[50] In *Mnésithé et Dieuchès*, ed. J. Bertier (Leiden, 1972).

[51] From Oribasius, *Medical Collections* 8.42, ed. Raeder, *CMG* 6.1.1 (Leipzig and Berlin, 1928), 292–3.

portion of his ideal day. Social life, unless in the gymnasium, and, still more, long journeys, are by implication 'off limits'. They must not interfere with the maintenance of health. The chief division, in this fragment, is not between the mobile and the sedentary: it is between the flatulent and the rest of us. I have saved mention of this fragment until now, yet it could well have been offered earlier, as a representation of fixity—and indeed as a depiction of the path to hypochondria, since anything less than healthy perfection in one's day must by definition bring on illness.[52]

Such contributions to regimen are part of the great 'confidence trick' that ancient Greek medicine first worked on the leisured and fastidious elite of the fifth and fourth centuries BC. Greek physicians persuaded this public that diet in the broad sense was a, if not *the*, key to health, its preservation and its restoration. A little like the expensive personal trainers of modern plutocrats, ancient doctors offered the illusion of autonomy to mask the reality of the patient's ultimate dependence on them for advice on every aspect of daily life, and the environment within which it is lived—every aspect from the gravest risk to a rumbling stomach. Regimens for travellers belong in the same expansionist, 'medicalizing', context as those for the different ages of life, from infancy onwards, or treatises on the properties of different foodstuffs: they are the spatial part of a supply-led movement towards extreme specialization in dietetics.[53]

Byzantine regimens have yet to be studied with any thoroughness: the accessible ones seem to vary regimen chronologically—month by month—rather than by degree of mobility or fixity.[54] I can better illustrate the fortunes of such material through the Middle Ages with glances at the Islamic

[52] Oribasius, *Medical Collections* 40, ed. Raeder, *CMG* 6.2.2, iv. 141–6. The fragment was the principal subject of L. Edelstein, 'The Dietetics of Antiquity', reprinted in translation in his *Ancient Medicine* (1967); abbreviated edn. (Baltimore and London, 1987), 303–16.

[53] Cf. Ibid. Wöhrle, *Studien zur Theorie*, 111–16; I. M. Lonie, 'A Structural Pattern in Greek Dietetics and the Early History of Greek Medicine', *Medical History* 21 (1977), 235–60.

[54] A. Delatte (ed.), *Anecdota Atheniensia et alia*: 2. *Texts grecs relatifs à l'histoire des sciences* (Paris, 1939), 455–99; J. L. Idler (ed.), *Physici et medici graeci minores*, 2 vols. (Berlin, 1841–2); repr. (Amsterdam, 1963), i. nos. XXVIII, XXIX, XXXI; ii. no. III.

and Latin European worlds. My underlying questions remain these. Is mobility represented as something special and separable from normal life? To what extent is it emphasized in the texts?

In an eleventh-century Arabic treatise on poisons can be found paragraphs attributed to Rufus of Ephesus about how travellers can protect themselves from reptiles and cold weather. These may have been taken from a fuller, even monographic, treatment of travel regimen that is listed as having been among his compositions. If this work once existed, however, it has left no trace in the Greek manuscript tradition and its influence must remain conjectural.[55] Oribasius was, more likely, the main link between antiquity and the Middle Ages. The fragmentary regimens for walkers and sea-voyagers that he preserved were translated, as part of his *Synopsis*, into Latin, and they were copied by the seventh-century Greek medical encyclopaedist Paul.[56] Thence they passed to the Arabs—or, if not these excerpts in particular, then the idea of including such regimens in more general guides to health preservation.

To take only the biggest names—those that, in translation, were later to dominate the Latin tradition: Ibn Sina (d. 1037) included in his *Canon of Medicine* a few pages for travellers on coping with fatigue and indigestion, extremes of heat and cold, changes of water supply, and seasickness (his advice on the last is simply 'ignore it').[57] If Ibn Sina is the most famous of the 'big names', Razi (d. 925) is the most interesting, and his writings offer the most variegated information. His vast, posthumously published, notebooks, the *Hawi*, give us, in their disorder, some hint of the progress of his reading and thinking on the topic of travel. He (or the students who published his work) placed the section on travel in the context of regimen for the aged and the obese.[58] This section runs through broadly the same topics that

---

[55] Ullmann, 'Neues', 39.

[56] Paul of Aegina, 1.50, 51, trans. F. Adams, *The Seven Books of Paulus Ægineta* (London, 1849), i. 76–9.

[57] Book I, 3rd fann, 4th talim, 1st jumla, in e.g. O. C. Gruner, *A Treatise on the Canon of Medicine of Avicenna, Incorporating a Translation of the First Book* (London, 1930).

[58] Abu Bakr Muhammas Ibn Zakariyya ar-Razi, *Kitab al-Hawi fi at-tibb* 23 (Hyderabad, 1974), 209–24. I am immensely grateful to Cristina

would later appear in the *Canon*, but displays its sources in Galen, Oribasius, and Muslim scholars. It also adds, in both its title and some of its jottings, a novel though obviously related subject: regimen for the army (where they should pitch camp, how they should protect their animals, etc.). A tidier, less alluring, version of all this was to appear in Razi's *Kitab al-Mansuri*, dedicated to the governor of his native Rayy.[59] Razi, however, affords us the chance to get behind the scenes of his formal treatises and come as close as we can get to the daily practice of a major Islamic physician. His *Kitab al-Tajarib* or *Casebook* contains records of almost 900 cases treated or supervised by him. We might expect the pathologies of travel to figure significantly in it. Not so. One traveller about to depart complains to him of dullness of vision in one eye. Another needs help because he has swallowed some coins while on a journey, presumably to avoid robbery, and cannot excrete them.[60] And that is all. The paucity raises uncomfortable questions about the bearing of regimen on reality, and not just in the Islamic context.

To Europe. Sections on travel are a relatively common feature of general regimen, both Latin and vernacular (though not, I think, in those associated with Salerno or in the Arabic work known in Latin as the *Tacuinum sanitatis*).[61] Most often their contents descend from Ibn Sina (Avicenna in the Latin West) or Razi (Rhazes). But they do so in subject matter—food, drink, weather, fatigue, seasickness—more than in detail: naturally there are local adaptations and individual touches. For example, in the earlier fourteenth century Maynus de Mayneriis says that the rich should prepare for a voyage by mixing sea water with their wine for several days beforehand, while the poor should drink the sea water neat. Both will thereby avoid

Álvarez-Millán for help with this text and for informing me of the contents of the manuscript cited in the next note.

[59] Escorial, Real Biblioteca del Monasterio, Arabic MS 858, fos. 73a–81a.

[60] C. Álvarez-Millán, 'Practice versus Theory: Tenth-Century Case Histories from the Islamic Middle East', *Social History of Medicine* 13 (2000), special issue, *Medical Practice at the End of the First Millennium*, ed. P. Horden and E. Savage-Smith, 298, 301.

[61] Though see Ibn Butlan, *Taqwim al-Sihha, Tacuini sanitatis*, ed. H. Elkhadem (Louvain, 1990), 217, 272. See further C. Thomasset, 'Conseils médicaux pour le voyage en mer au moyen âge', in C. Buchet (ed.), *L'homme, la santé et la mer* (Paris, 1997), 69–87.

seasickness.[62] It is a token gesture towards inclusiveness, reminiscent of the Hippocratic author who claimed to be writing for the great majority; and it goes well beyond the brief references to wine in the Muslim authorities. As well as such additions to the mainstream, there are also chronological developments. The most striking of these is the inclusion in travel regimens, from the close of the fifteenth century on, of measures to reduce the risk of contracting syphilis by avoidance of communal baths and by checking the bed linen wherever one stays.[63]

5. FREE-STANDING REGIMENS

I take the last example from an article of 1911 by the great Karl Sudhoff.[64] Besides publishing some short fifteenth- to sixteenth-century *consilia pro iter agentibus*, this paper has introductory material which remains, in some respects, the most recent synoptic view of its topic in print (despite two invaluable sections in the Catalan edition of Arnald of Villanova, to whom I return).[65] Sudhoff implicitly raises the question of whether the *Reiseregimen* is a distinct genre. We have seen it developing as a predictable presence in larger medical works. I should like to end by sharpening Sudhoff's question into this one: when, and in what circumstances, has travel regimen been the subject of a whole, free-standing, work? When has it been privileged by separate treatment and publication, at greater length than that of the *consilia* or the sections in handbooks and encyclopaedias?

From antiquity the answer is reasonably clear. There is no evidence that Diocles of Carystus wrote a whole book on the subject. Rufus of Ephesus, as we saw, is attested as having done that, but no one else. Who came next? From medieval Islam only two works of this kind are recorded and only one of them survives. The survivor is a strange production. Qusta ibn

---

[62] *Praxis medicinalis*, 2.30 (Lyons, 1586), 43, quoted by P. Gil-Sotres in *Arnaldi de Villanova Opera Medica Omnia*, vol. 10.1, ed. L. García-Ballester and M. R. McVaugh (Barcelona, 1996), 861 n. 112.

[63] K. Sudhoff, 'Ärztliche Regimina für Land- und Seereisen aus dem 15. Jahrhundert', *Archiv für Geschichte der Medizin* 4 (1911), 263–81, at 279–80.

[64] See ibid.

[65] *Arnaldi de Villanova Opera Medica Omnia*, 10.1, 384–94/851–61; 10.2, ed. M. R. McVaugh (Barcelona, 1998), 191–200. But also see Thomasset, 'Conseils médicaux'

Luqa's *Medical Regime for the Pilgrims to Mecca* is the only known medieval work with such a title.[66] Its author (d. *c*.912) wrote it for a secretary of the Caliph in Baghdad around the middle of the ninth century. Qusta was a Christian and so would not have made the hajj himself. Nor could he have been admitted to Mecca. He excuses himself, however, from accompanying his dedicatee on the ground that he must not leave his children. He identifies the need for a regimen as arising from the pilgrim's passing through 'a country where there is no doctor nor any required drug', yet he reassures himself by noting that the secretary will be accompanied 'by a doctor able to obtain whatever is necessary'.[67] He goes through what he takes to be the standard topics that any travel regimen should contain—food, fatigue, diseases caused by different winds, prophylaxis against vermin, etc. He then adds some topics which he thinks are especially necessary for the pilgrim to Mecca: improving contaminated water, quenching one's thirst, dust in the eye, and, lastly, dealing with the worst of Arabian parasites, the metre-long *dracunculus medinensis*, the Medina worm or guinea worm, which some Islamic authors unfortunately confused with a varicose vein.[68] On both kinds of topic, the pilgrim and the 'normal' travel regimen, Qusta is ultimately indebted to the Greek encyclopaedists Oribasius and Paul. He is not deploying local knowledge. One cannot imagine the secretary reading this work in his tent each night so as to anticipate the next day's risks. It seems more like a display of learning designed to impress a powerful patron.

The same is true of the two known medieval European examples of free-standing travel regimens. Pilgrimage remains the occasion of writing, but in Europe it is the armed pilgrimage of crusade. And the patrons are not less than royal. Beyond a short chapter in Vegetius (*Epitoma rei militaris* 3.2), no sus-

---

[66] *Qusta ibn Luqa's Medical Regime for the Pilgrims to Mecca: The Risala fi tadbir safar al-hajj*, ed. and trans. G. Bos (Leiden, 1992). See 5–6 for other writings in Arabic in the genre.

[67] Ibid. 16, 17.

[68] D. Bennett, 'Medical Practice and Manuscripts in Byzantium', *Social History of Medicine*, 13 (2000) (special issue, *Medical Practice at the End of the First Millennium*, ed. P. Horden and E. Savage-Smith), 289–90; M. Ullmann, *Islamic Medicine* (Edinburgh, 1978), 81–3.

tained writing survives from antiquity on the problems of keeping a field army healthy. Thus, when Adam of Cremona wrote a *Regimen iter agentium vel peregrinantium* to guide the Emperor Frederick II as he prepared to set off on his (as it turned out) disastrous expedition to the Holy Land in 1227, he had to turn to Arabic sources in translation.[69] His is indeed one of the earliest Latin works to make extensive use of the *Canon* of Avicenna (Ibn Sina). He does not seem to have had access to the Latin version of Rhazes's military advice. And what he borrowed from Avicenna was almost always the standard stuff of *individual* regimen: the health needs and problems of men *en masse* hardly occurred to him. As a church cantor writing for crusaders, he wanted to include spiritual advice too. This would have been a new departure in regimen, though one based on the inclusion of appropriate emotions among the 'non-natural' determinants of health. But Adam more or less forgot his religious task in the composition; the result is far more conventional than he intended.

A genuinely new departure was achieved by the next writer in this uneven sequence, the great Spanish physician Arnald of Villanova. His *Regimen castra sequentium* or *Regimen Almarie* belongs here because it is a free-standing treatise, albeit a very short one.[70] It is full of sensible, non-generic, advice, not all of it medical: 'When the army must move from one place to another, infantry shod with heavy-soled shoes should precede it by a mile or two, who will search in and around the route to see whether iron caltrops have been sown or scattered there ... And so that the army may be preserved from epidemic, let pits be dug everywhere outside its lines, like trenches, where animal waste and bodies can be thrown; and when they are half full

[69] Ed. F. Hönger, *Ärztliche Verhaltungsmassregeln auf dem Heerzug ins Heilige Land für Kaiser Friedrich II. geschrieben von Adam v. Cremona (ca.1227)* (Leipzig, 1913). For context see T. C. van Cleve, *The Emperor Frederick II of Hohenstaufen: Immutator Mundi* (Oxford, 1972), 316–17; M. R. McVaugh, 'Medical Knowledge at the Time of Frederick II', *Micrologus* 2 (1994), 12–13; McVaugh, 'Arnald of Villanova's Regimen Almarie (Regimen castra sequentium) and Medieval Military Medicine', *Viator* 23 (1992), 201–13, at 204–5.

[70] Ibid. and *Arnaldi de Villanova Opera Medica Omnia*, ed. McVaugh, 10.2. The quotation following is from para. 2.

cover them with earth.' And so on. It is rather a miscellany. And that doubtless reflects the circumstances of its composition. James II of Aragon had launched a crusade into the kingdom of Granada and was besieging Almería on the Mediterranean coast. In late 1309 or early 1310 he angrily summoned Arnald thither to explain the bizarre and undiplomatic statements he had reportedly been making at the papal court. Arnald seems to have composed the regimen as a peace offering en route from Sicily. By the time he arrived the campaign was virtually over, the Aragonese-Castilian alliance that underlay it having crumbled.

Ingratiation seems to be the leitmotif of these free-standing regimens. Failure of some kind also seems to be associated with all of them. As we have moved from ancient to medieval evidence, I have been suggesting that the confidence trick first attempted by the early Hippocratics—to the effect that thorough concern for regimen was essential to health—had a very uneven success rate. The regimens were designed to impress; and perhaps some did. How far they were actually implemented is, of course, another matter.

My final exhibit raises the question of purpose and effect in a slightly different form. We move from the world of crusades and military regimen into the Renaissance, with its systematic recovery of ancient dietetics. The pertinent texts of Celsus, Galen, and Paul are edited anew and commented upon.[71] Specialized treatises reappear, now of course in print: for example, *De arte gymnastica* (1569) of Girolamo Mercuriale, so all-embracing a work as to include gynaecological matters.[72] In this virtuoso context belongs the *Regimen omnium iter agentium* (1556) by Guglielmo Gratarolo (1516–68), a scarcely studied Renaissance physician.[73] In just under 200 pages he considers all the standard topics for those travelling on horseback, on foot, by ship, in a carriage, with an elegance and thoroughness that

---

[71] Mikkeli, *Hygiene in the Early Modern Medical Tradition* 23–32.

[72] V. Nutton, 'Les exercices et la santé: Hieronymus Mercurialis et la gymnastique médicale', in J. Céard, M.-M. Fontaine, and J. C. Margolin (eds.), *Le corps à la Renaissance* (Paris, 1990), 295–308.

[73] My knowledge of whom I owe to the kindness of Professor Ian Maclean, who plans a monograph on him.

befitted his status.[74] The book went through some twelve editions between 1556 and 1670 and was probably the most popular work of its kind in the early modern age. Educated in Padua, Gratarolo had fled to Basle around 1550. He secured a chair there some ten years later. He stressed in his preface the idea that I have seen as implicit in earlier regimens: that we are all travellers on the journey of life. Mobility is standard, not fixity. In his case the emphasis derived especially from contact with the Italian *Spirituali*. A rigorous Calvinist, he yet collected notes on incantations and defended alchemy. He wrote a modern physiognomy, and became famous for a book on repairing memory lapses.[75] The latter might endear him to scholars. Yet he has one further claim to their affection. Besides his regimen for travellers, perhaps inspired by an uncomfortable flight from his native land, he also wrote one in keeping with his profession. This was a regimen (later translated into English) for sedentary *literati*.[76] All others travel. Scholars alone are so immobile as to require special guidance on health.[77]

---

[74] I used *De regimine iter agentium, vel equitum, vel peditum, vel navi, vel curru seu rheda*, 2nd edn. (Strasbourg, 1563).

[75] Englished as *The Castel of Memorie* (London, 1573).

[76] Henrici Rantzouii *De conseruanda valetudine liber...Seorsim accessit Guilielmi Grataroli...De literatorum, & eorum qui magistratum gerunt, conseruanda valetudine, liber* (Frankfurt, 1591). Englished as *A Direction for the Health of Magistrates and Studentes* (London, 1574).

[77] Acknowledgements: beyond those thanked above, for unstinting advice and references I am grateful to Jim Adams, Sam Barnish, David Bennett, Vivian Nutton, Carole Rawcliffe, Emilie Savage-Smith, Philip van der Eijk, Heinrich von Staden, and Faith Wallis.

X

THE DEATH OF ASCETICS: SICKNESS AND MONASTICISM IN THE EARLY BYZANTINE MIDDLE EAST

HOW should an ascetic die? Aaron the presbyter knew how. He had always led an exemplary life. Born in Armenia, probably during the first quarter of the sixth century, he entered a Monophysite Syrian monastery in early youth. He there distinguished himself for his humility, his unremitting labour in the monastery's vineyard and guest-house, and his abundant zeal for the ascetic life. Frequently he would stand up all night. Only in old age did he consent to the luxury of a rug-covered plank as his bed.

Old age brought new trials however. Aaron's health deteriorated – to the evident alarm of John of Ephesus. John was an admirer, close friend and colleague of some thirty years' standing; he naturally included a brief account of the presbyter's career in his *Lives of the Eastern Saints*.[1] 'Once,' John writes of Aaron, 'he fell under a serious disease of gangrene in his loins;'

> and he bore this affliction with great discretion, until his loin was eaten up and mutilated and had vanished down to its root, and his disease began to enter his inner organs. But seeing that he was afflicted by a harsh malady and was cruelly rent in private, we besought him to tell what his illness was. But he for his part, until his wound had worsened severely, held fast – constant in prayer and filling his mouth with praise and thanksgiving to God.[2]

To pray and to endure: that, we might suppose, was the only decent course for a monk of Aaron's ascetic calibre during what seemed likely to prove his final illness. Asceticism is martyrdom

---

[1] c38, ed and trans E.W. Brooks *PO* 18 pp. 641–5. Aaron died in 560: see p. 644. John wrote the *Lives* in the late 560s: see *PO* 17 p. VII.
[2] *PO* 18 pp. 643–4 (trans Harvey: see n7 below).

continued by other means, an enslavement of the flesh that liberates the spirit. Like fasting and celibacy, like perching on a column or squatting manacled in a cage, the ravages of disease are simply one more extremity that will assist the holy man's soul on its path towards the ascetic ideal.[3] Treatment of a physical ailment is unnecessary; indeed it is spiritually damaging. Aaron might have endorsed the unambiguous response John of Ephesus attributes to Thomas, another Armenian ascetic, who was urged to let poultices be applied to the worsening sores on his feet:

> Then, when these feet are anointed with drugs, and are rubbed by many persons and cleansed with great care, someone would perhaps come and say, 'They have enough, now let them pay for the outward show with which they have been magnified, lest they be requited for it in hell.'[4]

Yet Aaron was in no position to adopt such a rigorist stance; and the matter was eventually taken out of his hands. John's account of his illness continues thus:

> Finally, when he could no longer pass water he was forced and so persuaded to reveal and make known his disease. Then the whole of his loin was found eaten away and consumed, so that the physicians contrived to make a tube of lead and placed it for the passing of his water, while also applying bandages and drugs to him. And so the ulcer was healed. Furthermore, Aaron lived eighteen years after the crisis of this test, praising God, and having that lead tube in place for the necessity of passing water.[5]

This striking passage has usually been noted as evidence of the history of surgery and of general Byzantine attitudes to medicine.[6] Only now is it beginning to attract the serious attention it warrants.

---

[3] Cf. among a vast literature P. Nagel, *Die Motivierung der Askese in der alten Kirche und der Ursprung des Mönchtums*, TU 95 (1966); [Arthur] Vööbus [*History of Asceticism in the Syrian Orient* 2 vols to date, CSCO sub 14, 17 (1958, 1960)].

[4] c21, PO 17 p. 292.

[5] PO 18 p. 644 (trans Harvey).

[6] H.J. Magoulias, 'The Lives of the Saints as Sources of Data for the History of Byzantine Medicine in the Sixth and Seventh Centuries', *BZ* 57 (1964) pp. 127–50 at p. 143; Peregrine Horden, 'Saints and Doctors in the Early Byzantine Empire: the Case of Theodore of Sykeon', *SCH* 19 (1982) pp. 1–13 at p. 10.

The Death of Ascetics

Susan Ashbrook Harvey argues that John's *Life* of Aaron is a document of much greater – although more local – significance than medical historians have supposed.[7] She contends that it points to 'an expedient alliance' between physicians and ascetics characteristic of the Monophysites in a time of troubles marked by warfare, plague, natural disaster and Chalcedonian persecution.[8] Aaron's operation was thus a pragmatic departure from the ascetic norm – prompted by circumstance and justified by success.

It is from the perspective of Dr Harvey's paper, and of the evidence she presents in it, that I wish to look once more at Aaron's touching history. I suggest that its diagnostic potential is not limited to Monophysite saints in John of Ephesus; that it perhaps divulges more about the way the ascetic life could be led in the early Byzantine empire than Dr Harvey allows.

If that suggestion has any force however, it is clearly not because the passage in question accords even with what we find elsewhere in John's hagiography. Thomas the Armenian after all conforms to expectation in equating submission to medical care with vainglory: a respect for the flesh which would entirely frustrate the ascetic's spiritual ambition. Nor does the resolution of Aaron's suffering accord with what we usually find in hagiographical works from the same tradition as the *Lives of the Eastern Saints* but dealing with other places, periods and ascetic styles. These works, too, apparently confirm our general presuppositions.

Benjamin, an octogenarian monk of Nitria in the fourth century and an unfailing healer, obviously accepted no remedy for the dropsy which bloated him so repulsively. 'Pray,' he said according to Palladius, 'that the inner man may not contract dropsy. My

---

[7] Susan Ashbrook Harvey, 'Physicians and Ascetics in John of Ephesus: an Expedient Alliance', forthcoming. I am most grateful to Dr Harvey for allowing me to see and profit from this paper, originally read to the Symposium on Byzantine Medicine at Dumbarton Oaks in 1983, in advance of its publication in the proceedings (in *DOP*). I am also indebted throughout to [H.] Chadwick ['John Moschus and his Friend Sophronius the Sophist', *JTS* 24 (1974)] pp. 41–74. Professor Hall, Jonathan Katz, Professor Wallace-Hadrill and Judith Wilson have kindly advised me on particular points.

[8] See also S. Ashbrook, 'Asceticism in Adversity: an Early Byzantine Experience', *Byzantine and Modern Greek Studies* 6 (1980) pp. 1–11; [S. Ashbrook] Harvey, 'The Politicisation of the Byzantine Saint' [*The Byzantine Saint* ed Sergei Hackel, Studies Supplementary to Sobornost 5 (1981)] pp. 37–43, and *Asceticism and Society in the Sixth Century Byzantine East* (forthcoming).

X

body did not help me when in good health, nor has it caused me harm when sick.' He lived only another eight months in immobile agony but continued as a healer of others right up to the end.[9] Attributing Benjamin's words to another ascetic in his *Spiritual Meadow* John Moschus even has him pray that his illness last a good while.[10] This was to ensure his salvation, not to prolong his life. In a passage which bears some resemblance to John's *Life* of Aaron, Moschus also reports the attitude to sickness of Barnabas, an anchorite who pierced his foot on a thorn when going down to drink from the Jordan. Barnabas refused to consult a doctor. His foot became so gangrenous that he had to give up his hermit's life and move to a lavra. The more the outer man suffered, he told visitors, the more the inner one flourished.[11]

'For this is the great asceticism: to control oneself in illness and to sing hymns of thanksgiving to God.'[12] Aaron's kind saw illness as deeply salutary, an advantageous opportunity for renewed self-discipline. To be in continuous good health for three years gave rise to anxiety.[13] Cure should come, if at all, from God rather than from physicians. Theodore of Sykeon, for example, was cured of two illnesses first through the intercession of Cosmas and Damian and later with the help of the Virgin, who in a vision offered him tablets and left him with the time-honoured advice to keep taking them.[14]

Less miraculous cures were to be avoided by holy men. God discerns the state of an ascetic's soul whereas physicians do not. And that distinction is crucial: illness is salutary in its aetiology as well as in its effects. The body is an index of sin. An affliction of the loins such as Aaron's would thus have been taken as a symptom of lust. Even with castration becoming relatively infrequent among ascetics there remained disease to cool the promiscuous. In Palladius's account of Heron the lapsed ascetic loses his genitals through

[9] Palladius [*Historia Lausiaca* ed G.J.M. Bartelink (Verona 1974)] c12. Cf. c55.
[10] Moschus [*Pratum spirituale*, PG 87. 3 coll 2851–3112] c8.
[11] Moschus c10. Cf. *Apophthegmata Patrum* [alphabetical collection, PG 65 coll 72–440] Daniel 4, trans [Benedicta] Ward [SLG, *The Sayings of the Desert Fathers* (London and Oxford 1975)] p. 52.
[12] *Apophthegmata Patrum* Syncletica 8, trans Ward p. 232.
[13] Moschus, ed Th. Nissen, *BZ* 38 (1938) p. 358, c5.
[14] *Vita Theodori* [*Syceotae* ed and trans A-J. Festugière, *sub hag* 48, 2 vols (Brussels 1970)] cc39, 77.

The Death of Ascetics

a severe ulceration consequent upon high living and unbridled desire. He is restored to health as a eunuch.[15]

The collective insistence of these texts seems plain. The monk should be indifferent to all physical suffering – whether he is a virtuoso of mortification like the elder Simeon, or a less celebrated solitary like Zoilus the reader, who lived in a verminous cell, did his own cooking and laundry, and earned a little money by calligraphy.[16] Illness is to be interpreted: it is always of the utmost spiritual significance. To seek to avoid the death of the body may be to risk the death of the soul. My body kills me, I kill it[17] – such is general ascetic philosophy.

It is in this light that the oddity of Aaron's cure has to be regarded. John's account is striking for two reasons. First it contains no interpretation of disease. No moral failing on Aaron's part is held responsible for either the gangrene or the retention of urine. He is not said to have been possessed, which is the hagiographer's usual alternative to sin as an explanation of disease. And no diminution of his ascetic worth and exemplary standing is implied in the operation's aftermath. His body did not die; yet neither did his soul. The illness was a test – but one which Aaron can hardly be said to have failed or shirked. For no pain is more excruciating than that of acute urinary retention: gangrene of the loins (necrosis, as doctors would now describe it) is mild in comparison. Aaron stoutly endured the lesser pain; no one can be expected to tolerate the greater.

John's account is striking, secondly, in that no supernatural intercession is reported to have brought Aaron's suffering to a close. God did not miraculously relieve his pain or spare him further torture by taking his life. Physicians were summoned instead, and summoned as a matter of course. They must have arrived quickly: the pain of retention comes suddenly, giving no advance warning, and is not to be borne for more than a few hours. Yet John does not even mention the physicians' arrival on the scene, let alone justify it. He clearly knew whom he could depend

---

[15] Palladius c26. Cf. Moschus c14. On castration see *The Sentences of Sextus* ed Henry Chadwick (Cambridge 1959) pp. 109–12; Vööbus vol 1 pp. 257–8.

[16] *La Vie et les miracles de Saint Syméon Stylite l'ancien* ed M. Chaîne (Cairo 1948) p. 18 (the Coptic *Life*); Moschus c171.

[17] Palladius c2.2.

upon and did not expect his readers to find anything untoward in that dependence. Aaron's problem was solved with bandages, drugs and a leaden tube. No eulogy of the physicians is forthcoming even though they performed the operation so well that the gangrene did not return – as well it might before the age of Lister – and the catheter continued to function.

How do we explain this seeming departure from the norm of ascetic conduct? Dr Harvey rightly suggests that it is John's behaviour as much as Aaron's which needs explaining. The way Aaron suffered in secret until the last possible moment could have been written up approvingly by Moschus or Palladius. 'Constant in prayer and filling his mouth with praise and thanksgiving to God,' he obviously knew the spiritual benefits that accrue from bodily infirmity. It was John, we may infer, who at last made him reveal the origin of a pain to which no amount of self-control was equal.

Dr Harvey has also emphasized that John wrote his *Lives* to honour ascetics who were for the most part devoted to practical philanthropy among stricken Monophysite communities. They had no time for accidie or sexual desire; and theirs was a world in which there was no miraculous escape from the hardships at hand.[18] If a moral is to be found in John's story it is the importance of Aaron's continuing ministry.

The problem here is that Aaron is by no means among the greatest of the philanthropists whom John presents to us.[19] It is hard on the presbyter to suppose his virtue to be merely a lack of opportunity. And John would surely not have thought Aaron's philanthropy was worth the price of his soul if that had been in question. Moreover if John's response to the sickness of ascetics was pragmatic, as Dr Harvey believes, it is still not clear why pragmatism should in a medieval context prompt a trust in physicians, rather than in God, and a lack of concern with the spiritual meaning of illness. Nor is it clear why dire circumstances should have been conducive to pragmatism of this sort. The hardships which form the sombre background to the *Lives of the Eastern Saints* are not so very much worse than those we glimpse in the *Spiritual Meadow*, a Chalcedonian work in which charity is just

---

[18] Harvey, 'The Politicisation of the Byzantine Saint', p. 40.
[19] *PO* 17 cc3, 12, 15; 18 cc34, 35.

The Death of Ascetics

as much a sign of sanctity as it is with John and whose author does not apparently share John's attitude to illness.[20]

At this point John's Monophysitism might be brought into play. Dr Harvey proposes that John's belief in the unity of the human and the divine in Christ would have had particular implications for his view of how God was present and active in creation. We do not yet know much about the effects of a particular Christology on everyday concerns in this period. But the work that has been done, say on the Christology of Severus of Antioch or Philoxenus of Mabbug, is far from indicating that their thought was conducive to that 'demythologizing' of disease of which John seems to have been capable.[21] And nothing strictly comparable to it can be found in the writings of other Monophysites such as John Rufus.[22]

A different approach is perhaps called for: one that gives less weight to the local conditions in which John wrote. For there is enough evidence that the type of cure Aaron enjoyed, though rare in hagiographical terms, is not unique. In Moschus for instance, an ascetic is advised by doctors to eat meat and, despite the horror of the rigorists, is defended for acting rightly.[23] In Theodoret one ascetic suffering from severe colic apparently resorts to medicine first and prayer afterwards.[24] And it is Theodoret himself who persuades another ascetic to accept minor alleviation of his distress during his first illness and a purgative during his second – a purgative he drinks only after hearing an emotive plea (such as we do not find in John) that he should stay alive and thus prolong his ministry.[25] There are also a number of apophthegmata which show that a sick ascetic might well receive quasi-medical assistance from his brothers. As long as he did so in the right spirit his behaviour remained exemplary.[26]

The departure from the norm which John's narrative of Aaron represents is therefore not without parallel. How then – to return to

[20] Cf. Chadwick pp. 61–3, 72–4.
[21] Cf. Roberta C. Chesnut, *Three Monophysite Christologies* (Oxford 1976) pp. 47–50, 70–75; André de Halleux, *Philoxène de Mabbog* (Louvain 1963) pt 3.
[22] *Plerophories* ed and trans F. Nau, *PO* 8 pp. 50–1, 65–7.
[23] Moschus c65.
[24] Theodoret (of Cyrus, *Historia Religiosa* ed and trans Pierre Canivet and Alice Leroy-Molinghen, 2 vols *SCR* 234, 257 (1977, 1979)] c22. 4.
[25] Theodoret c21. 8, 11. Cf. c2. 18.
[26] *Apophthegmata patrum* Aio, Arsenius 36, Theodore of Pherme 26, trans Ward pp. 16–17, 37, 77–8.

the principal question – do we set about explaining it? It is well to be precise about what requires an explanation here and what does not. The setting of Aaron's operation is Constantinople and we should not be surprised to find that highly skilled surgeons were available.[27] We should not be surprised, either, to find churchmen turning to doctors willingly and as a matter of course. John bishop of Hephaistu, for example, needed an excuse to go to the city to see the empress. What could have been more natural than for him to plead an appointment with his doctors when seeking permission from the patriarch? John of Ephesus at least reports the ruse without betraying disapproval or amazement.[28] We have been misled by the hagiographical topos, most frequent in the miracle books of urban shrines, by which doctors are condemned for their exorbitant fees and their patients are castigated for trusting them too much. The Church was far from rejecting their services. Holy men like Theodore happily passed on some of their clients to local doctors. Other saints, such as Sampson, had trained as physicians themselves and put their training to good use in the numerous ecclesiastically-controlled hospitals.[29]

This essentially favourable attitude to medicine was echoed in monasteries as well, and explanation can begin with them. By the standards of those singled out in John, Theodoret, Moschus or Palladius most Byzantine monks were not of course ascetic. Their resort to secular as distinct from spiritual medicine, whether in their monastery's own infirmary or privately with healers roundabout, was not thought incompatible with the minimal asceticism

---

[27] The technique of installing a catheter had been described in pseudo-Galen, *Introductio seu medicus, Claudii Galeni Opera Omnia* ed C.G. Kühn (Leipzig 1821–33, repr Hildesheim 1965) c19, vol 14 pp. 787–8. On medical schools see now N.G. Wilson *Scholars of Byzantium* (London 1983). Aaron died in 560 (cf. n1 above). John says that he lived for eighteen years after his operation, and eighteen sounds more precise than John's usual round figure of thirty (cf. *PO* 17 p. 291; 18 p. 626). The operation can therefore be dated to the early 540s, when we know John to have been generally in Constantinople. See *PO* 18 p. 643 and [Ernest] Honigmann, *Evêques et évêchés Monophysites d'Asie antérieure au VIe siècle*, CSCO sub 2 (1951) p. 208.

[28] *PO* 18 p. 536. On John of Hephaistu see Honigmann p. 165. Cf. Theodoret *Letters* 114, 115, ed Yvan Azéma SCR 40, 98, 111 (1964, 1965, 1982).

[29] *Vita Theodori* cc145–6. Mt Athos MS Philotheou 8 fol 198ᵛ.

The Death of Ascetics

that monastic seclusion implies.[30] A vast range of ascetic regimes was practised. Monks seeking to achieve the highest standard of asceticism would, as for example enjoined in one of the Macarian homilies,[31] have had nothing to do with doctors. The rest set their sights a little lower; and these were the ones unlikely to receive detailed hagiographical notice, especially in Syria where asceticism could be witnessed at its most horrifyingly inventive.

Aaron was conceivably one of the relatively few lesser lights in the ascetic firmament whose boundless courage, yet also whose eventual willingness to submit to treatment when in unbearable pain, has been recorded for posterity's edification. A pointer to the existence of others can perhaps be derived from the frequent instances in the hagiography where a bishop – John of Ephesus or Theodoret for example – is reported to have urged an ascetic to moderate his austerity. That the monk did so hardly proved that he was a poor ascetic or no ascetic at all: it rather showed that he was a sensible one. For what transpired between bishop and monk was hardly a clash between rival conceptions of monasticism – moderate Greek and rigorist Syrian for example.[32] It was a modest contribution to a less partisan debate about the nature and purpose of the ascetic life which cannot so easily be related to cultural geography. There were many reasons why ascetics should make minor adjustments to their self-imposed regime: to avoid a hubris bred of competition, to fulfil a pastoral obligation, or simply to survive.

That of Syrian fanatics apart, the ascetic way of life can be characterized under three headings. Each of them has some bearing

---

[30] Cf. *Barsanuphe et Jean de Gaza: Correspondance* trans Lucien Regnault *et al* (Solesmes 1972) cc225, 327, 508; Theodore of Petra, *Vita Theodosii Coenobiarchae* trans A-J. Festugière, *Les moines d'Orient* vol 3.3 (Paris 1963) c16; Palladius c7; *Syriac and Arabic Documents Regarding Legislation Relative to Syrian Asceticism* ed Vööbus (Stockholm 1960) pp. 16, 30, 175; Basil, *Regulae Fusius Tractatae* c55, *PG* 31 coll 1043–52; Diadochus of Photice, *Capita Gnostica* ed Edouard des Places *SCR* 5 (1955) c53.

[31] *Die 50 Geistlichen Homilien des Makarios* ed Hermann Dörries, Erich Klostermann and Matthias Kroeger, *Patristische Texte und Studien* 4 (Berlin 1964) c48. 3–6. Cf. Makarios/Symeon, *Reden und Briefe: Die Sammlung I des Vaticanus Graecus 694 (B)* ed H. Berthold, *GCS* (Berlin 1973) Logos 55. 3, vol 2 p. 168. I owe these references, and the final one in n30 above, to the kindness of Dr Chadwick. For a general, comparativist perspective see Vööbus vol 2 cc8, 9.

[32] *Pace* Vööbus. Cf. *Lives of the Eastern Saints*, *PO* 17 p. 181, 18 p. 627; Theodoret c21. 6.

on how we are to understand John's account of Aaron. First, if the ascetic should not strive officiously to keep alive then neither should he kill himself.[33] The evidence of John's *Lives*, if no other, shows that his attitude was not confined to 'Greek' monasticism. It had its 'Syrian' counterpart. Secondly the holy man was often the best judge of the state of his own soul and his physical condition. He generally foresaw his death. He knew which illness he might seek to ameliorate, which one should be endured because it was a sign of moral failure or a test of nerve, and which should be faced in the confidence that his work was done and his end was approaching.[34] Thirdly whatever the hagiographers say – and it could have suited their purpose to magnify the seriousness of holy men's ailments – the pathology of asceticism may not all the time have been as grave as it appeared. Endurance of sickness was not necessarily a supreme test.

It is time we ceased marvelling aimlessly at the physical stamina and frequent longevity of the great Byzantine ascetics. A more worthwhile perspective on their seeming immunity to degradation and disease is to be had from a comparison with recent Hindu ascetics whose mortifications frequently exceeded theirs and whose pathology can be studied with some closeness. I do not suggest that being a stylite was merely a way of working off surplus flab. But I do urge that we scrutinize the anthropology of asceticism – from which we may well learn that once an ascetic has absolutely conquered his body the illnesses he contracts are often comparatively minor and readily endured.[35]

Aaron's was of course no minor complaint: the generalization attempts to explain the habitual response rather than the particular challenge. Nor does it take us far enough. A favourable monastic and episcopal attitude to physicians; a flexibility of ascetic practice for the sake of survival; an ascetic's capacity to distinguish among illnesses and modulate his behaviour even more finely; the possibility that consummate ascetic technique enhanced rather than diminished health – these still do not necessarily make doctors welcome.

[33] Palladius c19; Vööbus vol 2 p. 293, with vol 1 pp. 154–5 on ascetic suicide.
[34] Cf. Theodoret c2. 18; *Historia Monachorum in Aegypto* ed A-J. Festugière *sub hag* 34 (Brussels 1961) bk 10 c17; *Vita Theodori* c39.
[35] John Campbell Oman, *The Mystics, Ascetics and Saints of India* (London 1903) remains a valuable ethnography. Joachim Friedrich Sprockhoff, *Saṃnyāsa: Quellenstudien zur Askese im Hinduismus* vol 1 (Wiesbaden 1976) is more a literary study.

The Death of Ascetics

There remain three ways in which their presence could have become spiritually palatable. The first was through the ascetic's achievement of a requisite perfection in accepting their attentions. If an ascetic can unsex himself to the extent that he remains indifferent to naked women (as some obviously could) he can learn the equivalent attitude to physicians.[36] Secondly, and alternatively, perhaps disease is not always 'psychosomatic' – the consequence of a particular sin, or of possession, or as a divine punishment or test. Even for a holy man it can have a more straightforwardly physical aetiology. There is evidence of such a view in Byzantine imperial legislation implicitly attributing ill health to poverty, in the literature of *Erotapokriseis* (or questions and answers) and in some of the hagiography.[37] John of Ephesus makes clear what is elsewhere presented obscurely. He saw, and perhaps Aaron was persuaded to see, that on this occasion gangrenous loins and retention of urine betokened nothing spiritual and that a remedy was close at hand.

Thirdly however, God's presence at the operation and His guidance of the scalpel is quietly implied in John's apparently factual description. To trust in physicians, and to hold that a naturalistic explanation can be given of some, but only some, diseases, is not to despair of supernatural aid. Byzantine surgery should be rated highly, but not too highly. John did not make that mistake. An operation on an ascetic was for him no ordinary operation. Compare his account of Aaron's cure with his description in the *Ecclesiastical History* of the moribund Justin II preparing for the removal of stones lodged in his bladder:

> When ... physicians came to cut them away, they requested him, after the usual cowardly manner of physicians, to take the lancet in his hand and give it to them; and he ... said, 'Fear not:

[36] Moschus cc3, 36, 194.
[37] Cf. pseudo-Justin (? Theodoret) *Quaestiones ad orthodoxos* c55, PG 6 col 1297; pseudo-Anastasius Sinaita, *Quaestiones* c94, PG 89 col 732. On *Erotapokriseis* see Gilbert Dagron, 'Le saint, le savant, l'astrologue: étude de thèmes hagiographiques à travers quelques recueils de "Questions et réponses" des Ve–VIIe siècles', *Hagiographie, Cultures et Sociétés IVe–XIIe siècles* (Paris 1981) pp. 143–55; *Theognosti Thesaurus* ed Joseph A. Munitiz CC Series Graeca 5 (1979) pp. CIX–CXXIII. See also Evelyne Patlagean, *Pauvreté économique et pauvreté sociale à Byzance 4e–7e siècles* (Paris 1977) pp. 101, 104–5 for the legislation and the hagiography. Passages such as the Greek *Vita prima* of Pachomius, ed F. Halkin *sub hag* 19 (1932) c52 might also be considered in this context.

even if I die, no harm shall come to you.' A deep incision was then made in both his groins, and the whole operation so barbarously performed that he was put to extreme torture.[38]

Aaron was spared such agony. His physicians were presumably not Chalcedonian bunglers. Yet that he survived the ordeal and lived another eighteen years can indeed, in modern eyes, be accounted a miracle.

[38] Pt 3 bk 3 c6, ed E. W. Brooks *CSCO* 105–6 (1935–6) trans P. Payne Smith (Oxford 1860) p. 177.

XI

SAINTS AND DOCTORS IN THE EARLY BYZANTINE EMPIRE: THE CASE OF THEODORE OF SYKEON

'HAVE done with doctors. Don't fall into their clutches: you will get no help from them. Be satisfied with this prayer and blessing and you will be completely restored to health.'[1] Theodore of Sykeon's obloquy and exhortation find numerous parallels in the social history of early Byzantine medicine. The hostility of holy men to doctors is a familiar theme. Less familiar may be that delegation of responsibility and spirit of cooperation suggested by another passage in the *Life* of Theodore:

> Again, if any required medical treatment for certain illnesses, or surgery or a purging draught or hot springs, this God-inspired man would prescribe the appropriate remedy to each like an experienced doctor trained in the art. He might recommend one to have recourse to surgery and would always state clearly which doctor he should employ. In other cases he would dissuade those who wished to have an operation or to undergo some other medical treatment, and would recommend rather that they should visit hot springs, and would name the springs to which they should go.[2]

Others, as the author of the *Life* goes on to relate, were deterred from visiting hot springs or taking the waters. The holy man would advise a purge, to be administered by his nominee. And to those who were wounded, or who wanted surgery for an abscess, he prescribed the application of specific plasters. In short, like an excellent doctor and a disciple of the true Master-physician, his prescriptions were always appropriate. All those who carried out his instructions recovered their health. Those who disobeyed him – through neglect, by using different treatment, or by turning to doctors other than

---

[1] [A-J. Festugière, *Vie de*] *Théodore* [*de Sykéon*], Greek text with French translation and commentary, Société des Bollandistes, *sub hag* 48, 2 vols (Brussels 1970) cap 156.

[2] *Ibid* caps 145-6.

those he had designated - found their illness incurable until they reverted to the prescribed course of action.

This extract requires comment. It offers a distinct and somewhat neglected perspective on Theodore's technique of healing and on popular attitudes to medicine. As Peter Brown noted in his classic exposition of the holy man's functions, relations with clients by no means always involved the miraculous.[3] What was important in daily village life was not the comparatively rare drama of exorcism and miracle. It was rather the more discreet or mundane manifestations of the ascetic's power: in leadership, patronage, mediation and arbitration. Since Brown wrote, some of the picture's shading has been altered. The urban saint has been isolated as a category.[4] And it has been emphasised that the geography of the Syrian countryside is not a sufficient explanation for the ideological formation of the holy man as *alter Christus*.[5] But Brown's deft outline of the saint as 'social worker' largely survives.

In all major respects Theodore of Sykeon conforms to type. Nevertheless, descriptions in early hagiographical sources of saints dispensing medical advice as he did, and despatching their clients to doctors or hot springs, are comparatively rare.[6] One roughly similar text may be found in the *Life* of Hypatios.[7] There the holy man summons an experienced doctor to cut off the fibula of a peasant with a gangrenous leg. The enthusiastic surgeon would prefer to amputate the entire leg below the knee. Hypatios is firm in his instructions. Though the peasant has to endure excruciating pain,

---

3   ['The Rise and Function of the] Holy Man [in Late Antiquity'], *JRS* 61 (1971) pp 80-101 at p 98.

4   See [Julia] Seiber, [*The Urban Saint in Early Byzantine Social History*], British Archaeological Reports, Supplementary Series 37 (Oxford 1977) for the analysis of a limited number of texts. Compare [Robert] Browning, ['The 'Low Level' Saint's Life in the Early Byzantine World'] in *The Byzantine Saint*, University of Birmingham Fourteenth Spring Symposium of Byzantine Studies, Studies supplementary to *Sobornost* 5 (Birmingham 1981) pp 117-27, a valuable composite image of the rural holy man.

5   Han J. W. Drijvers, 'Hellenistic and Oriental Origins' in *The Byzantine Saint* pp 25-33.

6   As noted by Browning p 122 and [Evelyne] Patlagean, *Pauvreté [économique et pauvreté sociale à Byzance]* (Paris 1977) p 103.

7   [Callinicus,] *Vita Hypatii* (Teubner 1895) translated by Festugière, *Les moines d'Orient* vol 2 (Paris 1961) cap 40. Hypatios died in 446. His pupil Callinicus wrote the *Life* 'wohl kaum vor dem 6. Jahrhundert'. See Beck p 404.

The Case of Theodore of Sykeon

the operation is a success. The *Life* does not imply that Hypatios frequently resorted to doctors in this way. Nor was his decision to have the fibula removed - naturally arrived at after prayer - made on the basis of the sort of medical wisdom ascribed to Theodore. He washed, put to bed, and cared for sick peasants he brought to his monastery.[8] Many had, predictably, been refused treatment by doctors because they could not afford the fees,[9] and no one else would approach them because of their foul smell. Hypatios did not use medicine, plasters, or any other remedies: he lacked medical skill and limited himself to prayer and poultices.[10]

There are then, in this respect, differences as well as similarities between Hypatios and Theodore. So it is unreasonable immediately to assume that the passage quoted from the *Life* of Theodore is entirely typical of a response of holy men to medical practice that many hagiographers simply omit to mention.[11] But a more moderate claim can be made: that holy men may often have acted, or been thought to act, in this way, and that their reasons for so acting are not entirely obscure. The claim can be strengthened by looking first at Theodore's own reputation and career more closely, then at the wider history of Byzantine medicine, and finally - with due regard for attendant dangers - at some passages from the literature of medical anthropology.

Before turning to Theodore himself, it would be well to look at the textual history of the *Life* on which we largely depend for our knowledge of his achievements. How widely known was it? More particularly, was the passage concerning him and doctors read? Fortunately, there is no doubting the enormous reputation Theodore posthumously enjoyed. Heraclius had his relics brought to the capital as additional protection against Persian attack. The translation, and the man, became the subject of a ninth-century encomium by Nikephoros Skeuophylax, monk and sacristan of the

---

[8]   *Vita Hypatii*, cap 40.
[9]   Compare *ibid* cap 44 where doctors appear even more corrupt and mercenary.
[10] *Ibid* cap 22.
[11] Compare Brown, 'Holy Man', p 98, adducing *Vita Hypatii*, cap 40, and commenting that 'the holy man appears far more often than we might at first sight suppose in a merely supporting rôle'.

church of Blachernae in Constantinople.[12] An eleventh-century manuscript of the miracles of Saint George has an epilogue referring to 'that great and famous Theodore, called the Sykeote, who I am aware is known to everyone.'[13]

However, these are only general indications of the saint's *Nachleben*. The longer version of the *Life,* as edited by Festugière, depends on two manuscripts, both menologies, of the tenth and early eleventh centuries respectively. It is noteworthy that, although one is dilapidated, both include the passage that is here of concern. Appropriately for a cult such as that of Theodore, there are other versions of the *Life*. One was intended for private monastic devotion and hence does not have the passage. Two others, of the eleventh and fourteenth centuries, again menologies though distinct from the three manuscripts already mentioned, are very much shorter and of no help here.[14] They must however be considered for a moment.

It has been argued[15] that the third and shortest manuscript of the long *Life* is not only derived from a better text than the other two manuscripts, but is much closer than they are to a homely and popular pre-metaphrastic original.[16] Some confirmation of the hypothesis is derived from the structure of the short lives and of the encomium. Its acceptance would entail regarding many passages to be found in the long *Life,* but not in the other texts, as rather late additions to a comparatively brief original.

The description of Theodore and the doctors might be reckoned among them. A new question would be raised: of why such an attitude to doctors was attributed to this most popular of saints - perhaps after the early ninth century, given the 'gaps' in the encomium? One suggestion has been made *à propos* a similar

---

12 On him, and for additional references in much of what follows see [Derek] Baker, ['Theodore of Sykeon and the Historians'], *SCH* 13, *The Orthodox Churches and the West* (1976) pp 83-96. The encomium was edited by C. Kirch from a twelfth-century manuscript in *An Bol* 20 (1901) pp 249-72.

13 Quoted by Festugière, *Théodore,* I pp xxiii-iv, from Paris MS Gr 1604. See also *Miracula S. Georgii,* ed J.B. Aufhauser (Teubner 1913) pp 40-1.

14 Full textual details and further references in *Théodore,* I pp xxiv-ix and Baker. Fresh examination of all the manuscripts is clearly called for.

15 By Baker.

16 On metaphrastic revision see Beck, esp pp 570-2, and Ihor Ševčenko, 'Levels of Style in Byzantine Prose', *Jahrbuch der Österreichischen Byzantinistik* 31 (Vienna 1981) pp 300-3.

The Case of Theodore of Sykeon

development in the *Miracles* of Cosmas and Damian.[17] Only in the last few miracles are Hippocrates, Galen, and contemporary physicians viewed at all favourably. The change is attributed to the belated effects of the transfer of the centre of medical studies from Alexandria to Constantinople.[18] This, it can be shown, is an unreal view of Byzantine medicine and tells us little about the medical reputations of Theodore or of Cosmas and Damian.[19] The passage in the *Life* of Theodore could belong to almost any period between the time of the initial composition by the saint's disciple, George Eleusios – that is, even before Theodore's death in 613 – and the final recension of the long *Life*. The entire *Life* will, on any account, have passed through a number of different versions.[20] Chapters dealing with Theodore and medicine form part of a slightly larger section on Theodore's work written in general terms without reference to individual cases; part summary, part extension, of what has gone before. It is most naturally read as having been introduced by George in one of his own revisions – to a text begun when he was less than eighteen years old.[21] Meanwhile, there seems to be enough corroborative evidence to show that detailed reports to be found in the long *Life* concerning the early years of Heraclius were in all probability written soon after the events described.[22]

The conclusion implied is, then, that Theodore's substantial and enduring reputation was, from the seventh century onwards, partly derived from diffusion of copies of the long version of his *Life*. The process of transmission is now completely hidden from us. But there is no reason to suppose that the earliest and most homespun versions did not include some reference to his medical prowess. This prowess was known and appreciated; it was not thought eccentric.[23]

---

[17] Seiber pp 88-9. [Festugière, *Collections grecques de miracles,* II *Miracles de SS.]Côme et Damien* (Paris 1971).

[18] On which see [Owsei] Temkin, 'Byzantine Medicine: [Tradition and empiricism'], *DOP* 16 (1962) pp 95-115.

[19] See below p 9-10.

[20] Baker p 94.

[21] *Théodore* cap 165.

[22] See W.E. Kaegi Jr, 'New Evidence on the Early Reign of Heraclius', *BZ* 66 (1973) pp 308-30; 'Notes on Hagiographic Sources for some Institutional Changes and Continuities in the Early Seventh Century', *Byzantina* 7 (Thessalonika 1975) pp 59-70; 'Two Notes on Heraclius', *REB* 37 (1979) pp 221-7. Compare Baker p 95. I am grateful to Michael Whitby for references and advice on this point.

[23] And hence would not have been noticed in the encomium. Compare Baker p 94.

Nor, of course, was it out of keeping with the holy man's more general function as omniscient director of rural, urban, or imperial affairs. Behind the feats of clairvoyance and prophecy attributed to the early Byzantine saints, there can be discerned enormous political and psychological acumen. The hagiographers ascribe a miraculous origin to this power. That is how Theodore learned the Psalter.[24] (The *Life* also tells us that he had already been quick to learn.)[25] Against this background, Callinicus's comment that Hypatios had no medical knowledge should perhaps be interpreted as a rather pointed one: he expected his readership to assume the contrary. After all, the application of poultices could have been taken to represent an elementary piece of folk medicine.

As for Theodore, he not only prescribed such folk remedies - plasters for example. He treated people quite directly, using similar skills. A severely contorted man, with a dislocated hip to add to his misery, has his limbs massaged; and the holy man then anoints his whole body with a salve made from wax. The aetiology of his disease could be called social: he has quarrelled with his abbot. Theodore's treatment fails until reconciliation has been achieved. Thereafter, the holy man guides his patient back to health, slowly and unmiraculously. He orders daily walks, helping the man to straighten his body by furnishing him with progressively longer walking sticks.[26]

The full version of the *Life* also has descriptions of acts of healing which seem to efface whatever imprecise boundaries we might care to draw between the medical and the miraculous. When Theodore has been poisoned, the Virgin appears to him in a dream and offers a purge - three castor-oil tablets, it seems - which he thinks he takes, and which do in some sense have the desired effect by the time of his awakening.[27]

Once again, there is nothing unusual here, even though we may be more used to reading about such cures in the miracle collections of 'medical saints' like Cosmas and Damian, or of Artemios, or of

---

24 *Théodore* cap 13. See further [Evelyne] Patlagean ['Ancienne] hagiographie byzantine [et histoire sociale'], *Annales* 23 (1968) pp 106-23, at pp 109-10.
25 *Théodore* cap 10.
26 *Ibid* cap 80b.
27 *Ibid* cap 77 with commentary II p 221. Compare cap 121, where the effects of a purgative are also achieved miraculously, and cap 124.

The Case of Theodore of Sykeon

Cyrus and John.[28] The holy man might even prefer to confuse the medical and the miraculous in an attempt to disguise his extraordinary powers. One of those eastern ascetics described by John of Ephesus is reluctant to interview a man whose wife is barren. Yielding eventually, he gives the man a clipping of his toe nail wrapped up for secrecy's sake. He is adamant that it is not what we might describe as a relic, but a herb. Like any folk doctor or village quack, he orders the man to hang the 'herb' round his wife's neck and to bring it back to him, still wrapped, when a son has been born.[29]

For all the blurring of distinctions with which the texts confront us, the question still ought to be raised of why Theodore (and other holy men) performed unmistakeable miracles on some occasions and acted like doctors on others. It is reasonable enough to recall that, as the *Life* of Hypatios stresses,[30] only God can cure certain afflictions, such as epilepsy and blindness from birth. Every Byzantine miracle worker had to be his own Christologist. His career, as represented by his hagiographer, follows, on one level at least, what Patlagean has identified as *le modèle scripturaire*.[31] But this sort of model, even reinforced by other Lévi-Straussian structures, seems insufficient as explanation. It does not explain why most Byzantine holy men were occupied as miraculous healers so frequently with demons or evil and unclean spirits, whereas western saints dealt with the paralysed and the blind far more often than they encountered possession.[32] Nor does it explain those peculiarities of technique which mark out one holy man from another, and one sphere of operation from its neighbour. The sources for a given group of cities can supply detail which enables the historian to tabulate the types of illness that holy men and 'dead' saints encountered, and the types of cure they

---

28 Some references collected by Seiber pp 87-93. See also [H.J.] Magoulias, ['The Lives of the Saints as Sources of Data for the History of Byzantine Medicine in the Sixth and Seventh Centuries'], *BZ* 57 (1954) pp 127-50, which is often very unreliable.

29 John of Ephesus, [*Lives of the Eastern Saints*], edited and translated by E.W. Brooks, *PO* 17 p 70.

30 *Vita Hypatii* cap 44.

31 Patlagean, 'Hagiographie byzantine', pp 112, 117.

32 See the statistics compiled, from a rather limited number of sources, by John Moorhead, 'Thoughts on Some Early Medieval Miracles', *Byzantine Papers* Byzantina Australiensia 1 (Canberra 1981) pp 1-11. On the larger question raised, [Peter] Brown, 'Eastern and Western Christendom [in Late Antiquity: A Parting of the Ways'], *SCH* 13 (1976) pp 1-24 is fundamental.

employed.[33] What such tabulation cannot reveal is the process by which the holy man diagnosed the social and moral origins of illness, and decided the seriousness of the case. Did it require simply a plaster; or an innocuous *placebo* charged with the holy man's blessing;[34] or something more vigorously demonstrative of his miraculous power? How the decision was taken is something we can only just begin to discern.

It was a decision complicated by an additional possibility: that of acting at a distance or at one remove. Theodore's *placebos* might be taken to neighbouring villages to be sprinkled over damaged crops.[35] Twice,[36] men are cured at a distance from him, on their way home after what they had taken to be an ineffectual meeting. And he will also produce 'secondary relics'. Dust from the area of a hollowed-out cave, in which he had spent the winter in order to drive out demons, becomes medicine for the sick when mixed with food or drink.[37]

However, Theodore is prepared to delegate, as well as to act at a distance. To his reformed grandmother, who had entered a convent, he sent children — especially girls — plagued by evil spirits. They were to receive care and instruction, so that those who wished to remain after they had been cured of their possession might become nuns in the same convent. Theodore did not himself perform the exorcisms.[38] Nor did he on three other, particular occasions mentioned in the *Life*. His deputy acted for him — because he was ill, because he desired seclusion, and because he could plead a prior commitment.[39]

That information offers one hint of the possible reasons why Theodore should send some of his clients off to doctors instead of healing or treating them himself. But there are other indications to be noted first. The obscure weighing of the merits (in all senses of the word) and needs of each case embraced several considerations: of whether it was really a matter for a doctor, just as much as the question of what sort of cure the holy man himself might offer. How

---

[33] Seiber pp 97-100. See further Patlagean, *Pauvreté*, pp 105-12 for many additional references.

[34] Brown, 'Holy Man', p 96.

[35] *Théodore* cap 145.

[36] *Ibid* caps 121, 122.

[37] *Ibid* cap 26a.

[38] *Ibid* cap 32.

[39] *Ibid* caps 60, 117, 143.

The Case of Theodore of Sykeon

he apportioned illnesses and cases – according to what medical or moral principles – can once more only be guessed at. There is not even the information for a rudimentary graph. One distinction can be made. Only saints like Artemios performed surgery during their patients' period of incubation.[40] Holy men did not shed blood; that is why Hypatios called in a surgeon. But why Theodore should despatch some to a doctor for a purging draught, when it is clear that he could prescribe them himself, is not so readily determined.

'Paradox' is one answer. Holy men were fond of the paradoxical. The *locus* of the holy, to borrow Brown's terminology, cannot easily be defined. Its coordinates are often unpredictable and shifting. The agent of cure, Brown is fond of reminding us, will not be the abbot but the redfaced monk with warts on his knees.[41] The insight can perhaps be extended. You find the man with the warts — and he promptly sends you off elsewhere bearing detailed instructions and someone's name and address. Theodore may have indulged in paradox from time to time, testing the faith of those who would not leave without being cured by him.[42] They came, as many patients do, with a clear idea of what treatment they should receive. The *Life* implies that not even the holy man could invariably convince them that they were mistaken.

Add now to Theodore's taste for paradox some practical considerations that may have affected his decision. He delegated exorcism because he was ill or busy.[43] He must have wished also to delegate the smaller task of healing minor ailments. Crowds followed him in hope of a cure. He could not attend to them all. But to send them to doctors? 'Have done with them', he had said, 'don't fall into their clutches'. When doctors appear in the *Life* of Theodore it is as failures. Whether summoned to treat the emperor Maurice's son for elephantiasis, or an imperial secretary with an intestinal disease, or a hydroptic man bearing the marks of surgical incision all over his body,[44] the physicians are unambiguously presented as having laboured in vain.

The message of this and similar texts is plain. Doctors are

[40] See for example *Miracula S. Artemii*, ed. A. Papadopoulos-Kerameus, Varia graeca sacra (St. Petersburg 1909), nos. 25, 44.

[41] Brown, 'Eastern and Western Christendom', p 15; 'Holy Man', p 95.

[42] See above n 36.

[43] Compare *Théodore* cap 143, where the visit of an official prevents his going to a disaster-stricken village.

[44] *Ibid* caps 97, 121, 156.

ineffectual, even positively harmful. They charge too much, draining a patient of his resources. The patient's condition only improves when he turns to a saint. The despair of doctors, in cases where the saint eventually triumphs, becomes a *topos* of hagiographical invective.[45] It is inevitable that the hagiographers should castigate those who place more trust in human than in holy physicians, and should stress the impotence of doctors in order to exalt the miraculous power of the saints. Yet these *topoi* may show something of the truth. The miracles of the saint are indeed the last resort. It is natural first to consult a doctor, and if he fails, to try another one. This is the banal reality which gave rise to such colourful abuse from those recording the miracles of saints like Cyrus and John or Artemios.[46] Generally in or close to the major cities, the cults of these 'medical' saints were, by the same token, too close for comfort to the big centres of the medical profession. Their picture need not be accepted as the only one possible.[47]

Doctors have often over-charged for their services, anxious to preserve respect for their profession. Complaint at the scale of their fees is older than Christianity.[48] Yet if we move away from hagiographical to, say, patristic sources, we find a more appreciative view of the efforts of medical practitioners.[49] There is justification for that view. The achievements of Byzantine medicine were considerable. John of Ephesus describes the case of an Armenian monk who came to Constantinople with gangrene of the loins. Apart from treating him with plasters and drugs, the physicians were able to insert a leaden tube so that he could urinate. The man

---

[45] See for example *La Vie ancienne de S. Syméon Stylite le Jeune*, ed Paul van den Ven, Societé des Bollandistes, *sub hag* 32, 2 vols (Brussels 1962, 1970) cap 102 and editor's note.

[46] See for example *Miracula S. Artemii* no 23 on the 'braggarts' Hippocrates and Galen, and the miracles of Cyrus and John *passim*, in the new edition of Natalio Fernandez Marcos. *Los 'thaumata' de Sofronio. Contribución al estudio de la 'incubatio' Cristiana* (Madrid 1975).

[47] Compare Magoulias, justly criticized by Patlagean, *Pauvreté*, p 103.

[48] See most recently Owsei Temkin, 'Medical Ethics and Honoraria in Late Antiquity', *Healing and History. Essays for George Rosen*, ed Charles E. Rosenberg (Folkestone 1979) pp 6–26.

[49] See for example the useful collection of references in Hermann Josef Frings, *Medizin und Arzt bei den Griechischen Kirchenvätern bis Chrysostomos* (Bonn 1959). Basil and Sampson were not the only saints to whom medical knowledge was ascribed.

The Case of Theodore of Sykeon

lived for another eighteen years. There is no derogation of that achievement in the text.[50]

Byzantine society knew a whole range of doctors from court physicians and the municipal *archiatri*[51] to itinerant free-lancers, village quacks and local folk healers.[52] Not all were in any sense qualified. Gregory of Nyssa relates the *curriculum vitae* of Aetius, who began as a tinker, became the assistant of an itinerant quack, was taken on by a wealthy man as his personal physician, took part in medical conferences, moved from them to theological debates and went on to outstrip Arius himself.[53] But local Byzantine doctors were not all such charlatans. It was with the lesser, reasonably competent members of the breed that Theodore had to deal. He knew the ones in whose abilities he could trust, and was prepared to name them for the benefit of his clients.

There is insufficient evidence to describe these people. Few of them will have gained their knowledge from professional teachers or from access to large, well-written medical manuscripts. Indeed the general dependence of Byzantine medical culture upon such manuscripts has been grossly exaggerated. Clinical experience was the starting point of medical education, not its goal. The impressive manuscripts which have come down to us will often have been compiled from simple lists of remedies, pinned up in hospitals or consulting rooms, and forming part of a much more diffuse medical inheritance that embraced magical and folk healing. One text is quite plain about this.[54] Outside the great centres of medical excellence, the really important manuscripts for the practice of medicine were the small *iatrosophia:* muddled, ephemeral, unappealing compilations, many of which for that reason have still to find their editor.[55] The doctors with whom Theodore was acquainted

---

[50] *PO* 18 pp 643-4.
[51] See now Vivian Nutton, 'Archiatri and the Medical Profession in Antiquity', *Papers of the British School at Rome* 45 (London 1977) pp 191-226.
[52] Some references, not always adequately interpreted, in Halina Evert-Kappesowa, 'The Social Rank of a Physician in the Early Byzantine Empire', *Byzance et les Slaves Mélanges Ivan Dujčev* (Paris ? 1980) pp 139-64.
[53] *Contra Eunomium, PG* 45 cols 260C-261D.
[54] E. Jeanselme, 'Sur un aide-mémoire thérapeutique byzantin contenu dans un manuscrit de la Bibliothèque National de Paris (Suppl. Gr. 764). Traduction, notes et commentaire', *Mélanges Charles Diehl*, 1 (Paris 1930) pp 147-70.
[55] Temkin, 'Byzantine Medicine', p 113. See further Charles Daremberg, *Notices et extraits des manuscrits médicaux grecs, latins et français* (Paris 1853) pp 22 seq.

XI

depended either on them for their medical knowledge or on related oral traditions. Each of them will have perhaps had his own following and sphere of activity. It may be that in sending clients to specific doctors Theodore was respecting important lines of demarcation. The doctors for their part will have respected his special abilities, referring cases to him when they thought it necessary, rather as doctors can occasionally be seen 'referring' cases to Cosmas and Damian in the record of their miracles.[56]

Concluding his published lectures on *The Cult of the Saints*,[57] Peter Brown draws a distinction between two types of healing: that of Saint Martin of Tours and that to be found in the *De medicamentis* of the physician Marcellus of Bordeaux.[58] He notes 'the studious absence in the therapeutic system of Marcellus of a high-pitched idiom of relationships of dependence.' But unlike most of his colleagues, Marcellus was, as Brown admits, offering the means to self-help.[59] He is not typical and the distinction is unreal. The difference between the saint and the doctor was not one which turned on personal relationships.[60] When they sought medical advice, clients who were referred by a doctor to Theodore or *vice versa*, would not have felt they were passing between a personal and an impersonal system of healing. The problem was not that. There were hard decisions to be made, about whom to consult first, whose instructions to follow. Fine judgement was required.

Medical anthropology has shown how comparable decisions are made in a wide variety of cultures, wide enough to suggest some universal features of 'illness behaviour'.[61] Where there is more than one type of healer available, this 'behaviour' exhibits a 'hierarchy of resort', first to the advice of members of the family and to folk medicine, but then also to healers of all kinds, doctors and saints, local or distant. Not only is there a hierarchy of resort; in addition,

[56] For example *Côme et Damien* nos 27, 32.
[57] (London and Chicago 1981) pp 113 *seq.*
[58] ed M. Niedermann, translated by J. Kollesch and D. Nickel, *Corpus Medicorum Latinorum* 5, 2 vols (Berlin 1968).
[59] *De medicamentis, praef,* 3, vol 1, p 2.
[60] Compare Brown, 'Holy Man', p 100: 'the holy man was thought of as having taken into his person, skills that had previously been preserved by society at large'.
[61] See Lola R. Schwartz, 'The Hierarchy of Resort in Curative Practice: The Admiralty Islands Melanesia' *Journal of Health and Social Behaviour* 10 (New York 1969) pp 201-9. See further George M. Foster and Barbara Gallatin Anderson, *Medical Anthropology* (New York 1978) pp 248-9.

The Case of Theodore of Sykeon

there is often a very clear idea of what technique or which healer is most appropriate for any given illness. One knows where to start.[62] Seen in this perspective, which may have been that of his clients too, the holy man becomes one healer among many, prominent in the medical landscape of his area, but not, as a source of medicine or medical advice, wholly different from local physicians. Though Brown would remove him from society (by stressing his detachment, his status as an outsider),[63] he is brought firmly back into it.

Early medieval 'illness behaviour' should not be characterized by reference to Marcellus of Bordeaux. If there is to be a western example, let it be from a revealing account of a miracle. A girl's father is recorded as having taken her about among doctors *and* holy places — *per medicos et per loca sancta* — in search of health.[64] The priority is unclear. Competition between sources of healing could sometimes be stiff. The holy man was not too exalted to cooperate with the doctors. For, as the Egyptian monk Copres put it to some visitors: 'what wonder if we...perform the little things that we do, healing the lame and the blind, which the physicians also accomplish by their skills'.[65]

[62] See Vincent Crapanzano, *The Hamadsha. A Study in Moroccan Ethnopsychiatry* (Berkeley and Los Angeles 1973) pp 178-83, for a striking case study.

[63] 'Holy Man', pp 91-3.

[64] Cited from Ronald C. Finucane, *Miracles and Pilgrims: Popular Beliefs in Medieval England* (London 1977) p 67.

[65] *Historia Monachorum in Aegypto*, Greek text ed Festugière, Société des Bollandistes, *sub hag* 34 (Brussels 1961) cap 10. 24; I follow the translation of Norman Russell, *The Lives of the Desert Fathers*, introduced by Benedicta Ward (London and Oxford 1980) p 85.

XII

Responses to Possession and Insanity in the Earlier Byzantine World

I

The sixth-century Syrian stylite Maro, as reported by John of Ephesus in his *Lives of the Eastern Saints*, was unusual in refusing to heal the sick and possessed.[1] If he were to do so, he claimed, demons would at once seize 'women and girls and many persons' merely to create the opportunity of mocking him.[2] Once their victims had been brought to Maro the demons would deliberately withdraw, just as if they had been cast out. A gratifying outcome for the possessed but a spiritual disaster for the saint. Imagining himself a successful exorcist, he would become puffed up and arrogant. His asceticism would thus be compromised. To avoid this, Maro feigned dementia and had himself bound to a stone in his monastery. 'To myself the madman and man of evil life why do you come?'[3]

If Maro was unusual among early Byzantine ascetics he was not unique.

---

[1] Throughout the preparation of this paper, I have been indebted to the conversation and writings of the late Michael W. Dols. The paper can indeed be regarded as both pendant to, and debate with, his major posthumous work: *Majnūn: The Madman in Medieval Islamic Society*, D. E. Immisch (ed.) (Oxford, 1992).

[2] John of Ephesus, *Lives of the Eastern Saints*, 4, E. W. Brooks (ed. and trans.) *Patrologia Orientalis*, XVII (Paris, 1923), 64–9.

[3] Quoted from S. Ashbrook Harvey, *Asceticism and Society in Crisis: John of Ephesus and 'The Lives of the Eastern Saints'* (Berkeley, 1990), p. 51.

The monk Jacob for instance, also one of John's eastern saints, attended to the throng of the possessed only 'under great pressure' and sought – unsuccessfully – to elude them by moving to another village.[4] Yet stories of such comparatively rare individuals, precisely because they show holy men attempting to deny what were widely held to be their obligations, articulate a common assumption: that exorcism was the most typical resolution to the plight of the possessed. The demons themselves acknowledge the teleology implied in John's narrative: they are driven toward confrontation with the saint. Possession and exorcism seem inextricable.

That assumption, although open to challenge, is none the less compelling. It is naturally so from the point of view of the hagiographer, interested in possession because the inevitably triumphant exorcism manifests the virtue and power of his saint.[5] It has also been compelling to the modern historian. I think here particularly of the writings of Peter Brown, for whom the phenomenon of possession is to be condensed into a *psychodrame* enacted in the presence of a saint.[6] This psychodrama is a sharply-contoured, searing process. Those who approach the saint may not know that they are possessed, as in the story of Maro; for possession usually takes the form either of a state of ecstasy or dissociation, or of a recognized illness.[7] Alternatively, the saint's clients may not, initially, be possessed at all: they may come to the saint in order to *achieve* or *induce* possession – and to 'work through', and perhaps dissolve, whatever underlying torment has disposed them to this exigent condition. In either event it is the encounter with the quasi-judicial *praesentia* of the saint, living or dead, that is crucial. In the case of a living saint, there then follow exchanges of insults between demon and exorcist, physical aggression on the saint's part, rites of exorcism in some form, a demonic admission of saintly power, the collapse of the possessed individual, the departure of the demon, and the final prolonged decrescendo of the victim's

[4] John of Ephesus, *Lives*, 15, *Patrologia Orientalis*, XVII, pp. 223–4. Harvey, *Asceticism*, p. 48. For the more usual behaviour of ascetics, see J. Moorhead, 'Thoughts on Some Early Medieval Miracles', in E. and M. Jeffreys and A. Moffat (eds.) *Byzantine Papers* (Canberra, 1981), pp. 1–11.

[5] E. Patlagean, 'Ancienne hagiographie byzantine et histoire sociale', *Annales: Economies, Sociétés, Civilisations* (1968), 106–26. S. Hackel (ed.) *The Byzantine Saint*, Studies supplementary to *Sobornost*, 5 (Birmingham, 1981), especially the contributions by Patlagean and R. Browning. C. Mango, *Byzantium* (London, 1980), pp. 248–9. Compare C. Stancliffe, *St. Martin and his Hagiographer: History and Miracle in Sulpicius Severus* (Oxford, 1983), chapters 8, 22.

[6] P. Brown, *The Cult of the Saints: Its Rise and Function in Latin Christianity* (London, 1981), pp. 106–14. Compare *idem*, *Society and the Holy in Late Antiquity* (London, 1982), pp. 123–6.

[7] A personal selection from a vast bibliography. General historical orientation: M. Eliade (ed.) *Encyclopedia of Religion*, 14 (London and New York, 1987), pp. 12–19 (s.v. 'Spirit possession'); T. Klauser et al. (eds.) *Reallexikon für Antike und Christentum*, IX (Stuttgart, 1976), coll. 546–798 (s.v. 'Geister (Dämonen)'). Historical studies: D. P. Walker, *Unclean Spirits: Possession and Exorcism in England and France in the Late Sixteenth and Early Seventeenth Centuries* (London, 1981); G. Levi, *Inheriting Power: The Story of an Exorcist* (Chicago, 1988). Social anthropology: I. M. Lewis, *Ecstatic Religion: An Anthropological Study of Spirit Possession and Shamanism* (Harmondsworth, 1971); E. Bourguignon, *Possession* (San Francisco, 1976); V. Crapanzano and V. Garrison (eds.) *Case Studies in Spirit Possession* (New York, 1977); F. D. Goodman, *How about Demons? Possession and Exorcism in the Modern World* (Bloomington, 1988).

recovery. 'It was, indeed, the liberating precision of exorcism that com-
mended itself so strongly to late antique men. It was a deeply reassuring
drama for men anxious about themselves and their society.'[8]

Understanding of the psychodrama of exorcism has come to historians very
much through acquaintance with anthropological studies of spirit mediumship
and shamanism as well as of a variety of possession states. These studies have
shown that the broad phenomenon of possession is not to be conceived as a
marginal superstition, but rather may be integral to the management of
relations between society at large and the individual. Yet, like hagiographers
and historians, social anthropologists have also tended to concentrate on the
peculiar ritual or drama toward which possession has seemed directed, to the
exclusion of the phenomenon's numerous other aspects.[9]

In what follows I propose an alternative, less narrowly-focused view of
responses to the possessed in the earlier Byzantine world. To challenge the
assumption that possession and exorcism were inextricable, attention will be
drawn to those unable to benefit from any psychodrama; and their history
will be set in what may be a more appropriate context, that of responses to
the insane.[10]

To many, if not most, of the possessed in Byzantium the possibility of
exorcism was, I suspect, remote. Despite our best critical efforts, we have
perhaps taken the hagiographers too much at their word, failing to question
their recurrent implication that saints were readily available to those in need.
Because we have tended to underestimate the degree of mobility frequently
achieved by ancient Mediterranean peoples,[11] we have in effect operated with
too localized a conception of the geography of exorcism. We have supposed
that the arrival of the sick and possessed before the saint – or his tomb –
required no tremendous effort: there were so many saints that only short
distances would have been involved in visiting them. I suggest rather that the
Byzantine world did *not* pullulate with ascetics, that there *were* villages
complete without a holy man, a resident 'outsider' who would resolve
conflicts and cast out devils.[12] A visit to such a figure required a particular

---

[8] Brown, *The Cult of the Saints*, p. 110. For the psychoanalytic background to the notions of
'working through' and 'psychodrama', see A. Rousselle, 'Jeunesse de l'antiquité tardive: les leçons
de lecture de Peter Brown', *Annales: Economies, Sociétés, Civilisations* (1985), 525–6. *Reallexikon*,
VII (1969), coll. 44–117 (s.v. 'Exorzismus').

[9] See for example L. M. Danforth, *Firewalking and Religious Healing: The Anastenaria of Greece
and the American Firewalking Movement* (Princeton, 1989), to which I am especially indebted; C.
Stewart, *Demons and the Devil: Moral Imagination in Modern Greek Culture* (Princeton, NJ, 1991),
chapter 8; R. P. Werbner, *Ritual Passage, Sacred Journey: The Process and Organization of Religious
Movement* (Washington, 1989), chapter 2; V. Skultans, 'The Management of Mental Illness among
Maharashtrian Families: A Case Study of a Mahanubhav Healing Temple', *Man*, new ser. XXII
(1987), 661–79.

[10] I omit consideration here of the exorcism involved in baptism, on which see H. A. Kelly,
The Devil at Baptism: Ritual, Theology, and Drama (Ithaca, NY, 1985).

[11] P. Horden and N. Purcell, *The Mediterranean World: Man and Environment in Antiquity and the
Middle Ages*, I: *The Corrupting Sea*, Oxford, forthcoming, part 5.

[12] Compare Brown, *Society and the Holy*, pp. 103–52.

decision and effort, and often a considerable journey. For very many of the possessed it was, in consequence, only rarely feasible. Some saints would, moreover, have gained a greater reputation as successful healers than others; the geography of 'revealed preference' may have been rather more limited than that of supply, and the distances involved correspondingly deterrent.

As in classical antiquity or medieval Islam, therefore, so in Byzantium: the destinies of the unhinged may have been far more various than the prevailing scholarly emphasis on exorcism would imply.[13] The presiding image on which I shall settle as most appropriate to the present enquiry is not that of Maro or Jacob shunning the possessed or reluctantly performing their triumphal rites. It is rather of Maro tied to his stone – Maro 'the madman', simulating a *chronic* mental disturbance that no psychodrama could alleviate.

To confirm the appropriateness of that image I shall first concentrate on a single, though substantial, hagiographical source; well-known, frequently cited and glossed – the *Life* of Theodore of Sykeon, who became Bishop of Anastasioupolis in Asia Minor and died in 613; a saint who, like Maro, feared that his curative excesses would lead him to commit the sin of pride.[14]

II

Here certainly, in this *Life* written by the saint's disciple George, are saintly diagnoses of possession where none had previously suspected them, and numerous dramatic confrontations with demons (involving, perhaps unlike those attributed to Maro, more men than women[15]).

Then he tortured them by the divine grace of Christ and by the sign of the holy Cross and by beatings on his chest, and after offering up prayers for a long time he bade them come out of the people and return to their own abode. They uttered loud shouts and tore the garments which covered the sufferers and threw them down at his feet and then came out of them . . .[16]

Theodore's hagiographer, as we should expect, is true to his purpose: the possessed are prominent in his narrative largely because their exorcism glorifies God and His saint. But thanks to the fullness of the *Life*, and the

[13] Antiquity: G. Rosen, *Madness in Society: Chapters in the Historical Sociology of Mental Illness* (New York and Evanston, 1969), chapters 2–3, has not been replaced as a general sociological account. Islam: Dols, *Majnūn*, Introduction.

[14] A.-J. Festugière (ed. and trans.) *Vie de Théodore de Sykéōn*, Subsidia hagiographica, 48, I (Brussels, 1970), with cap. 161 (p. 141). Compare the somewhat contemptuous brief account of the demonic elements in the *Life* by Festugière, 'Epidémies "hippocratiques" et épidémies démoniaques', *Wiener Studien*, LXXIX (1966), 157–64.

[15] A rough count of individually described possession cases in the *Life* of Theodore: 26 males, 11 females. On the particular susceptibility of women to possession in modern societies that anthropologists have observed, see Skultans, 'Management of Mental Illness', pp. 661–2; Werbner, *Ritual Passage*, pp. 76–81.

[16] *Vie de Théodore*, 43 (p. 38), translation quoted from E. Dawes and N. Baynes, *Three Byzantine Saints* (London, 1977), p. 119. Compare Brown, *Society and the Holy*, p. 126.

extent to which it sheds unusual light on the curative history of Asia Minor around 600, there are other aspects of possession that the hagiographer apparently feels no qualms about revealing.[17]

First, however rapid the rough and tumble of exorcism, possession was recognized as potentially chronic. At the sight of Theodore a woman's demons levitated her, and then made her lick the dust at the entrance of the sanctuary to which the saint had been invited. Such was the holy man's power: demons responded dramatically to his proximity as to that of no other human being. Less to be expected is that the possessed woman should have been bedridden with her affliction for many years, ignorant of the true cause of her numerous illnesses and attacks.[18]

Chronic possession could, however, be rather more obvious – and it could be salutary. Theodore left a young and apparently undisciplined monk to endure the terrible suffering of being possessed throughout his adolescence.[19] The longest period of possession mentioned in the *Life* is still greater, however: twenty-eight years. Like the levitated woman, the slave girl in question did not know that she was possessed: she needed the saint's diagnosis.[20] But the hagiographer finds nothing surprising in the length of time that she had endured; the detail merely accentuates the praeternatural insight of the saint. Nor does the *Life* imply that only ascetics like Theodore could recognize chronic possession when they saw it. It may be presumed that not all such cases required specialist diagnosis. Lay people clearly formed their own opinions on these matters, as can be seen from a debate briefly recorded in Theodoret's *Historia Religiosa*. The lady in question was bulimic: twenty chickens a day would not satisfy her. Some attributed her condition to possession; others saw in it a purely somatic infirmity.[21]

Secondly, if the possession might be chronic, so might the holy man's response to it. The psychodrama, if there was one, could be considerably spun out. In one case Theodore offered only temporary alleviation – so that the harvest could be gathered – rather than cure.[22] The healing of a man whose arm had been swollen by a demon took three days.[23] Another demon proved so recalcitrant that the saint had to abandon his task for several hours in order

[17] Patlagean, 'Ancienne hagiographie', and for Theodore's attitude to doctors, P. Horden, 'Saints and Doctors in the Early Byzantine Empire: the Case of Theodore of Sykeon', *Studies in Church History*, 19 (1982), 1–13.

[18] *Vie de Théodore*, 71 (pp. 58–9).

[19] Ibid. 46 (p. 41). Compare a near-contemporary text, *The Arabic Life of S. Pisentius*, 24, De L. O'Leary (ed. and trans.) *Patrologia Orientalis*, XXII (Paris, 1930), 397: a five-year possession (quoted Dols, *Majnūn*, p. 205).

[20] *Vie de Théodore*, 84 (pp. 70–1).

[21] Théodoret de Cyr, *Histoire des moines de Syrie*, XIII, 9, P. Canivet and A. Leroy-Molinghen (eds. and trans.) *Sources chrétiennes*, 234 (Paris, 1977), pp. 490–2. Cf. Dols, *Majnūn*, pp. 200–21, on conflicting diagnoses of the Prophet.

[22] *Vie de Théodore*, 35 (pp. 31–2).

[23] Ibid. 91 (p. 75).

to keep a prior appointment with the patriarch.[24] Several days' prayer and repeated blessings were needed in other cases.[25] In the *Life* of Hypatius, to turn briefly to another piece of early Byzantine hagiography, a process of 'depossession' (perhaps a more suitable general term than exorcism) required the sufferer to spend forty days in a monastery. In another case described in the same *Life* a man who had apparently been successfully exorcised by Hypatius in fact found no permanent relief. Rather, through lack of self-discipline, he had to endure several relapses spread over a four-year period.[26]

Thirdly, in contrast, possession could manifest itself in distinctly minor matters: the scurrying of rodents, a swollen hand, a mouse-like lump under the skin, a fit of quasi-intoxication, a cache of bad meat, a phase of refractoriness in a camel.[27] Again, not the obvious constituents of a psychodrama.

Fourthly, the *Life* of Theodore encourages a possible revision of the often-cited recommendation of Norman Baynes: that the burden of ancient belief in demons can be captured if we imagine that the myriad bacilli around us are each inspired by a conscious will to injure man.[28] This analogy makes early Byzantine people sound like exemplary Freudian neurotics, in the grip of perpetual fears.[29] I prefer to strengthen my previous point – that possession can be a minor matter – by emphasizing not the ubiquity of demons but rather their scarcity, the limited number of 'ecological niches' that they occupy. In the fourth-century *Life* of St Antony, demons had inhabited an aerial realm, below the heavens, which left them at the mercy of the winds.[30] For Theodore's hagiographer, by contrast, there is a precise demonic *geography*; a geography that can to a certain extent be mastered, in order to reduce human interaction with it to a minimum.[31]

---

[24] Ibid. 93 (pp. 76–7). For a comparable episode in the *Acta* of St Anastasius the Persian (H. Usener (ed.) (Bonn, 1894), pp. 14ff.) see C. Mango, 'Diabolus Byzantinus', *Homo Byzantinus: Papers in Honor of Alexander Kazhdan*, A. Cutler and S. Franklin (eds.) *Dumbarton Oaks Papers*, 46 (1992), 215–23, at p. 221.

[25] *Vie de Théodore*, 94, 103, 110, 122 (pp. 77–8, 82–3, 87–8, 98–9).

[26] Callinicos, *Vie d'Hypatios*, XL, 5–15, G. J. M. Bartelink (ed. and trans.) *Sources chrétiennes*, 177 (Paris, 1971), pp. 234–7.

[27] *Vie de Théodore*, 43, 91, 123, 132, 143, 160 (pp. 39, 75, 99–100, 105, 113, 137–8). Mango, 'Diabolus Byzantinus', pp. 216–17, drawing on the *Life* of Hypatius. Compare Stancliffe, *St. Martin*, pp. 194–5, on the mentality perhaps underlying such diabolical attribution.

[28] Dawes and Baynes, *Three Byzantine Saints*, p. xii.

[29] Compare E. R. Dodds, *Pagan and Christian in an Age of Anxiety* (Cambridge, 1965), with the comments of R. Lane Fox, *Pagans and Christians* (Harmondsworth, 1986), chapter 3. Festugière, 'Epidémies'; Brown, *Society and the Holy*, p. 145. The random, frightful, nature of demonic possession according to Byzantine belief is, however, re-emphasized by Mango, 'Diabolus Byzantinus'. See also V. I. J. Flint, *The Rise of Magic in Early Medieval Europe* (Oxford, 1991), pp. 101–8.

[30] J. Daniélou, 'Les démons de l'air dans la "Vie d'Antoine"', *Antonius Magnus Eremita, 356–1956*, *Studia Anselmiana*, 38 (1958), 136–47.

[31] This conception of a religious geography is developed in Horden and Purcell, *The Corrupting Sea*, part 4. A Constantinopolitan comparison: C. Mango, 'Antique Statuary and the Byzantine Beholder', *Dumbarton Oaks Papers*, XVII (1963), 53–75. Compare also Festugière, *Les Moines d'Orient*, I (Paris, 1961), chapter 1 ('Le moine et les démons), for further geographical reflections, and Stewart, *Demons and the Devil*, p. 211, for quiet routine exorcisms, and ibid. pp. 216–19, for characteristic *times*, as well as places, of demonic assault.

This geography is presented most forcefully in the *Life* of Theodore when the demons of Gordiane protest that they are tougher than the demons of Galatia and that, in effect, the saint enjoys no jurisdiction over them.[32] Perhaps, then, each area had its own demons. But, at the local level, there was far more to demonic geography than that. There were, in Byzantine eyes, knowable areas where demons had been 'bottled up', areas often associated with paganism or buried treasure. There were also areas simply acknowledged as demonic haunts, for example that deliberately chosen by one of Theodore's ascetic followers as the site of his wooden cage.[33] If some imprudent act should release a pent-up gaggle of demons, their subsequent movements were far from randomly aggressive. They occupied frontiers, routes, and specific houses; they destroyed granaries – all in true military fashion. ('Spirits are organized men', as Blake observed.[34]) They also took on the appearance of migrations of wolves and mice.[35]

Their course might further be directed by magic. Sorcerers, who appear on several occasions in the *Life* of Theodore, could clearly be called upon for maleficence. An amulet could be inscribed for protection.[36] And, at the eastern end of Theodore's world, in Mesopotamia and Iran, magic bowls could be deployed: a single one left upside down or a pair placed rim to rim might even, conceivably, have served as a domestic 'demon-trap'.[37]

Finally, the movements of demons were determined, in a manner of which the details are now mostly lost but the outline is imaginable, by relations within and between families; by the seemingly petty local strains and hostilities (perhaps expressed in a curse) that the social anthropology of medicine has shown to be of such importance in disease aetiology.[38] Here the findings of anthropologists may have been anticipated by common Byzantine belief. How many clues does Theodore's hagiographer actually offer in the apparently incidental details of his miracle stories? Whether an individual or a whole household is involved in the trauma of possession, whether the victim is a slave girl or an imperial silentiary, whether he or she is brought to the saint by a

---

[32] *Vie de Théodore*, 43 (p. 38); compare ibid. 161 (p. 144). Mango, *Byzantium*, p. 162.

[33] *Vie de Théodore*, 48 (p. 42). Mango, 'Diabolus Byzantinus', pp. 216, 219–20.

[34] *Vie de Théodore*, 43, 114, 161 (pp. 38, 89–90, 143). W. Blake, *A Descriptive Catalogue of Pictures* (1809), in G. Keynes (ed.) *Blake: Complete Writings* (Oxford, 1966), p. 577.

[35] *Vie de Théodore*, 8, 161 (pp. 8, 145).

[36] Ibid. 35, 37 (pp. 31, 32). R. Kotanski, 'Incantations and Prayers for Salvation on Inscribed Greek Amulets', in C. A. Faraoni and D. Obbink (eds.) *Magika Hiera: Ancient Greek Magic and Religion* (New York, 1991), pp. 107–37. J. G. Gager, *Curse Tablets and Binding Spells from the Ancient World* (New York and Oxford, 1992), provides an introduction to the wider context. For Syrian magic, see H. Gollancz (ed. and trans.) *The Book of Protection, being a Collection of Charms* (London, 1912), a (?)sixteenth-century collection containing much older material, e.g. codex A, no. 46 (pp. lii, 28), with Dols, *Majnūn*, pp. 206–8.

[37] J. Naveh and S. Shaked, *Amulets and Magic Bowls: Aramaic Incantations of Late Antiquity* (2nd edn.) (Jerusalem, 1987), especially p. 15.

[38] For example *Vie de Théodore*, 86, 92, 103, 129, 160, 162 (pp. 72, 75, 82, 103, 136, 148). Brown, *Society and the Holy*, pp. 124–5. Cursing: Palladio, *La Storia Lausiaca*, XXIV, 2, G. J. M. Bartelink (ed.) and M. Barchiesi (trans.) (Milan, 1974), p. 216. G. M. Foster and B. G. Anderson, *Medical Anthropology* (New York, 1978), chapter 3.

relative: to the original intended audience of the *Life* of Theodore, information on such matters could have given signals as clear as those reports of divisions between villagers – between rich and poor, one neighbour and another – that form the background to stories of demons accidentally let loose by excavation.[39]

Demons are not, therefore, as ubiquitous and unpredictable as bacilli: though sometimes invisible they move along recognizable paths, according to discernible patterns. A small society such as that pictured for us in the *Life* of Theodore can come to terms with its demons. It can learn how to maintain a sort of ecological balance that mitigates their disturbing impact, a balance comparable to that achieved by certain modern African societies which thus keep at bay potentially epidemic diseases, or, on a quotidian scale, comparable to that of the more fastidious inhabitants of contemporary Asia Minor, who may placate the *jinn* by prefacing numerous activities with the expression 'destur' ('excuse me').[40]

The *fifth*, and summational, point is that, from this prominent Byzantine saint's *Life*, possession emerges as what it has also been found to be in more recent cultures: as much an *idiom* for describing, and making intelligible, sometimes quite lengthy processes as a short-lived *state* of trance or ecstasy.[41] It is too variable in quality for the medieval holy man to be seen as its inevitable focus. I can attempt to support this point by proceeding to the question of how, again according to the *Life* of Theodore, the possessed were cared for or treated in Byzantium.

The holy man as exorcist was by no means their only recourse. There are hints in the *Life* that other forms of treatment could have been of equal if not greater importance. The sorcerer offered one such, although the hagiographer is at pains to describe the penalties incurred by those who consulted him in preference to the holy man.[42] Saint Michael was another. In one instance some possessed people crowded into the Church of the Archangel that Theodore had built. They were waiting for a cure, certainly; but it is not at all clear from what the hagiographer writes that an exorcism by Theodore was to be their prize, as against a slow recovery obtained by regular prayer and wrought through the intercession of the Archangel.[43] That the holy man himself might indeed consider the rite of exorcism to be inappropriate in certain cases is suggested by another story in the *Life*. Theodore had one villager who was possessed of an uncontrollable demon attached to a stake for

---

[39] *Vie de Théodore*, 114, 116 (pp. 89–90, 92–3).

[40] O. M. Oztürk, 'Folk Treatment of Mental Illness in Turkey', in A. Kiev (ed.) *Magic, Faith and Healing: Studies in Primitive Psychiatry Today* (New York and London, 1964), p. 351. G. Prins, 'But What was the Disease? The Present State of Health and Healing in African Studies', *Past and Present* , no. 124 (1989), 166–72. An early medieval application: Horden, 'Disease, Dragons and Saints: The Management of Epidemics in the Dark Ages', in T. Ranger and P. Slack (eds.) *Epidemics and Ideas: Essays on the Historical Perception of Pestilence* (Cambridge, 1992), pp. 45–76.

[41] Danforth, *Firewalking*, pp. 59–60. Patlagean, *Pauvreté économique et pauvreté sociale à Byzance, 4e–7e siècles* (Paris, 1977), pp. 106–7.

[42] *Vie de Théodore*, 35, 37, 38, 159 (pp. 31, 32–4, 139).

[43] Ibid. 40 (p. 36).

a fortnight. Nothing more dramatic – and nothing less potent – than the saint's daily prayer was required before the demon could be burned out of its victim.[44]

Those who benefited from Theodore's intercession may have constituted the minority among the possessed who are referred to in his *Life*. The rich, we learn from an account of an epidemic of possession, could be too ashamed of the afflicted members of their families to do other than keep them in their homes. There, we may surmise from other stories in the *Life*, it was not thought unreasonable to whip the devil within the body of the possessed.[45] As for the treatment available to the humble, it is noteworthy that the local hospice or hospital appears several times in the *Life*. But it does not here seem to have been conceived as an institution to harbour the chronically possessed, ecclesiastical sanctuary or the home being preferable. Theodore's hagiographer does report that demons caused illnesses in some of their victims precisely so that they would be taken into the hospital; but this was only a ruse to distance themselves from the power of the saint. Their victims were presumably not recognized as suffering from possession.[46]

III

Thus far I have confined discussion almost exclusively to the *Life* of Theodore. And I have studiously avoided defining the Byzantine idea of possession, merely indicating some of the contexts in which possession was discerned. For if, as I have proposed, possession is best conceived by historians as an idiom that could be adopted according to precise but varying circumstances, then clearly, in human beings, it was an idiom appropriate to a considerable range of both physical and mental conditions. And almost all of these conditions could, in Byzantine eyes, have had non-demonic causes: sin, some flaw in personal relations, divine test or punishment, old age, environment.[47]

The remedy for confusion may be to envisage a spectrum of possibilities. At one extreme would lie organic conditions for which the idiom of possession could on occasion have been suitable: epilepsy and paralysis for example.[48] At the other extreme would lie severe forms of mental illness that today are categorized as psychoses.

---

[44] Ibid. 103 (p. 83).
[45] Ibid. 161, 18, 116 (pp. 138, 15, 92).
[46] Ibid. 156, 161 (pp. 127, 143), *pace* Dols, *Majnūn*, pp. 194–5.
[47] E.g. *Vie de Théodore*, 81 (p. 68). Patlagean, *Pauvreté*, pp. 104–5. G. Dagron, 'Le saint, le savant, l'astrologue: étude de thèmes hagiographiques à travers quelques recueils de "Questions et réponses" des Ve–VIIe siècles', in *Hagiographie, Cultures et Sociétés, IVe–XIIe siècles* (Paris, 1981), pp. 143–55.
[48] E.g. *Vie de Théodore*, 85, 102, 107 (pp. 71, 82, 85). Patlagean, *Pauvreté*, pp. 105, 107, 109. On epilepsy, O. Temkin, *The Falling Sickness* (Baltimore, 1945), is the classic exposition: see especially pp. 84–9 (I have not seen the second edition of 1971).

186

It should be emphasized at this point that by no means all serious mental disorders and defects would have been interpreted as demonic in character. At least some late antique and Byzantine observers could distinguish possession from mental disease or incapacity. Their criteria wavered, and were ultimately more sociological than psychiatric in character. Status, that is, perhaps counted for more than symptoms, although the sufferer's age and general demeanour would clearly have been important in the diagnosis of chronic cases. None the less the distinction between possession and madness could be made.[49]

Witness John Chrysostom's readiness to distinguish possession from 'endogenous' depression (*athumia*); or Augustine's avowal that, although some might think a febrile and delirious patient to be possessed, he could in truth (and here Augustine used a medical term) be simply *phreneticus*.[50] Witness the plague of madness, the outbreak of collective hysteria, that struck Amida in the time of John of Ephesus, attributed to the devil's work but not obviously a case of mass possession.[51] Witness the ascetic Maro's own description of himself as a madman (Syriac *sania'*), rather than as possessed (*daiwana*); or the sixth-century Saint Theodosius's provision in his Jericho monastery for demented, because over-zealous, ascetics.[52] Witness the various legal texts, for instance the West Syrian *Synodicon*, that apparently differentiate possession from insanity; or those, such as a *Novel* (new law) of Leo the Wise, that envisage derangement (in a wife) either as having no obvious cause or as being inflicted, without demonic intermediary, through sorcery. Witness again the more informal literary sources, such as the thirteenth-century collection of 'laughable stories' by Gregory Barhebraeus, that imply the same distinction.[53] Witness, finally, the vigour of the whole Galenic tradition in medical thought, a tradition that set what we now distinguish as mental illnesses firmly in the context of somatic diseases, and analysed them as an imbalance of humours or spirits – sometimes, as in Posidonius, pseudo-Theophanes Nonnus or

[49] Contrast V. Nutton, 'From Galen to Alexander: Aspects of Medicine and Medical Practice in Late Antiquity', *Dumbarton Oaks Papers*, XXXVIII (1984), 9; Dols, *Majnūn*, p. 191. See also Temkin, *Falling Sickness*, pp. 84ff. and *idem*, *Hippocrates in a World of Pagans and Christians* (Baltimore and London, 1991), chapter 15.

[50] Chrysostom, *Ad Stagirium a daemone vexatum*, II, 1, J.–P. Migne (ed.) *Patrologiae Cursus Completus . . . Series Graeca*, XLVII (Paris, 1863), coll. 447–8; Augustine, *De Genesi ad Litteram*, XII, 17, 35 (and cf. 36), J.–P. Migne (ed.) *Patrologia . . . Series Latina*, XXXIV (Paris, 1865), col. 468. For explicit reference to the medical origins of the term *phreneticus*, see Gregory the Great, cited in n. 63 below. Galen's discussion of *phrenitis* is summarized in Dols, *Majnūn*, pp. 30–31; see also n. 55 below.

[51] Ashbrook Harvey, *Asceticism and Society*, pp. 64–5.

[52] Theodore of Petra, *Life* of St Theodosius, XVII, A.–J. Festugière (trans.) *Les moines d'Orient*, III/3 (Paris, 1963), p. 125. Compare Palladio, *La Storia Lausiaca*, XXV, 5 (p. 136): mad ascetic restrained in irons for a year.

[53] A. Vööbus (ed.) *The Synodicon in the West Syrian Tradition*, Corpus Scriptorum Ecclesiasticorum Orientalium, Scriptores Syri, 161 (Louvain, 1975), no. 16, questions 2–4, pp. 140–1. P. Noailles and A. Dain (eds. and trans.) *Les Novelles de Léon VI le Sage* (Paris, 1944), Novel CXI, pp. 360–7. For the larger legal context, a useful compendium is R. C. Pickett, *Mental Affliction and Canon Law* (Ottawa, 1952). A less formal example: Gregory Barhebraeus, *The Book of Laughable Stories*, E. A. Wallis Budge (ed. and trans.) (London, 1897), chapters 16–17.

Michael Psellus, explicitly in opposition to alternative aetiologies involving diabolical interference.[54] This is by no means a negligible body of evidence.[55] It is the middle of the spectrum – between the organic and the psychotic – that presents the greatest conceptual problems. Medical anthropologists have encouraged us to recognize the frequency of 'folk illnesses', highly localized conditions, psychosomatic in origin, that evade western diagnostic categories. They have also prompted recognition of the larger phenomenon of *somatization*, the expression of dysphoria in the idiom of somatic symptoms.[56] Possession enters the picture at this point as yet a further available idiom: a means of coping with stress or neurosis. We should perhaps also be on the alert for the related phenomenon of what might conveniently be labelled *antipossession*: the avoidance of the idiom of possession, because of the stigma or the difficulty associated with it, in favour of a purely somatic presentation of symptoms, a recognized illness. It may be that in this category we can find an explanation for those cases of latent possession masquerading as chronic physical illness that Theodore encountered and rediagnosed.

Now the saints of Byzantium, like some of their modern Middle Eastern counterparts, may have been able to choose the points on the above spectrum at which they would practise their exorcisms (for example, leaving psychoses and organic disorders well alone[57]). But historians of Byzantium cannot be so selective. They must attempt to envisage the entire range of cases for which the idiom of possession might have seemed proper: latent as well as manifest cases, organic as well as functional disorders.

[54] Dols, *Majnūn*, part I, includes an excellent introduction to the Byzantine medical tradition, anticipated in *idem*, 'Insanity in Byzantine and Islamic Medicine', *Dumbarton Oaks Papers*, XXXVIII (1984), 135–48. For the explicit rejection of demonic aetiologies of, respectively, nightmare, epilepsy, and 'possession' in Posidonius, pseudo-Theophanes Nonnus, and Michael Psellus, see O. Temkin, *Hippocrates*, p. 201; *idem*, 'Byzantine Medicine: Tradition and Empiricism', *Dumbarton Oaks Papers*, XVI (1962), 109–10; and P. Ioannou, *Démonologie populaire – démonologie critique au XIe siècle: la Vie inédite de S. Auxence par M. Psellos* (Wiesbaden, 1971). For Psellus, see further J. Grosdidier de Matons, 'Psellos et le monde de l'irrationel', *Travaux et Mémoires*, VI (1976), 325–49; and, for his wider context, R. P. H. Greenfield, *Traditions of Belief in Late Byzantine Demonology* (Amsterdam, 1988). A medieval western parallel: P.-A. Sigal, *L'Homme et le miracle dans la France médiévale (XIe–XIIe siècle)* (Paris, 1985), pp. 236–9. For some idea of the ways in which humoral and supernatural pathologies can interact in a modern Middle Eastern society, see B. Greenwood, 'Cold or Spirits? Choice and Ambiguity in Morocco's Pluralistic Medical System', *Social Science and Medicine*, 15 B (1981), 219–35.

[55] The equivalents of madness, lunacy, possession, and so forth in the various relevant languages still await a proper comparative philological examination (of the sort that I have neither space nor competence to undertake here). Compare A. Rousselle, *Croire et guérir: la foi en Gaule dans l'antiquité tardive* (Paris, 1990), chapter 10, for an exploration of a western part of the terrain; D. Krueger, 'Cynics, Christians, and Holy Fools: The Late Antique Contexts of Leontius of Neapolis' *Life of Symeon the Fool*' (unpublished Ph.D. thesis, Princeton University, 1991), pp. 81ff. for the Greek terms *salos* and *mōria*; and Dols, *Majnūn*, chapter 8.

[56] R. Simons and C. Hughes (eds.) *The Culture-Bound Syndromes: Folk Illnesses of Psychiatric and Anthropological Interest* (Dordrecht, 1985). On somatization, see A. Kleinman, *Social Origins of Distress and Disease: Depression, Neurasthenia, and Pain in Modern China* (New Haven, 1986); *idem* and B. Good (eds.) *Culture and Depression: Studies in the Anthropology and Cross-cultural Psychiatry of Affect and Disorder* (Berkeley and Los Angeles, 1986).

[57] Compare V. Crapanzano, *The Ḥamadsha: A Study in Moroccan Ethnopsychiatry* (Berkeley, 1973), pp. 4–5.

XII

Approached in this way, the Byzantine response to possession clearly cannot be equated with any one category such as exorcism. It has to be seen in the immediate context of the treatment of organic disease on one hand and mental illness (insanity of the non-demonic variety) on the other. In what follows I shall, however, leave aside such cases of latent possession as could not be distinguished from somatic disorders, for that would take the discussion into comparatively well-charted terrain. Instead, taking my cue from the work of Michael Dols,[58] and extending the enquiry beyond the *Life* of Theodore in just one of several promising directions, I shall assemble scattered evidence for the fate in Byzantium of those thought to be chronically possessed or insane: those whose condition was serious enough to bring them to the attention of contemporary writers but for whom exorcism could provide no deliverance.

IV

The extremes of treatment could be severe. Some of the possessed were imprisoned.[59] Worse, from the anonymous collection of fourth- to fifth-century, possibly Messalian, Syriac sermons known as the *Liber Graduum* comes the implication that the 'righteous' (by whom the preacher means ordinary Christians as distinct from the 'perfect') might well kill off their frenzied and demented instead of restraining them.[60] Others, the more charitable, were presumably relieved when their prayers for the release from suffering of someone violently possessed were answered in the victim's death.[61]

At the other end of the range of conceivable responses lies hospitalization. The *Life* of Theodore lends no support to the notion that the possessed or insane might enter a hospital. And the tenor of the relevant modern historiography is that such hospitalization was not to be available until the foundation of *bimaristan* in the medieval Muslim world. For although *bimaristan* were initially just places for the sick, as the meaning of their originally Persian designation implies, they soon developed specialized facilities for the care of the mentally ill. These acquired such prominence that by the later Middle Ages the term *bimaristan* had become virtually equivalent to 'insane asylum'.[62]

There are, however, possible interpretations of Byzantine sources that

---

[58] Dols, *Majnūn*, especially chapter 7, offers both Byzantine references (often my starting point in what follows, although our conclusions differ) and parallels from the Islamic world (with which I am not here generally concerned).

[59] I know only one piece of evidence to support Dols's conjecture (*Majnūn*, pp. 199, 464) that violent or dangerous madmen were imprisoned in Byzantium: the commentary of Balsamon on the canon of the Council *in Trullo* cited below, n. 83. On Byzantine prisons, see the brief entry *sub verbo* in A. P. Kazhdan (ed.) *The Oxford Dictionary of Byzantium*, 3 vols. (New York and Oxford, 1991), III, 1723.

[60] M. Kmosko (ed.) *Liber Graduum*, VII, 15, *Patrologia Syriaca*, III (Paris, 1926), col. 173. For bibliography on this text, see D. Krueger, 'Cynics, Christians and Holy Fools', p. 69, n. 19.

[61] *The History of Rabban Hormizd*, V, Wallis Budge (ed. and trans.) *The Histories of Rabban Hormizd the Persian and Rabban Bar-Idta* (London, 1902), pp. 31–2.

[62] Dols, 'The Origins of the Islamic Hospital: Myth and Reality', *Bulletin of the History of Medicine*, LXI (1987), 367–90.

deserve mention in this context, and that may help to answer the question of why Muslim hospitals catered so extensively for the demented. Taken together, these sources perhaps reflect a tradition of hospitalizing the insane. It would not have been a tradition peculiar to the Eastern Christian world. Writing in the 590s, Gregory the Great for example includes in his *Dialogues* a short account of the miraculous cure of a madman (*freneticus*) who was a patient in a 'house of the sick'.[63] The tradition may, none the less, have been at its most vigorous in Byzantine Syria and its Persian hinterland.

An early, eastern manifestation of it might be detected in the 'monastery within a monastery' that St Theodosius established for deranged monks in sixth-century Jericho. More impressive testimony is to be found in the correspondence of Timothy, patriarch of the Nestorian Church in Baghdad from 780 to 823. A letter from Timothy datable to around 790 and relating to his ecclesiastical foundations in the Persian capital, Seleucia-Ctesiphon, mentions that he has built a *xenodocheion* or hospital for those who are 'bodily or spiritually sick', presumably including the mentally ill or possessed.[64] Tenth-century Muslim geographers also mention what they understood to be an asylum for the insane, dating from before the Arab conquest, within the Ezechial or Heraclean Monastery in Lower Mesopotamia. The establishment may have been atypical but it was not, apparently, unique.[65]

An indication of the degree of specialized care for which Syrian monks could earn a reputation can be derived from the geographer and chronicler al-Muqaddisi's report of one monastery that dealt in cases of rabies.[66] The aetiology of the disease was widely recognized to be completely different from that of possession or mental illness, but some of the symptoms – especially hydrophobia – and even some of the cures were similar to those of insanity in the Byzantine medical tradition.[67] Finally, and to race forward several more centuries, as is inevitable with the scattered and sporadic evidence for this subject, there is an item in the 'laughable stories' of Gregory Barhebraeus in which a possessed man appears chained up in a hospital.[68]

Barhebraeus was a learned Syrian bishop; so the hospital to which he referred was presumably a Christian foundation. The means of restraint was, however, also commonly to be found in Islamic hospitals of the central Middle Ages. In 1185, for example, Ibn Jubayr observed in the hospitals of Damascus 'a system of treatment for confined lunatics, and they are bound in

---

[63] *Dialogues*, III, 35, 3–4, A. de Vogüé (ed.) *Les Dialogues de Grégoire le Grand, Sources chrétiennes*, 251, 2 vols. (Paris, 1979), II, 404–6.

[64] Quoted in Dols, 'Origins', p. 379. I am grateful to Sebastian Brock for linguistic advice. See also Dols, *Majnūn*, p. 114.

[65] Dols, 'Insanity in Byzantine and Islamic Medicine', p. 142. *Idem, Majnūn*, p. 203, with nn. 121–3.

[66] Vööbus, *Einiges über die karitative Tätigkeit des syrischen Mönchtums*, Contributions of Baltic University, 51 (Pinneburg, 1947), p. 21.

[67] J. Théodoridès, 'Rabies in Byzantine Medicine', *Dumbarton Oaks Papers*, XXXVIII (1984), 155.

[68] Barhebraeus, *Book*, pp. 156, 127 (no. 624); compare pp. 161, 134 (no. 643).

190

chains'.[69] It might therefore be argued that the evidence just reviewed for the hospitalization of the insane reflects contemporary Islamic influence on Christian institutions, rather than Byzantine tradition. But in that case the nature of the Islamic model would itself require explanation: why was such prominence accorded in the Islamic *bimaristan* to the care and treatment of lunatics?

Part of the answer may be that exorcism was not, apparently, a valued function of Muslim saints, who might be expected to have provided a powerful alternative explanation and source of treatment for insanity.[70] And a still greater part of the answer must certainly reside in the contrast between the predominantly secular character and Galenic orientation of Muslim hospitals and the ecclesiastical administration and Christian purpose of Byzantine philanthropic institutions. The derivation of so much Islamic medicine from the Galenic corpus; the consequent absorption by Muslim physicians of Galen's theories of mental disorder as explicable in the same humoral terms as were other kinds of disease; the close association between medical education and hospital practice in medieval Islam – all these features reveal why a *non-demonic* aetiology of insanity should have been favoured in *bimaristan*; and they contrast with the emphasis on *divine* therapeutics in a good many Byzantine hospitals.[71] Also, the quantity and vividness of the evidence for the treatment of the mentally ill in Islamic hospitals far outstrips that assembled above from Greek and Syrian sources. Nevertheless, if Islamic hospitals effectively 'Galenized' insanity, still it cannot be said that Byzantine thought had previously 'demonized' it. Byzantium did not entirely place the mentally ill beyond the scope of medical and hospital care.

Perhaps, then, the argument that sees the *bimaristan* as deeply rooted in the soil of Eastern Christian charity ought to be pressed a little further. Instead of counting Islamic wards for the insane as an exception to the generalization that Islam owed its idea of the hospital to Byzantium, we should admit the possibility that the indebtedness of Islam to Byzantium was, in this respect, all-embracing. Undeniably, there were differences of emphasis: Byzantine hospitals were never potent centres of Galenism, nor did they *regularly* accommodate the possessed and insane. Yet, on the other hand, it would be rash to assume that the treatment offered to mental patients in *bimaristan* was wholly without precedent in the Byzantine world.

A context that would make such Byzantine precedent intelligible is supplied by the hospital-like services – not always too gentle – offered at monasteries and shrines. Monastic instances that impressed Muslim authorities have already been noticed. In these monasteries, the help afforded to demoniacs had perhaps grown to such an extent that special housing was necessary. Elsewhere, we may envisage possessed figures restrained in or near the

---

[69] R. J. C. Broadhurst (trans.) *The Travels of Ibn Jubayr* (London, 1952), p. 296. Dols, 'Insanity and its Treatment in Islamic Society', *Medical History*, XXXI (1987), 1–14.

[70] *Idem, Majnūn*, p. 230.

[71] *Idem*, 'Insanity in Byzantine and Islamic Medicine', p. 143.

sanctuary of a saint. This too has already been encountered, in the *Lives* of Maro and Theodore. St Anastasia's was only one of a number of churches in Constantinople to receive so many demoniacs that it functioned virtually as a lunatic asylum.[72] A sixth-century western parallel could be drawn with the story, related by Gregory of Tours, of a man from Périgueux who lost his mind; he had to spend four months at the shrine of St Martin, abstaining from meat and wine, before he could depart cured.[73] There is also a scatter of other texts, mostly Syrian, that include vignettes of possessed and manacled figures.[74]

The practice of chaining was, indeed, to have a long history. In the early years of this century, Gertrude Bell was shown a collar and chain attached to the wall of a monastery chapel in the Tur 'Abdin, for the sake of 'men who were afflicted with fits or madness'; and yet more recent instances of the remedy have been reported, often linked to the cult of St George.[75] The proximity of the enchained to the tomb of a saint indicates the kind of relief that was, in theory, expected for them. But, if their possession was chronic, the care presumably offered by the monks might in practice hardly have differed from that available in a hospital. It is a possibility at least worth entertaining.

V

Failing the institutional support of hospital or sanctuary, the possessed and mentally ill might be left to their own devices, or they might of course look to their family and friends. The fullest description of such domestic care to survive in Byzantine sources is that of John of Ephesus in his *Ecclesiastical History*. It concerns the possession, by an evil angel, of the later sixth-century emperor, Justin II. The common report in Constantinople was that the emperor, filled with agitation and terror, had to be managed by strong young attendants, who would by turns tie him up, frighten him into submission, and divert him with music or a ride in a little wagon. Bars were also placed on the windows in his part of the palace. Varied treatment indeed; more so

---

[72] J. O. Rosenqvist (ed.) *The Life of St Irene Abbess of Chrysobalanton* (Uppsala, 1986), pp. 62–3, 68–9. For a general reference to the possessed in other churches in the city, see the *Miracles* of St Artemius, A. Papadopoulos-Kerameus (ed.) *Varia Graeca Sacra* (St Petersburg, 1909, repr. Leipzig, 1975), no. 18, p. 20.

[73] *Libri de virtutibus sancti Martini episcopi*, IV, 44, B. Krusch (ed.) *Gregorii Episcopi Turonensis, Miracula et Opera Minora, Monumenta Germaniae Historica, Scriptores Rerum Merovingicarum*, vol. I, part II (Hannover, 1885, repr. 1969), p. 210.

[74] Palladio, *La Storia Lausiaca*, XXV, 5 (p. 136), XLIV, 2 (p. 216). Vööbus, *Synodicon*, no. 16, question 15 (p. 143). A. Palmer, *Monk and Mason on the Tigris Frontier: The Early History of Tur 'Abdin* (Cambridge, 1990), p. 93. J.–B. Chabot (ed. and trans.) 'Vie du moine Rabban Youssef Bousnaya', *Revue de l'Orient Chrétien*, III (1898), 92, 96. Barhebraeus, *Book*, pp. 156, 127 (no. 624).

[75] G. L. Bell, *Amurath to Amurath* (London, 1911), pp. 313–14. V. Rochcau, 'Saint Siméon Salos, ermite palestinien et prototype des "Fous-pour-le-Christ"', *Proche-Orient Chrétien*, XXVIII (1978), 214, n. 8.

than that later forced upon George III. But, at least in John's censorious and far from wholly reliable account, no exorcist was summoned. To those around him, perhaps, the emperor's condition appeared simply incurable.[76] Stray references shed an intermittent light on the everyday life of the more humble demoniac or madman in the Byzantine world. This, for example, from Epiphanius in the fourth century: 'there was a madman in the city who roamed the town, I mean Tiberias, naked. If he was dressed he would often tear his clothing apart, as such people will'.[77] But the nearest that we can reach to the characteristic predicament of such figures may be anecdotes preserved in the *Lives* of the holy fools, fools for the sake of Christ.[78] We must, of course, proceed cautiously in deriving an image of mental illness from these works, since we are at two removes from the reality that we seek: first, the role-playing of the saint, whose foolery was not inevitably intended to suggest derangement;[79] second, the literary shaping of his hagiographer, who was not particularly concerned with the symptoms or sociology of dementia. It is, none the less, hard to resist the impression created by the ensemble of relevant *Lives* that the chronically insane or possessed might easily find themselves in the dregs of society. Symeon of Emesa and Mark of Alexandria consorted with beggars, snatching food and warmth where they could, liable to attack from children, seemingly capable of only menial employment.[80] Two brief stories set down by John Moschus in the early seventh century could also be adduced, even though only the first of them concerns a holy fool.

Visiting the Church of St Theodosius in Alexandria, John and his friend Sophronius met a bald man dressed in sackcloth and apparently mad. He took money from Sophronius as a beggar would. He then showed his true colours by putting the money on the ground, prostrating himself before God, and departing. The implication of the tale is, however, that a mad beggar cut a plausible figure outside a church. In the second Moschan narrative, a hermit is warned to serve an apprenticeship with a spiritual guide; otherwise he could find himself wandering dementedly from city to city like the possessed.[81]

---

[76] E. W. Brooks (ed. with Latin trans.) *Iohannis Ephesini historiae ecclesiasticae pars tertia, Corpus Scriptorum Christianorum Orientalium, Scriptores Syri*, 54–5 (Louvain, 1952), III, 2–3, trans. pp. 88–91. Contrast I. Macalpine and R. Hunter, *George III and the Mad Business* (London, 1969). On the burden of familial care of the insane, see Skultans, 'Management of Mental Illness'; R. H. Blum and E. Blum, *Health and Healing in Rural Greece* (Stanford, 1965), chapter 9.

[77] F. Williams (trans.) *The Panarion of Epiphanius of Salamis Book I (Sects 1–46)*, II, 10, 3, p. 127.

[78] For context and bibliography, see Krueger, 'Cynics, Christians, and Holy Fools'; and L. Rydén, 'The Holy Fool', in S. Hackel (ed.) *The Byzantine Saint*, pp. 106–13.

[79] John of Ephesus, *Lives*, 52, *Patrologia Orientalis*, XIX, 164–79: a pair of holy fools masquerading as mime-actors. On this theme of concealed sanctity, see Krueger, 'Cynics, Christians, and Holy Fools', pp. 89ff.

[80] Krueger, 'Cynics, Christians, and Holy Fools', includes as an appendix a translation of Leontius' *Life* of Simeon. For Mark, L. Clugnet (ed.) 'Vie et récits de l'Abbé Daniel, de Scété', *Revue de l'Orient Chrétien*, V (1900), 60–2; Patlagean, *Pauvreté*, p. 112.

[81] *Pratum Spirituale*, 111, J.-P. Migne (ed.) *Patrologia . . . Series Latina*, LXXXVII, pt. 3 (Paris, 1865), col. 2976; Th. Nissen, 'Unbekannte Erzählungen aus dem Pratum Spirituale', *Byzantinische Zeitschrift*, XXXVIII (1938), no. 7 (p. 360). For context, see H. Chadwick, 'John Moschus and his Friend Sophronius the Sophist', *Journal of Theological Studies*, new ser. XXV (1974), 41–74.

Circumstantial details of this type cannot be mere hagiographical fancy. The bishops assembled in 691–2 at the Council *in Trullo* decreed that anyone pretending to be possessed should be subject to the same harsh treatment as genuine demoniacs.[82] Unfortunately, the Council's objective here cannot be recovered. It was, most likely, castigating those who feigned possession in order to beg. Alternatively, as Theodore Balsamon would conjecture in the thirteenth century, the bishops may have had in mind those who simulated frenzy to profit from soothsaying. In either case, the fact that the bishops were moved to devote a separate canon to the topic perhaps gives some indication of the extent to which both the possessed and their imitators constituted a social nuisance.[83]

Adequate support was not even to be relied upon in a monastery. From the early fifth century, Palladius tells the distressing tale of a nun in an Egyptian convent who, convincingly simulating possession, lived like an outcast in the kitchen, eating crumbs and leftovers, subject to beatings and humiliation by her fellows. In a narrative concerning the late sixth century presumably modelled on that of Palladius, another apparently pathetic figure is shown sprawling on the ground in the middle of the monastery's courtyard, where she is 'revived' with a pailful of water; she is later found sleeping by the latrines.[84]

No dramatic release through exorcism was reportedly offered to such apparent unfortunates. Other types of cure might have been attempted, however. The *Life* of Andrew the Fool, whatever its date and purpose, has the merit of showing us one such attempt; and if its saint is fictional its circumstantial touches may well reflect the likely fate of the possessed in Constantinople. The slave Andrew was supposedly sent to the Church of St Anastasia by his master, who thought his behaviour indicative of possession. Andrew spent four months shackled in the church. The guards looking after him, ignorant of course that he was feigning, then declared that his condition had worsened rather than improved. His master ordered Andrew's release. The saint spent the remainder of his life on the streets of Constantinople.[85]

[82] Canon 60, in J. D. Mansi (ed.) *Sacrorum Conciliorum nova et amplissima collectio*, XI (Florence, 1765), col. 969; or in G. A. Rhallis and M. Potlis, *Syntagma tōn theiōn kai hierōn kanonōn*, II (Athens, 1852), 440–1.

[83] Patlagean, *Pauvreté*, p. 111. Commentary of Balsamon, Rhallis and Potlis, *Syntagma*, pp. 441–2, including a report of the imprisonment of those caught infringing the canon. See also F. R. Trombley, 'The Council in Trullo (690–2): A Study of the Canons relating to Paganism, Heresy, and the Invasions', *Comitatus*, IX (1978), 6. In a hitherto neglected discussion, J. Wortley, 'The Sixtieth Canon of the Council *in Troullo*', *Studia Patristica*, XV (1984), 255–60, interprets the canon as directed against 'some abuse or distortion of the practice of holy folly', possession feigned for material rather than spiritual profit.

[84] Palladio, *La Storia Lausiaca*, XXXIV, 1–2 (pp. 164–5); L. Rydén, 'The Holy Fool', p. 106. S. P. Brock and S. Ashbrook Harvey, *Holy Women of the Syrian Orient* (Berkeley, 1987), pp. 144–5.

[85] J.–P. Migne (ed.) *Patrologia . . . Series Graeca*, CXI (Paris, 1863), coll. 637–48. S. Murray, *A Study of the Life of Andreas, the Fool for the Sake of Christ* (Borna and Leipzig, 1910), includes a useful summary of the *Life*. Dols, 'Insanity in Byzantine and Islamic Medicine', p. 146. Controversy over the date of the text is summarized and taken a step further by Rydén, 'The "Life" of St Basil the Younger and the Date of the "Life" of St Andreas Salos', in C. Mango and

VI

I end this survey of the plight of the insane in Byzantium with a small incident from an East Syrian verse panegyric of an early eighth-century saint, John of Daylam. It concerns sorcery rather than possession, but makes a pertinent point.[86]

There was a handsome deacon in Basra whose speech had been impaired by sorcerers for eight years. His mother had first taken him to a monastery, but he received no healing 'either from the monastery or from anyone else'. She then took him to Galenic doctors, then to some sorcerers, and to 'the wicked whom the demons had deceived'. Of course, none of these could alleviate the impediment. Finally she heard about John, who happened to be visiting the city. The rest can be surmised. The following Sunday the handsome deacon read the Epistles in church, to universal astonishment. On this occasion, then, a cure proved possible. But it was a 'close-run thing'. Without John's chance visit the deacon would have remained mute. What is of interest about the 'hierarchy of resort' exhibited in the mother's choice of successive healers is that the monastery comes first – and fails – and that physicians and sorcerers are also included.[87]

Reading such a panegyric, we know that the saint will eventually triumph. I would suggest that for those not so blessed as to encounter their saint at the right moment, the picture would have looked rather different, and the possibility of escape from demonic or mental impairment rather more distant. As in medieval Islam, there is a great deal more to the history of possession than descriptions of triumphant exorcism. We should give the saints of Byzantium their due – but no more than that.

Acknowledgements

Earlier versions of this paper were presented at conferences or seminars in Madrid, Oxford, and Princeton. I am most grateful to all participants, but especially to Peter Brown, John Gager, and Judith Herrin for generous advice and valuable references.

O. Pritsak (eds.) *Okeanos: Essays presented to Ihor Ševčenko, Harvard Ukrainian Studies,* VII (1983), 568–86. An edition by Rydén of the *Life* of Andrew is forthcoming. I have not seen P. Cesaretti (ed. and trans.) *I santi folli di Bisanzio: Vita di Simeone Salos, Vita di Andrea Salos, Uomini e religioni,* 53 (Milan, 1990).

[86] S. P. Brock, 'A Syriac Life of John of Daylam', *Parole de l'Orient,* X (1981–82), 166–7.

[87] On the notion of the hierarchy of resort, Horden, 'Saints and Doctors', pp. 12–13.

XIII

Disease, dragons and saints: the management of epidemics in the Dark Ages

Dragons exist. Let us begin with the effort of imagination necessary to make that assertion plausible. Let us entertain the idea that never having seen a dragon may reflect only narrowness of experience. Others have, if not encountered the beast, at least come close to doing so. Here is the opening of a paper by the anthropologist Dan Sperber, appropriately entitled 'Apparently Irrational Beliefs'. It takes the form of a quotation from his field diary:

> [*Dorze, Southern Ethiopia*]
> *Sunday 24 viii* 69
>
> Saturday morning old Filate came to see me in a state of great excitement: 'Three times I came to see you, and you weren't there! ... Do you want to do something? ... If you do it, God will be pleased, the Government will be pleased. So?'
> 'Well, if it is a good thing and I can do it, I shall do it.'
> 'I have talked to no one about it: will you kill it?'
> '*Kill*? Kill what?'
> 'Its heart is made of gold, it has one horn on the nape of its neck. It is golden all over. It does not live far, two days' walk at most. If you kill it, you will become a great man!'
> And so on ... It turns out Filate wants me to kill a dragon. He is to come back this afternoon with someone who has seen it, and they will tell me more ...[1]

Filate did not return – to the anthropologist's embarrassed relief.

I am grateful to Edward Hussey, Emily Kearns, Gwyn Prins, Nicholas Purcell, Richard Smith and Ian Wood for advice and references on various matters. I am particularly indebted to Peter Brown for commenting on my draft.
[1] D. Sperber, *On Anthropological Knowledge* (Cambridge and Paris, 1985), p. 35.

XIII

A report of another dragon narrowly missed can be found in
Carlo Levi's classic *Christ Stopped at Eboli*, a description of his exile
by the fascist government to a remote Lucanian village. In a nearby
hillside church with a miraculous Madonna 'were preserved the
horns of a dragon which in ancient times had infested the region'.

> Everyone ... had been to see these horns, but unfortunately I
> could not fulfil my wish to do so. The dragon, they told me, once
> lived in a cave near the river; it devoured the peasants, carried off
> their daughters, filled the land with its pestiferous breath, and
> destroyed the crops, until life ... became impossible.

Only the effort of a mighty prince emboldened by an apparition of
the Madonna enabled the villagers to return to their homes. In the
mid-1930s peasants still made pilgrimages to gaze at the vanquished
monster's horns. 'Nor would it be strange if dragons were to appear
again today before the startled eyes of the country people.'[2] For
them as for old Filate – and doubtless for numerous others still –
dragons exist. They are a part of nature: a cause of environmental
disaster. In addition, as part of some divinely created order, they
may bear a weighty symbolic charge. They may have to be interpreted as well as slain. For Sperber's and Levi's informants, however, the brute fact of dragons' natural existence seems to be
primary. The heroes who slay them may please God or the government. But their achievement is above all to have made normal life
possible once again – by removing an ecological hazard.

I

I begin in the recent past, with identifiable individuals and their
ostensibly uncluttered beliefs, as an attempted corrective to the
habitual procedure of those who study dragons academically. It is
all too easy to dismiss Filate or the Lucanian villagers as simply the
passive beneficiaries of a vast and diverse heritage of legend accumu-
lated over millennia – as if nothing in their immediate experience
could have contributed to the formation of their beliefs.[3] Such easy

[2] *Christ Stopped at Eboli* (Harmondsworth, 1982), pp. 110–11. Cf. F. Huxley, *The Dragon: Nature of Spirit, Spirit of Nature* (London, 1979), p. 5.
[3] Huxley, *The Dragon*, is an attractive compendium. Useful collections of references, and full bibliographies, can be had from *Reallexikon für Antike und Christentum*, IV (Stuttgart, 1959), *s.v.* 'Drache', and the briefer entries in *Lexikon des Mitte-lalters*, III (Munich and Zurich, 1986), *s.v.* 'Drache', and *Encyclopedia of Religion*, IV (New York and London, 1987), *s.v.* 'Dragons'.

dismissal permits historians to ignore particular circumstances in favour of a large, undifferentiated 'background' of world mythology, and to indulge in a superficial comparativism. It also encourages them to treat notions about dragons far more as part of the history of symbolism than as an aspect of the history of science, of everyday ideas about nature. Such beliefs, like other manifestations of apparent irrationality, can then be summed up in one or more of the ways that philosophers and anthropologists have variously proposed: as pre-logical, as expressive or metaphorical, as semi-propositional, culturally relative, and so on – not to be taken entirely seriously.[4] The most absurd and otherwise inexplicable ideas can be allocated to folklore – as if, for the remoter past, that term possessed any sociological precision or explanatory power.[5]

In what follows, comparative mythology cannot wholly be avoided. But I hope to rescue at least one associated group of recorded dragons from this undisciplined realm and restore them to a possible local context – which I shall, at this preliminary stage, crudely describe as the malarial (or at least miasmatic) swamp. I want to envisage these dragons less as symbols with meanings than as animals with effects. I want to take seriously the epithet 'pestiferous' that, in Lucania and elsewhere, has so often been applied to them, and to ask what consequences so doing may have for our appreciation of the role of heroic dragon-slayers. And, so far as is possible when considering the early Middle Ages, I want to evoke the immediate ideological and material surroundings in which belief in pestiferous dragons might be sustained. These ambitions do not entail a positivist confidence that the genesis of myths or legends can be adequately accounted for by reference to specific historical events. Instead, they involve an attempt at what has (rather suitably for present purposes) been dubbed an 'epidemiology of representations' – an attempt to see why certain images or ideas prove more

---

[4] M. Hollis and S. Lukes (eds.), *Rationality and Relativism* (Oxford, 1982). See also D. Sperber, *Rethinking Symbolism* (Cambridge, 1975); and D. Sperber, 'Is Symbolic Thought Prerational?', in M. Foster and S. Brandes (eds.), *Symbol as Sense* (New York, 1980), pp. 25–44. Contrast C. R. Hallpike, *The Foundations of Primitive Thought* (Oxford, 1979), ch. 4; P. Veyne, *Did the Greeks Believe their Myths?* (Chicago and London, 1988).

[5] For the variety of folklorists' approaches to hagiography, from which much of the evidence for what follows here is drawn, see W. W. Heist, 'Hagiography, Chiefly Celtic, and Recent Developments in Folklore', in *Hagiographie, cultures et sociétés IVe–XIIe siècles* (Paris, 1981), pp. 121–41.

'contagious' than others and become part of a community's common stock.[6]

I do this as a way of advancing three general propositions, albeit to unequal extents. The first – admittedly hard to defend using medieval evidence – is that malaria has yet to be given due prominence by historians of morbidity and crisis mortality. After a long period in historiography during which the disease was invoked to explain far too much – the decline of states, the vicissitudes of the economy and the like – we have only quite recently settled down to an appreciation of its complex ecology, its more subtle demographic effects and the conditions under which its incidence may grow to epidemic proportions.[7] The second and third propositions are interrelated, and provide the justification for my subtitle, 'the management of epidemics'. The second proposition is that while much attention has been given to the iconography of medicine, too little has been devoted to representations of disease. Historical notions of contagion have been discussed, but not ideas of the diseases being transmitted. There is a history here that has yet to be examined in more than desultory fashion. It would begin in antiquity with such arresting items as the Greek personification of diarrhoea possibly referred to by (?pseudo-)Empedocles, the Roman *Dea Febris* and Robigo, and the beggar who embodies disease in the *Life* of Apollonius of Tyana. And it would continue right through to

[6] D. Sperber, 'Anthropology and Psychology: Towards an Epidemiology of Representations', *Man*, n.s., 20 (1985), pp. 73–89. On the perils of adducing historical evidence for dragon combats, see F. W. Hasluck, 'Dieudonné de Gozon and the Dragon of Rhodes', *Annual of the British School of Athens*, 20 (1913–14), pp. 73–6; L. Dumont, *La Tarasque* (Paris, 1951), pp. 13–14, on the 'rationalising' of processional dragons. See more generally F. Graus, *Volk, Herrscher und Heiliger im Reich der Merowinger* (Prague, 1965), pp. 11ff, 28ff.

[7] Examples of those who invoke malaria to explain too much: W. H. S. Jones, *Malaria and Greek History* (Manchester, 1909); A. Celli, *The History of Malaria in the Roman Campagna from Ancient Times* (London, 1933); C. Laderman, 'Malaria and Progress: Some Ecological and Historical Considerations', *Social Science and Medicine*, 9 (1975), pp. 587–94; L. Bruce–Chwatt and J. de Zulueta, *The Rise and Fall of Malaria in Europe* (Oxford, 1980). Correctives: L. W. Hackett, *Malaria in Europe* (London and Oxford, 1937); P. A. Brunt, *Italian Manpower* (Oxford, 1971), appendix 18; P. Toubert, *Les Structures du Latium Médiéval*, 2 vols. (Rome, 1973), II, pp. 363–4; M. D. Grmek, *Diseases in the Ancient Greek World* (Baltimore and London, 1989), pp. 275–83. Historical demographers have unfortunately done little work on the disease. There are few European equivalents to the publications of M. J. Dobson. Cf. '"Marsh Fever": The Geography of Malaria in England', *Journal of Historical Geography*, 6 (1980), pp. 357–89; 'Mortality Gradients and Disease Exchanges: Comparisons from Old England and Colonial America', *Social History of Medicine*, 2 (1989), pp. 259–97.

relatively modern times.[8] This history might be thought to constitute evidence of the management of epidemics in a *conceptual* sense. A potent image, pre-eminently such as that of the dragon, provides a means of reducing to a single 'contagious' representation an involved aetiology that is perhaps barely accessible to modern experimental science.[9] The third proposition, to which I can return only briefly at the end, concerns the management of epidemics at a *practical* level. It is that the means of controlling a potentially epidemic disease (such as malaria) may in the past have been less formal, less medical or technological in character than has usually been supposed – at least by medievalists and ancient historians.

II

I have introduced dragons and the management of epidemic disease. I must now present my saints. As with the dragons in question, I shall focus on one particular saint and adduce others more briefly for clarification. The principal is in some respects not the one who best exemplifies my argument. But I shall begin and end with him (turning to other saints in between) both because he has already

---

[8] Three types of disease (dry, putrefactive, wet) haunt 'the meadow of disaster': H. Diels and W. Krantz, *Die Fragmente der Vorsokratiker*, 6th edn, 3 vols. (Berlin, 1951), I, p. 360, B121; three types of fever (presumably quotidian, tertian and quartan) appear as three women in the autobiography of Guibert of Nogent, *Self and Society in Medieval France*, ed. J. F. Benton (New York and Evanston, 1970), p. 141; cholera, smallpox and plague as three demons in modern Athenian folklore: J. C. Lawson, *Modern Greek Folklore and Ancient Greek Religion* (Cambridge, 1910), pp. 21ff. The spirit of an epidemic apparently takes the form first of a beggar then of a huge rabid hound in Philostratus's *Life* of Apollonius of Tyana, IV, 10 (Loeb edn, I, pp. 362-6). Other ancient disease personifications: Roman *Dea Febris* and Robigo, see G. Wissowa *et al.* (eds.), *Paulys Real-encyclopädie der classischen Altertumswissenschaft*, *s.vv.* 'Febris', 'Robigalia'; Greek equivalent: K. Deichgräber, 'Parabasenverse aus Thesmophoriazusen II des Aristophanes bei Galen', *Sitzungsberichte der Deutschen Akademie der Wissenschaften zu Berlin: Klasse für Sprachen, Literatur und Kunst* (1956), no. 2, pp. 34-8. Pestilence as tornado-like column of vapour: 'Life of St. Teilo', *The Text of the Book of Llan Dav*, ed. J. G. Evans and J. Rhys (Oxford, 1893), p. 107. S. Thompson, *Motif-Index of Folk Literature*, 2nd edn, 6 vols. (Copenhagen, 1955-8), III, pp. 131-2, F493. An Indian comparison: E. C. Dimock Jnr, 'A Theology of the Repulsive: The Myth of the Goddess Sītalā', in J. S. Hawley and D. M. Wulff (eds.), *The Divine Consort: Rādhā and the Goddesses of India* (Boston, Mass., 1982), pp. 184–203.

[9] Cf. M. Last, 'The Importance of Knowing about Not Knowing', *Social Science and Medicine*, 15 B (1981), pp. 387–92, on the preferred absence of systematic knowledge in a traditional medical culture. Sperber, 'Anthropology and Psychology', pp. 85–6.

50

been the subject of an influential study and because his sphere of operation can be mapped with relative clarity. He takes his place in a long line of dragon-slayers and tamers of whom the Babylonian god Marduk is perhaps the oldest, St George is the best known and the anthropologist Dan Sperber is (in a sense) the most recent. His name was Marcellus and he probably became bishop of Paris during the first part of the fifth century, dying in about 436. (The ecclesiastical historian must tread cautiously here because there is a little room for doubt about the saint's historicity. Dragons exist, but bishops may be mythical creatures.[10]) In the present context, however, it is the later representation of Marcellus rather than the original reality that is mainly important. For information about this we must turn to his sole biographer.

Venantius Fortunatus, himself a bishop as well as a major poet and hagiographer, was commissioned to write a *Life* of Marcellus by one of the saint's successors as bishop of Paris, Germanus.[11] Since Fortunatus dedicated his work to Germanus, he must have completed it by the time of Germanus's death in 576. He was thus writing well over a century later than the events that he describes, and in somewhat different cultural surroundings. (During the sixth century much of Gaul passed under the political control of the Merovingian Franks.) Also, he was clearly short of material. The *Life* of Marcellus fills no more than six pages in the standard edition.[12]

There was an additional source of embarrassment. Marcellus was

[10] M. Vieillard-Troiekouroff *et al.*, 'Les Anciennes Eglises suburbaines de Paris (IVe–Xe siècles)', *Paris et Ile-de-France*, 11 (1960), p. 122; E. Griffe, *La Gaule chrétienne à l'époque romaine*, rev. edn, 3 vols. (Paris, 1964–6), I, p. 305.

[11] On Fortunatus, see W. Wattenbach and W. Levison, *Deutschlands Geschichtsquellen im Mittelalter: Vorzeit und Karolinger*, 2 vols. (Weimar, 1952), I, pp. 96–9; P. Godman, *Poets and Emperors: Frankish Politics and Carolingian Poetry* (Oxford, 1983), ch. 1; J. M. Wallace-Hadrill, *The Frankish Church* (Oxford, 1983), pp. 82–8. See also R. Collins, 'Observations on the Form, Language and Public of the Prose Biographies of Venantius Fortunatus in the Hagiography of Merovingian Gaul', in H. B. Clarke and M. Brennan (eds.), *Columbanus and Merovingian Monasticism*, British Archaeological Reports international ser. CXIII (Oxford, 1981), pp. 105–31. On Germanus the essential references are collected in R. Van Dam (trans.), *Gregory of Tours: Glory of the Confessors* (Liverpool, 1988), p. 93 n. 99. On possible reasons for the promotion of Marcellus's cult, A. Lombard-Jourdan, 'Du nouveau sur les origines chrétiennes de Paris: une relecture de Fortunat', *Paris et Ile-de-France*, 32 (1981), pp. 125–60.

[12] *Vita Marcelli*, *Monumenta Germaniae Historica* (hereafter *MGH*), *Auctores Antiquissimi* (hereafter *AA*), IV, 2, ed. B. Krusch (1885), pp. 49–54. General context: Wallace-Hadrill, *Frankish Church*; R. Van Dam, *Leadership and Community in*

of humble origin (born to 'mediocris parentibus'). And by the sixth century it had become widely abhorrent that a future prince of the church should not (in Lady Bracknell's phrase) 'rise from the ranks of the aristocracy'. Indeed, for such a common fellow as Marcellus to have clawed his way up the ecclesiastical hierarchy could only be accounted a miracle.[13] But that, of course, exactly fitted the hagiographer's requirement. Marcellus was to be portrayed as a saint. The performance of miracles before or after death was, and remained, the one essential sign of sanctity. The personal details of the man's life were less important than his conformity to type.[14]

I shall briefly survey Marcellus's few recorded miracles. The last of these is the one that is of particular interest here. But the character of the others provides a useful hint of things to come. The miracle that heralds Marcellus's entry into the priesthood occurs when the saint is challenged by a smith to determine the weight of a piece of red-hot iron. Marcellus takes it in his hand and volunteers a very precise measurement – which is later proved accurate. Such scientific know-how and immunity to extreme physical discomfort are what we have learned to expect of the early medieval holy man.[15] The second miracle resembles that wrought by Christ at the marriage of Cana. Marcellus is drawing water from the Seine. He offers some to his bishop so that he can wash his hands. The water promptly turns to wine. Although the bishop uses it to give communion to all present, the quantity of wine remains undiminished. Many of those who have tasted it, moreover, are subsequently cured of their ailments. Some time later the same bishop is struck dumb when he orders the flogging of a disobedient priest. Marcellus's intercession enables him to regain the power of speech. Who better, then, to

Late Antique Gaul (Berkeley, Los Angeles and London, 1985); P. J. Geary, *Before France and Germany* (New York and Oxford, 1988).

[13] *Vita Marcelli*, 4 (p. 50). On the attempted aristocratic monopoly of bishoprics and sanctity in Merovingian Francia see Graus, *Volk*, pp. 362ff; M. Heinzelmann, *Bischofsherrschaft in Gallien*, Beihefte der Francia V (Zurich and Munich, 1976); Collins, 'Venantius Fortunatus', p. 114; Geary, *Before France and Germany*, pp. 123ff.

[14] Gregory of Tours, *Liber Vitae Patrum*, preface, *MGH, Scriptores Rerum Merovingicarum* (hereafter *SRM*), I, ed. Krusch *et al.* (1885), p. 662 (for the various writings of Gregory, all subsequent page references are to this edition). Wallace-Hadrill, *Frankish Church*, p. 79.

[15] *Vita Marcelli*, 5 (p. 51). Background: P. Brown, *Society and the Holy in Late Antiquity* (London, 1982), pp. 103–52. For Roman Gaul and Francia, see C. Stancliffe, *St Martin and his Hagiographer* (Oxford, 1983); Van Dam, *Leadership and Community*.

succeed the man as bishop on his death? While bishop, Marcellus performs those miraculous deeds of patronage and protection that the age expected from its heroes. For example, a prisoner is miraculously released from his chains and then, absolved by Marcellus, he is freed from the greater bondage of sin.[16]

What is striking about these miracles is that they mostly involve mastery of nature. Marcellus can turn the water of the Seine into health-giving wine, an easier feat in his time than it would be now but admirable nonetheless. Such an achievement benefits the whole community, not just select individuals. From Marcellus this community learns to expect a quasi-scientific expertise, a swift and practical solution to problems, an enhancement of corporate well-being. That much is confirmed by Marcellus's last miracle, 'illud triumphale mysterium'.

This is the story as Fortunatus tells it.[17] A noble woman of sullied reputation dies blind and is placed in her tomb. A dragon or monstrous snake (draco, serpens inmanissimus, belua) sets about devouring her body. Members of her family, still nearby, hear the noise and rush to the tomb. They see a huge monster leave the tomb, uncoiling itself and whipping the air with its tail. Terrified, they abandon the place – even to the point of migrating from their homes ('de suis sedibus migraverunt'). When Marcellus is informed, he gathers the people of Paris together. He orders them to stand within sight of the tomb and marches forward to do battle. The dragon comes out of the wood (to which it has presumably retreated) and returns to the tomb; Marcellus prays; and the dragon approaches him with bowed head and trailing tail to ask pardon. Marcellus subdues it by striking its head three times with his pastoral staff and putting his stole around its neck. 'Thus,' Fortunatus writes, 'in a spiritual theatre [or perhaps arena], with the populace looking on, he alone fought with the dragon.' Amazed by his performance, the audience of this theatre runs up to have a closer look at the captured enemy. Then, with the bishop leading, almost three thousand people form a procession with the dragon at its head and they celebrate the monster's exequies. Marcellus then reprimands the somehow still

---

[16] *Vita Marcelli*, 6 (p. 51), 8–9 (pp. 52–3). On the liberation of prisoners, see F. Graus, 'Die Gewalt bei den Anfängen des Feudalismus und die "Gefangenenbefreiungen" der merowingischen Hagiographie', *Jahrbuch für Wirtschaftsgeschichte*, 1 (1961), pp. 61–156; E. James, ' "Beati Pacifici": Bishops and the Law in Sixth-Century Gaul', in J. Bossy (ed.), *Disputes and Settlements* (Cambridge, 1983), pp. 33–6.

[17] *Vita Marcelli*, 10 (pp. 53–4).

living beast, and tells it to stay either in the desert or in the sea. The dragon disappears.

This edifying tale has been analysed before. Most influentially, Jacques Le Goff made it the subject of a substantial paper that he originally published in 1970.[18] As in a number of his other works, Le Goff was here concerned to elaborate a distinction between clerical culture and popular culture. The clerical culture of the early Middle Ages portrays the combat with the dragon in relatively simple terms, as involving an embodiment of the Devil or of paganism. In doing so, this culture is attempting to transform, as Le Goff puts it, 'a monster that had formerly carried one of the most complex symbolisms in the history of culture'. Popular culture, for Le Goff, embraces this complexity. The people in Marcellus's spiritual theatre had 'invested the same symbol with an ambiguous value as a result of a long series of contaminations and metamorphoses'. The potential sources of these are vast. Le Goff ranges from China to Ireland, across what he distinguishes as Germano-Asiatic, Graeco-Roman and autochthonous dragon lore. He then writes confidently: 'underlying all these traditions, do we not find the quasi-universal serpent-dragon common to all primitive beliefs and myths? Was not the Merovingian dragon above all a monster of folklore which had resurfaced during an interregnum between two beliefs, when pagan culture was fading before the Christian cultural system had really taken root?' And he concludes that the story of Marcellus's taming of the dragon is essentially a foundation myth. The bishop's victory represents the subjugation of the hostile forces of nature. Marcellus's miracle makes possible both cultivation and settlement.[19]

My purpose is far more to supplement this analysis than to quarrel with it. There is much to command immediate assent. First, Le Goff notes that two different stories involving dragons appear to have been run together in the narrative of the saint's last miracle.

---

[18] 'Ecclesiastical Culture and Folklore in the Middle Ages: Saint Marcellus of Paris and the Dragon', first published in L. de Rosa (ed.), *Ricerche Storiche ed Economiche in Memoria di Corrado Barbagallo*, 3 vols. (Naples, 1970), II, pp. 51–90. I have for convenience used the translation: *Time, Work, and Culture in the Middle Ages* (Chicago and London, 1980), pp. 159–88. In what follows it will be clear that I am overwhelmingly indebted to Le Goff's piece as an abundant source of references and ideas, and also that I am not concerned with the second half of his paper (pp. 174ff), on the later medieval cult of Marcellus.

[19] Le Goff, 'Marcellus', pp. 162, 172.

54

The opening story – of the adulteress whose entombed corpse the monster devours – has a history of its own that need not be pursued here.[20] We should certainly register the implied correspondence between the various elements in Fortunatus's paragraph: between the woman's loss of moral and sexual integrity, the violation of her tomb (which should have been a place of order and repose), and the disruption of the whole pattern of settlement.[21] Yet it is the dragon as communal enemy rather than individual nemesis that dominates the narrative and demands attention. Secondly, Le Goff rightly points out that in the later of the two stories Fortunatus hardly represents his hero's dragon as diabolical in character. There is not, perhaps, 'a total absence of symbolic interpretation'.[22] Fortunatus after all emphasises the 'spiritual' aspect both of the weapons that the saint deploys – prayer, crook and stole, frail fingers – and of the context in which he performs – a theatre or arena. In the saint's injunction to the monster to confine itself to the desert or the sea, moreover, there is a strong hint of a formula of exorcism.[23] Yet, overall, the dragon-slaying saint does appear 'in his worldly role as chief of an urban community'. Thirdly, when seen in the widest context, the dragon is certainly a 'polyvalent' creature. Late antique and early medieval Christianity could not avoid bearing the imprint of a number of traditions in which Marcellus's combat is foreshadowed. And these traditions do imply the freeing for human occupation of an initially unpromising site and the taming of natural forces.[24]

There are, however, two aspects of Le Goff's analysis that seem to me to hinder understanding of the significance of the saint's dragon-taming for sixth-century Parisians. The first of them is the sheer number of dragon legends that we are offered by way of background. There are no established criteria of relevance to Fortunatus's

---

[20] *Ibid.*, p. 162 nn. 12, 28. Cf. 'Apocalypse of Paul', *New Testament Apocrypha*, ed. E. Hennecke and W. Schneemelcher, 2 vols. (London, 1963–5), II, p. 783 n. 4.

[21] I owe the point to Peter Brown.

[22] Le Goff, 'Marcellus', p. 164.

[23] Cf. the prayer of exorcism (misattributed to St Basil) quoted by C. Mango, *Byzantium* (London, 1980), p. 160, from J. Goar, *Euchologion sive Rituale Graecorum* (Paris, 1647), pp. 730–1; A. Franz, *Die kirchlichen Benediktionen im Mittelalter*, 2 vols. (Freiburg im Breisgau, 1909), II, pp. 547ff.

[24] Cf. P. Boglioni, 'Il Santo e gli Animali nell'alto medioevo', *Settimane di Studio . . . Spoleto*, 31, 2 (1985), pp. 970ff. Contrast H. Delehaye, 'Euchaïta et la Légende de S. Théodore', in W. H. Buckler and W. M. Calder (eds.), *Anatolian Studies Presented to Sir William Ramsay* (Manchester, 1923), p. 131.

text. It is not therefore clear that, say, the Egyptian Seth or Cadmus of Thebes exerted any great pressure on the minds of sixth-century Franks. Nor can we be confident that Asiatic dragons were beginning to make a discernible impact on the Franks' repertoire of monstrous imagery during the Merovingian period.[25]

The second difficulty arises from the sharp distinction that Le Goff draws between his two cultures, and his tendency to represent each of them as homogeneous. Perhaps there was a determinate clerical culture in the early Middle Ages – a culture that derived its ideas about dragons from the Bible, the Fathers and the earliest hagiography. But if so, it was far from speaking with one voice on the subject. As Le Goff himself reveals, there was for example a tradition of scientific thinking about monsters in which the indebtedness to antiquity is as striking as the absence of diabolical symbolism.[26] A satisfactory definition of popular culture proves even more elusive. For Le Goff it seems to be, on one hand, the residue of ancient mythology, a collection of 'quasi-universals' that survive more or less unchanged across millennia until they can be recorded by folklorists. On the other hand, it is apparently so amorphous that it must be defined in negative terms. It is non-clerical – which means that it is what cannot be found in the standard encyclopaedias of Christian thought. It is not literate – so that it breaks surface in the historical record of the early Middle Ages only when the repressive culture of the dominant class (clerical culture) is in disarray, and drops its literary guard.

Everything that we have learned in recent years from historians of cult practice, of language, of 'lay literacy', of the interaction between the written and the oral, of clerical and monastic taste in supposedly folkloric material, suggests that this Marxian typology is inadequate.[27] I would prefer to conceive Fortunatus's account of Marcellus

[25] Cf. Gregory of Tours, *Liber in Gloria Martyrum*, preface (p. 487); *Liber de Passione et Virtutibus Sancti Juliani Martyris*, 5 (pp. 566–7). E. Salin, *La Civilisation mérovingienne*, 4 vols. (Paris, 1949–59), IV, pp. 207ff, 241ff.

[26] Le Goff, 'Marcellus', pp. 166–7; *Reallexikon für Antike und Christentum*, *s.v.* 'Drache', cols. 226–7; Collins, 'Venantius Fortunatus', p. 97.

[27] P. Brown, *The Cult of the Saints* (London, 1981), ch. 1; R. McKitterick, *The Carolingians and the Written Word* (Cambridge, 1989); B. Stock, *The Implications of Literacy. Written Language and Models of Interpretation in the Eleventh and Twelfth Centuries* (Princeton, 1983); P. Wormald, 'Bede, "Beowulf" and the Conversion of the Anglo-Saxon Aristocracy', in R. T. Farrell (ed.), *Bede and Anglo-Saxon England*, British Archaeological Reports XLVI (Oxford, 1978), pp. 32–95.

56

less as a focus of tension between two widely differing cultures than as a point on the single spectrum of possible beliefs about monsters that formed part of the essentially unitary culture of Merovingian Francia. On this spectrum there is certainly room for the use of the dragon as pure symbol (metaphor rather than metonymy, to recall Jakobson's antithesis[28]). But at the heart of most propositions involving dragons is an acceptance of their material existence. In preparing his *Life* of the saint, Fortunatus needed oral testimony, for he had little or nothing in writing on which to base his narrative.[29] But there is no evidence that his informants were mainly the old Filates of sixth-century Paris. Nor are there any clear signs that he found his information ideologically repugnant – even though he was among the most educated men of his day. Recounting Marcellus's final miracle, he moves back and forth between the metaphorical and the metonymic within the space of two lines of text. His *Life* of the saint was, like all his hagiography, designed for both clerical and lay consumption. It would have been read annually to Parisian congregations, perhaps as part of the liturgy, on the day commemorating Marcellus's death. Its audience formed what has usefully been called a textual community. That community should, I believe, provide our frame of reference.[30]

III

I now wish to propose a reading of Fortunatus's text that takes its cue less from supposed universals of myth and folklore or models of cultural conflict than from a shared sense of locality between saint and populace, hagiographer and audience. The case that I hope to make cannot be properly supported in even the limited fashion with which medievalists must generally be content. As far as Marcellus is concerned, I have to go beyond, though I trust not against, the evidence. I cannot hope for 'glory' according to Humpty Dumpty's wilful definition – that is, 'a nice knock-down argument'. I certainly do not propose a complete revaluation of all early medieval dragons

---

[28] R. Jakobson, 'Two Aspects of Language and Two Types of Aphasic Disturbance', in R. Jakobson and M. Halle (eds.), *Fundamentals of Language* (The Hague, 1956), pp. 55–82.

[29] *Vita Marcelli*, 2 (p. 50). Does the mention of the date of the saint's death at the very end of the text suggest access to an episcopal list?

[30] Collins, 'Venantius Fortunatus', pp. 107–8; Stock, *Implications of Literacy*.

or even of the few on which I shall concentrate, but, rather, a hint of one particular pressure exerted upon those who spoke or wrote about them: the pressure of an epidemic upon an idea.

Recall first, from his earlier miracles, Marcellus's ability to assess the capacity of nature and turn possible harm to certain benefit. Recall in addition the report that the dragon whips the air with its tail, and that its ferocity compels Parisians to abandon their homes. Fortunatus identifies these Parisians as the dead woman's *familia*, but that may have been a device to harmonise the two stories that he or his informants had conjoined. Certainly by the end of his account the monster has become the 'public enemy'. The dragon seems to appear on the outskirts of the city. When it has left the woman's tomb it retreats to the woods. After subduing it, however, Marcellus banishes it to either desert or sea ('aut deserta . . . aut in mare'), in effect to water or wasteland. Thereafter, not even traces (*indicia*) of it are to be found.

To begin to clarify the possible implications of these ecological touches, we must look for analogues. An immediate comparison is suggested by Fortunatus himself, who concludes that 'Gaul should admire Marcellus as Rome does Silvester'.[31] The legend of Pope Silvester has usually been studied in connection with that renowned forgery, the Donation of Constantine. There is one version of the legend in which the pope manages to subjugate a dragon that lives in a rocky cave under the Capitol. When the heathens see that the monster really has at last been overcome, they convert to Christianity. The pope's battle with the dragon appears in this context to be equivalent to his victory over paganism. But there is another version of the legend, apparently favoured within Rome, according to which Silvester's dragon was a giant serpent washed ashore when the Tiber flooded. The pope's task becomes one of leadership in the response to natural disaster, the consequence of flooding.[32] Something of the perceived extent of the challenge is revealed by events in Rome in the time of Pope Gregory the Great.

Gregory of Tours, writing only a few years after the occasion that he purports to describe, recounts what his deacon told him on returning from Rome in 590. In November of the previous year the Tiber had flooded the city, destroying the papal granaries and a number of churches. 'A great school of water snakes swam down the

---

[31] *Vita Marcelli*, 10 (p. 54).   [32] Le Goff, 'Marcellus', p. 168 with nn. 45–7.

river to the sea, and in their midst was a tremendous dragon as big as a tree-trunk, but these monsters were drowned in the turbulent salt waves of the sea and their bodies were washed up on the shore.' An epidemic ensued – of plague. The first to succumb was Pelagius, the reigning pontiff. His successor, Gregory the Great, led the people in penitential processions. There was no dragon to combat: it had already died. But the association of dragons with the linked disasters of flooding and pestilence is noteworthy. (According to Gregory, torrential rains were among the signs preceding the arrival of plague in Gaul.)[33]

To determine Fortunatus's sources for the *Life* of Marcellus is not my aim. But it is a useful connection to make, a check on relevance, that he might have known Gregory's account. He might also have known the story, much later preserved by Isidore of Seville, about Donatus, a bishop of Epirus who would have been a near-contemporary of Marcellus. This bishop was said to have slain an enormous dragon whose breath and body turned the air putrid.[34]

Fortunatus's own work provides a further illuminating analogue of his story of Marcellus. It comes from his *Life* of St Hilary. The saint is passing the island of Gallinara, which lies opposite Albenga on the Ligurian coast. Coastal dwellers tell him of the innumerable serpents that infest the island, making settlement impossible. Although it is within sight of the mainland, its inaccessibility makes it seem further away than Africa. The serpents flee, however, at the sight of the saint. Hilary uses his episcopal staff as a marker to divide the island into two parts. The serpents are restricted to one sector, and cannot again trouble the other, even though a portion of the island – including, presumably, some of the sector now available for settlement – 'is not so much land as water' – lake or swamp. In contrasting Hilary with Adam, the hagiographer does here gloss these serpents as diabolical. But he emphatically ends this chapter in his narrative with the assertion that Hilary has opened up the island for human occupation.[35] And we might add, in a gloss of our own, that he has done it through some kind of technological insight. He

---

[33] *Libri Historiarum*, X, 1 (pp. 406–7); X, 23 (p. 435); quotation adapted from the translation by L. Thorpe, *Gregory of Tours: History of the Franks* (Harmondsworth, 1974), p. 543. Cf. Gregory the Great, *Dialogi*, III, 19, ed. A. de Vogüé, Sources Chrétiennes, 3 vols. (Paris, 1978–80), II, pp. 346–8.

[34] *Chronicon*, 107, ed. J.-P. Migne, *Patrologia Latina*, LXXXIII, col. 1051; Le Goff, 'Marcellus', p. 167.

[35] *Vita Hilarii*, 10, ed. Krusch, *MGH, AA*, IV, 2, p. 5.

manages the threat posed by the snakes; he knows where to draw the line between the safe and unsafe parts of the island.

After such analogues, it will be asked, what of St George? A late version of his career, preserved in the *Golden Legend*, has the saint living in a great swamp near the town of Silene in Libya. The inhabitants are daily being killed by the dragon's breath, and the survivors offer up their children to appease it until none is left but the king's daughter. The rest of the story is now familiar. But it would not have been so in the sixth century. The cult of George had indeed spread to Gaul – despite papal prohibition. But his fight with the dragon was apparently not then part of his legend.[36]

If we must exclude St George, there are nonetheless other Frankish hagiographical dragons that can helpfully be set alongside the one challenged by Marcellus. In the story of the conversion of the martyr Afra, a Carolingian text, a dragon is to be found living near a spring in the Julian Alps. It allows no one to drink there; indeed its breath kills all who approach. It is not simply a manifestation of the Devil, for only a ruse of Narcissus, the bishop involved, transfers into its body the demon that has been possessing Afra.[37] The pestilential quality of the monster is not always so explicit. But the dragons or serpents (it would be a mistake to distinguish between them too carefully) that are quite often reported as infesting wells or other sources of water are clearly capable of a variety of harms: they can do more than coil and bite.[38]

Gregory of Tours, for example, includes in his anthology of local saints, the *Book of the Life of the Fathers*, the curious tale of the hermit Caluppa. He is one day confronted in his cave by two enormous dragons. Gregory pronounces one of them stronger than the other and thus 'the very chief of every temptation', the Devil. While the saint is conquering this animal with the power of the cross, the second monster entwines itself around his legs. It too is expelled from the cave (by prayer). But as a parting shot it lets out 'a formidable noise from its rear end', filling the little cell with a great stink. For Gregory, such eructation must, again, be a sign of the Devil's work: he appears far more reluctant than Fortunatus to

---

[36] *Reallexikon für Antike und Christentum*, cols. 245–6; Gregory of Tours, *Liber in Gloria Martyrum*, 100 (pp. 554–5).

[37] *Conversio Afrae*, 7, ed. Krusch, *MGH, SRM*, III (1896), p. 60. Contrast the allegorical interpretation in *Reallexikon für Antike und Christentum*, col. 248.

[38] Cf. *Vita Iohannis Abbatis Reomanensis*, 2, ed. Krusch, *MGH, SRM*, III (1896), p. 507: serpent infests a well.

accept the metonymic character of his sources, even though the hermit was his near-contemporary and, at the end of the story, the reader is left wondering why two diabolical dragons, unequal in strength, should have been included.[39] The dragon's lingering stench may have been differently construed by those who transmitted the story. Gregory himself, moreover, is happy elsewhere to adopt a naturalistic account of a giant serpent that inhabits a field. It has been devastating an entire region, causing widespread panic and depopulation. The saint who deals with it is no less than the Apostle Andrew. As the serpent dies, it coils itself around an oak tree, and vomits a river of blood – and poison. The apostle goes on to bring back from the dead one of those whom the serpent has smitten.[40]

In another piece of hagiography, ostensibly Merovingian but perhaps a Carolingian forgery, the young St Amand frees a whole island from imminent danger by miraculously compelling a huge snake to retreat to its cave.[41] In this account the nature of the threat is not specified at all. But some idea of its possible consequences may perhaps be gained from a different part of the *Life*, where the 'ingens plaga' ('great disaster' – or perhaps 'great plague') visited upon those who ignore the saint's preaching is described with a certain vividness: 'houses collapsed, fields were made into solitudes, even small towns and forts were destroyed, and hardly anyone remained in these regions of those who had despised the preaching of the man of God'.[42] The two episodes in the *Life* are not directly connected – unless, that is, one ignores the naturalistic tone of the author and interprets both as signs of the Devil's work. But the second one (just quoted) does show us that the hagiographer envisaged the saving power of the saint in terms of corporate material well-being. And his evocation may suggest, to the incautious, nothing so much as the aftermath of some epidemic.

---

[39] *Liber Vitae Patrum*, XI, 1 (pp. 709–10), trans. E. James, *Gregory of Tours: Life of the Fathers* (Liverpool, 1985), pp. 88–9. *Libri Historiarum*, V, 9 (p. 199). Cf. Wallace-Hadrill, *Frankish Church*, pp. 81–2.

[40] *Liber de Miraculis Beati Andreae Apostoli*, 19 (p. 837). On the matter of authorship, and the original that was adapted, see K. Zelzer, 'Zur Frage des Autors der Miracula B. Andreae Apostoli und zur Sprache des Gregor von Tours', *Grazer Beiträge*, 6 (1977), pp. 217–41.

[41] *Vita Amandi*, 2, ed. Krusch, *MGH, SRM*, V (1910), p. 440, trans. J. N. Hillgarth, *Christianity and Paganism, 350–750* (Philadelphia, 1986), p. 140. On the question of authenticity, see I. N. Wood, 'Forgery in Merovingian Hagiography', *Fälschungen im Mittelalter*, MGH Schriften XXXIII (Hanover, 1988), V, pp. 371–2.

[42] *Vita Amandi*, 19 (p. 443), trans. Hillgarth, *Christianity*, p. 146.

I must clearly not urge too strongly a purely nosological explanation of this cluster of sources. But a loosely connected group of recurrent images can be said to have emerged. The dragon makes its home in fields or standing water of some kind. It prevents access to the pure spring. Its insides or its exhalations are lethal. It is in the strict sense of the word epidemic, affecting not just individuals.[43] It can cause widespread depopulation. Sometimes it is an embodiment of the Devil – though that need hardly make it any the less pestiferous, for the Devil is quite capable of causing epidemics, whatever form he assumes.[44] The texts invoked present something rather different from foundation myths, partly because in some there is already habitation in the area where the dragon wreaks its destruction, partly because the making available of an area of land that occurs in others does not apparently signify the origin of a determinate settlement. The dragon-slayer is the figure who renders safe a whole route or area, who demarcates the waste and the habitable, contains the environmental hazard and, it can be added, given the dragon's noxious breath, makes the area salubrious.

This attempt to capture the implications of the hagiography may be strengthened by looking at evidence that does not specifically relate to dragon-slaying. One form of dragon is a monstrous snake. It is we, not early medieval commentators, who make a distinction of terminology (and ontology) between the two. Snakes, of whatever size, can obviously be harmful, both individually, as the remedies for snake bite in the medical texts of the early Middle Ages remind us,[45] and collectively. The image of snakes infecting the whole world with their poison goes back at least to the Emperor Diocletian's Edict against the Manichaeans.[46] And we can perhaps relate to it one of the more curious anecdotes in the *Book of Histories* by Gregory of

---

[43] Cf. *Lacnunga*, 80, ed. J. H. G. Grattan and C. Singer, *Anglo-Saxon Magic and Medicine* (London, 1952), pp. 152–5: origin of diseases in pieces of serpent smitten by Woden.

[44] Gregory of Tours, *Liber Vitae Patrum*, XVII, 3–4 (pp. 730–1).

[45] See Marcellus Burdigalensis, *De Medicamentis Liber*, XXXV, 8, ed. M. Niedermann and E. Liechtenhan, Corpus Medicorum Latinorum V, 2 vols. (Berlin, 1968), II, pp. 588–90; W. Bonser, *The Medical Background of Anglo-Saxon England* (London, 1963), ch. 20. Cf. Sulpicius Severus, *Dialogi*, I, 25, ed. C. Halm, Corpus Scriptorum Ecclesiasticorum Latinarum, I (1866), p. 177.

[46] P. Brown, *Religion and Society in the Age of Saint Augustine* (London, 1972), p. 95. Cf. Eusebius, *Historia Ecclesiastica*, VII, 31. The image's subsequent history is examined in P. Courcelle, 'Le Serpent à face humaine dans la numismatique impériale du Ve siècle', in R. Chevallier (ed.), *Mélanges d'archéologie et d'histoire offerts à André Piganiol*, 3 vols. (Paris, 1966), I, pp. 343–53.

62

Tours. The discovery in the mud blocking a drain of a snake and rat, fashioned in bronze and presumably pagan cultic objects, heralds the infestation of the city by large numbers of both animals, and a 'plague' of fires.[47]

A further passage in Gregory's writings deserves consideration in this context.

> In the territory of Javols there was a mountain . . . that contained a large lake. At a fixed time a crowd of rustics went there and, as if offering libations to the lake, threw [into it] linen cloths and garments that served men as clothing. Some [threw] pelts of wool, many [threw] models of cheese and wax and bread as well as various other objects . . . They came with their wagons; they brought food and drink, sacrificed animals, and feasted for three days.[48]

The models may have been votive offerings of the kind that had long been an established feature of cultic practice in Gaul. And the whole episode is frequently cited as an example of how cunningly bishops in Francia dealt with enduring instances of rural paganism.[49] For the bishop simply diverted the revellers into a church that he had built nearby. But his mildly ungrammatical exhortation, 'nulla est religio in stagnum' – literally and most effectively translated as 'there is no religion in a lake' – can perhaps be taken as an indication of a more general problem that the Frankish church had to confront: an awareness of the potentially dangerous forces – dragons certainly among them – that could issue from standing water and that would require propitiation. Without reverting to Le Goff's interpretation of dragon combats as no more than symbols of the church's victory over paganism, we could nonetheless see Marcellus's great victory as another way of proclaiming: 'nulla est religio in stagnum'. The destructive power of waste or water could be far more effectively dealt with by a bishop than by a model made of cheese. The celebrations could signal not just temporary appeasement of that power (as in Gregory's vignette) but its permanent negation.

[47] *Libri Historiarum*, VIII, 33 (pp. 349–50).

[48] *Liber in Gloria Confessorum*, 2 (p. 750), trans. Van Dam, *Glory of the Confessors*, p. 19. Cf. Brown, *Cult of the Saints*, pp. 125–6, with discussion but mistaken reference.

[49] S. Deyts, *Les Bois sculptés des sources de la Seine* (Paris, 1983); Wallace-Hadrill, *Frankish Church*, ch. 2, esp. p. 29. Cf. G. Traina, *Paludi e Bonifiche del Mondo Antico* (Rome, 1988), pp. 120–4.

I have set out evidence to support the proposal that we envisage some of the monsters infesting the pages of Merovingian and related early medieval hagiography as dragons of epidemic disease, and therefore that we recognise in some feats of dragon-slaying a means of restoring salubrity. This is, I submit, at least a possible interpretation of the sources. To demonstrate that it is a possibility quite clearly capable of being realised in medieval hagiography, whatever our final assessment of the Merovingian evidence, I turn to another corpus of texts not entirely remote from those already reviewed.

IV

'If we take the Celtic world as a whole,' Le Goff noted, 'certain areas are swarming with dragons.'[50] A good many of them are aquatic monsters. They emerge from standing water. A certain amount of what we initially find is, indeed, familiar, particularly in Irish sources (both Latin and vernacular). St Molua saves two young swimmers from a beast pursuing them across a lake, and then, when the monster attempts to climb on to dry land, orders it to return to the lake and stay there – rather as Marcellus despatched his dragon. St Samthanne confronts another lacustrine beast, dangerous to men and animals alike. The Latin *Life* of Abbanus is more detailed than most. Here, the saint first causes a poisonous leonine monster that is terrorising the area literally to lie down and die. He is then besought by the people to deal with the equally poisonous beasts living in the lake that have already killed one hundred men and as many animals. Much like Marcellus he goes forward with the people to the place of danger. He then enters the water alone. The beasts are overcome by the sight of his angelic countenance. He orders them to go with him deep into the lake, and establishes a particular habitat for them there, binding them that they remain in it until the end of the world. It is no surprise, then, that the saint should subsequently chain to the edge of a lake a monstrous and fiery cat that he has 'domesticated'. Such beasts have to be kept within aqueous confines.[51]

The Old Irish *Life* of Colman Ela presents us with a rather unusual, explicitly pestilent, enemy: 'a small pointed gaping appari-

[50] Le Goff, 'Marcellus', p. 171. Cf. Graus, *Volk*, pp. 231–2.
[51] *Vita Moluae*, 25, ed. C. Plummer, *Vitae Sanctorum Hiberniae*, 2 vols. (Oxford, 1910), II, p. 213; *Vita Samthanne*, 8 (ed. Plummer, II, p. 255); *Vita Abbani*, 15–16, 18 (ed. Plummer, I, pp. 12–13, 15).

tion in the shape of a woman' with 'short bushy hair, unwashed and unkempt'.[52] And the various *Lives* of Coemgen bring out the connection between the taming or containment of such a beast and the improvement of health. In the Latin *Life*, the saint is found praying at night in the freezing water of a lake, where he is threatened by a horrid beast. One of the Old Irish *Lives* adds some detail:

> There was a horrible and strange monster in the lake, which wrought frequent destruction of dogs and men ... Coemgen ... drove the monster from him into the other lake. That is to say, the lesser lake, in which the monster [originally] was, is the place where help of every trouble is wrought both for men and cattle; and they all leave their sicknesses there, and the sicknesses and diseases go into the other lake to the monster, so that it does not injure anyone.

A verse *Life* clarifies this account a little. The saint 'expelled ... the drop-poison of the monster from the lough', so that, far from being a source of harm, its function was, as it were, reversed, and 'plagues were removed from the kine of the Gaels'.[53]

These examples are all drawn from Plummer's editions of Irish saints' *Lives*. The Latin versions are apparently the earliest, and none of them is very ancient. (One of the first monsters in Celtic hagiography, the seventh-century ancestor of the Loch Ness monster that is subdued by St Columba in Adomnan's *Life* of him, does not belong here, because the monster remains in the water and bites, shark-like, at its victims.[54]) The identifiable individuals who appear in Plummer's texts can generally be dated to the sixth or seventh centuries. But the impulse toward their composition may have been the reconstitution of many monasteries that followed the coming of the English in the twelfth century. Very little can be said about the prior elaboration of the traditions on which they depended, except by adducing parallels and comparisons from other literary genres.[55]

---

[52] *Betha Cholmain Eala*, 1, 2, ed. C. Plummer, *Bethada Náem Nérenn: Lives of the Irish Saints*, 2 vols. (Oxford, 1922), I, pp. 168–9 (text); II, pp. 162–3 (trans.).

[53] *Vita Coemgeni*, 18 (ed. Plummer, *Vitae Sanctorum*, I, p. 243); *Bethada Caoimhgin* (I) 8, (II) 3b (ed. Plummer, *Bethada*, I, pp. 126, 135; II, pp. 122, 131).

[54] *Vita Columbae*, II, 27, ed. A. O. and M. O. Anderson, *Adomnan's Life of Columba* (Edinburgh, 1961), pp. 386–8.

[55] Plummer, *Vitae Sanctorum*, I, p. clxxxvii. Since the above was written, R. Sharpe, *Medieval Irish Saints' Lives* (Oxford, 1991), has shown that base-texts from around 800 may be postulated for some of the Latin hagiography.

(One such comparison is the extraordinary image to be found in the twelfth-century *Vision* attributed to the peasant Tnugdal. A fire-breathing bird-like monster sits on a frozen swamp digesting the souls of sinners and excreting them as dung on the ice.[56]) It seems reasonable, however, to suppose, with Plummer, that the *Lives* contain much earlier, and 'sometimes primitive', materials – dating from the ninth or tenth centuries, if no earlier.[57] The saints may therefore not be quite as remote in time from the world of Marcellus (and Adomnan) as the textual history of their *Lives* would suggest.

Less remote in a geographical sense is a late ninth-century text, the *Life* of St Paul Aurelian (Paul of Léon in Brittany) by the monk Wrmonoc. A monster, described with extraordinary physiological exactitude, is terrorising the coastal area of an island, the Ile de Batz, causing man and beast to expire with, among other attributes, its pestiferous breath. The saint confronts it with the question, 'what are you up to here, you sower of a malign, pestiferous crop?', and then proceeds to harangue it at some length. He subdues the monster by tying his stole around its neck and then, in a phrase strikingly reminiscent of Fortunatus's narrative, banishes it 'to the inaccessible wastes of the sea'.[58] No mere dragon-tamer, moreover, the saint has already proved adept at turning back the forces of nature to appointed confines. His sister planned to establish a religious house on the coast of their native Britain, but the sea continually encroached on the narrow strip of available land. Paul took her to the edge of the water at low tide and told her to dispose pebbles in two rows as a boundary marker. The pebbles immediately grew into huge stone columns – still visible in Wrmonoc's day. The sea never thereafter crossed the boundary. And the land thus reclaimed became the most fertile in the nunnery's possession.[59]

Samson of Dol should also be allowed his contribution at this point. According to his early Breton hagiographer, this saint confines a giant fire-spitting serpent within a circle that he has drawn on

[56] *Visio Tnugdali: Lateinisch und Altdeutsch*, ed. A. Wagner (Erlangen, 1882), pp. 27–9 (cf. pp. 16–17); trans. J. M. Picard and Y. de Pontfarcy (Dublin, 1989), p. 130. On the work see H. Spilling, *Die Visio Tnugdali* (Munich, 1975).

[57] Plummer, *Vitae Sanctorum*, I, p. xc.

[58] 'Vie de Saint Paul de Léon en Bretagne', ed. C. Cuissard, *Revue Celtique*, 5 (1881–3), pp. 447–9 (*cap.* 18).

[59] Ed. Cuissard, pp. 434–6 (*cap.* 10). Cf. the parallel anecdote (of St Illtud) on pp. 422–3 (*cap.* 14); also G. H. Doble, *Lives of the Welsh Saints*, 2nd edn (Cardiff, 1971), pp. 146–61, for topographical speculations.

the ground. (The monster gives up its venom as it dies.) He also deals with a poisonous snake that has depopulated two villages and, significantly in the present context, lives beyond a river in a cave. A similar beast, 'afflicting with a severe pestilence' according to a late version of Samson's *Life*, is made to cross the Seine and remain under a stone.[60]

'Possibly some of the many stories of the destruction of monsters are to be explained in this way': Plummer had two grounds for the explanation that he cautiously offered in a footnote.[61] One was the frequency with which monsters such as those now described are said by the hagiographers to be spreading pestilence. The second was the small number of texts in which the apparent implication of the others is made quite explicit and the monster does indeed embody some epidemic. I have already noticed the unprepossessing female apparition in the *Life* of Colman Ela. I now present two other monsters, neither of which, unfortunately, can confidently be said to derive from any early tradition.

The first moves us from Ireland and Brittany to Wales. Among the legends of the death of Maelgwn, the king of Gwynedd so prominent in Gildas, is one that has him hiding from an epidemic in a church not far from his court. 'And Maelgwn Gwynedd beheld the Yellow Plague through the keyhole in the church door and forthwith died.' What he is supposed to have seen is described in the verse attributed to the renowned bard Taliesin in the 'Hanes Taliesin' that Lady Charlotte Guest included in her pioneering translation of the *Mabinogion*: a beast with golden eyes, teeth and hair that has come, again significantly, from a marsh.[62]

---

[60] *Vita Samsonis*, I, 32, 50, 58, ed. R. Fawtier, *La Vie de Saint Samson*, Bibliothèques de l'Ecole des Hautes Etudes, Sciences Historiques et Philologiques, 197 (1912), pp. 129–31, 145–6, 152–3; *The Text of the Book of Llan Dav*, ed. Evans and Rhys, p. 23. For the various versions of the *Life* see E. R. Henken, *Traditions of the Welsh Saints* (Woodbridge, 1987), ch. 8. On the date of the early version, P. Ó Riain, 'Samson alias San(c)tán', *Peritia*, 3 (1984), pp. 320–3; Wood, 'Forgery', pp. 380–4.

[61] Plummer, *Vitae Sanctorum*, I, p. cxi n. 1. Cf. p. cxxxix.

[62] T. Williams (ed.), *Iolo Manuscripts* (Llandovery, 1848, repr. 1888), pp. 78 (text), 467 (trans.). *Mabinogion*, ed. Lady C. Guest, 3 vols. (London, 1849), III, p. 377. On the legend of Maelgwn, in Gildas's *De Excidio Britanniae* and elsewhere, see *Trioedd Ynys Prydein: The Welsh Triads*, ed. R. Bromwich (Cardiff, 1961), pp. 437–41. On the 'Yellow Plague' see the divergent accounts and diagnoses in Bonser, *Medical Background*, pp. 64ff; J. C. Russell, 'The Earlier Medieval Plague in the British Isles', *Viator*, 7 (1976), pp. 65–78; G. Twigg, *The Black Death: A Biological Reappraisal* (London, 1984), pp. 38–42.

A more extensive account of such a monster of plague is to be found in the *Life* of the somewhat mercenary and unpleasant saint Mac Reiche. The historical existence of this figure is described by Plummer as 'extremely shadowy' and the *Life* of him as 'utterly unhistorical'.[63] First we meet the Crom Conaill, a beast which, one reads, 'is' the plague. Later in the *Life*, however, we learn of a variety of beasts, each of which attacked a different area of Ireland during the pandemic (of the sixth century?). One of these is the Broicsech, the badger monster, that apparently survived in local tradition in the 1920s. Like Columba's beast, it came from a loch:

> a monster most vehement, strong, malignant, unwearied, with its bestial rage upon it; and it wreaked great slaughters throughout the land generally ... it would open its ravenous raging maw like a mad dog, with its jaws all on fire, and emit a broad terrifying stream of harsh magical breath ... and every man whom that poisonous breath touched and every animal died a premature and sudden death ... and this was the extent of their losses, to wit, men and women to the number of sixty every day.

The *Life* goes on to describe an agonised assembly where the people debate what should be done (and which the monster itself infiltrates), the collective fasting and the eventual summoning of the saint who uses his staff to force the monster back into its loch, and then contains it with a skull cap when it reappears.[64]

V

I have relied on the presumed continuities of the various Celtic traditions as a licence to extend the search for pestilent dragons into the central and later Middle Ages. I shall not take the same chronological liberty with other traditions. Instead, I come back to Marcellus. Now that the *ideological* context of his legend has been offered for inspection (principally in the form of hagiographical analogies), I turn to its *material* context, the environs of Merovingian Paris.

---

[63] *Miscellanea Hagiographica Hibernica, Subsidia Hagiographica* XV, ed. C. Plummer (Brussels, 1925), p. 8.

[64] *Bethe Meic Creiche*, 9, ed. Plummer, *Miscellanea*, pp. 18–19 (text), 58–9 (trans.); 14–18 (pp. 36–51, 75–90); quotation from pp. 36, 76; 'survival' of monster in local tradition, p. 11.

The backdrop against which we should visualise Marcellus's encounter with his dragon can be reconstructed in surprising detail.[65] By the time that Fortunatus wrote, Marcellus's name had come to be associated with the territory of a particular suburban village, later the Faubourg Saint-Marcel. This faubourg covers the lower valley of the Bièvre, a small confluent of the Seine that once joined it in the region of the Gare d'Austerlitz. Something of the area's aboriginal character can still be seen in low-lying parts of the present-day Jardin des Plantes. Because it rests on a base of soft impermeable clay, the soil of Paris has always been poorly drained, and the rivers have, until modern times, easily spilled over into marshes. One of the most frequently flooded and marshy areas of the Left Bank was the confluence of the Seine and the Bièvre. Not far from such marshes lay the edge of the forest, of which the Bois de Boulogne and the Forest of Vincennes are the modern remnants. Pollen analysis reveals the ancient abundance of this forest. In the spaces remaining here for agriculture and settlement, cultivation had to be quite intensive to make the best of limited resources. For marshes that stretched in a barely interrupted arc from the site of the Bastille to the Champ de Mars prevented extensive colonisation of the Right Bank.[66]

There were other reasons why the area that concerns us became important. In Roman and sub-Roman times the main road to Sens and Lyons ran through it, parallel to the Left Bank. Marcellus's suburb, the oldest of those around Paris, grew up beside this road. Along it, stone from the nearby quarries could, of course, easily be transported. (The stone of the public buildings of Roman *Lutecia* is nearly all of local provenance.) Saint-Marcel was, then, in all likelihood a Roman faubourg of masons and artisans. Along its main road, also, came Christianity from the south. This suburb is indeed the oldest area of Christian settlement in Paris. From the end

---

[65] In what follows I have relied on: P.-M. Duval, *Paris antique des origines au troisième siècle* (Paris, 1961); M. Roblin, *Le Terroir de Paris aux époques gallo-romaine et franque*, 2nd edn (Paris, 1971); M.-L. Concasty, 'Le Bourg Saint-Marcel à Paris des origines au XVIe siècle', in *Ecole Nationale des Chartes: position des thèses 1937* (Nogent-le-Rotrou, 1937), pp. 26–37. Cf. Le Goff, 'Marcellus', pp. 162, 172–3. It is not clear what evidence permits Le Goff to assert so confidently (pp. 160–1) that 'the site of [Marcellus's] last miracle was the location of his tomb'.

[66] See A. Lombard-Jourdan, *Paris – genèse de la 'ville': la rive droite de la Seine des origines à 1223* (Paris, 1976).

of the third century, Christian cemeteries spread out on either side of the main road. And during the fifth century, tombs began to cluster around the doubtless modest sanctuary where Marcellus was – or was later thought to be – buried.[67] Such was the area to which the saint lent his name. Its topography corresponds to what we find mentioned in the *Life*. The scene there is suburban. There is a cemetery, but also settlement. Forest, wasteland and water are not far off. But for some conception of the hazards of life in the faubourg we have to turn to evidence of a later date. The floods seem to have posed the greatest clearly identifiable danger. Gregory of Tours records what is perhaps the earliest one of known date in Paris. That of 1196 was, so a seventeenth-century report had it, equal in volume to Noah's. Exactly a century later, the Bièvre flooded so destructively that Philip the Fair had to order the hasty construction of pontoon bridges. And the early fifteenth-century *Journal d'un Bourgeois de Paris* creates a vivid impression of the terrible impact of recurrent inundation on city life generally.[68]

To read Richard Cobb's *Paris and its Provinces* is to gain the perhaps not wholly misleading impression that the ecology had not changed fundamentally by the time of the Revolution. Eighteenth-century Paris remained encircled by woodland. Trees lined the major roads leading into the city to within two leagues of its centre. The Left Bank was still periodically flooded. Narrower than the Seine, the Bièvre burst its banks more easily, covering wide areas of Saint-Marcel with pestilential mud and adding to the continual stench produced by the Gobelins. In the early nineteenth century, to turn from Cobb to Louis Chevalier, fevers and consumption remained the occupational hazards of the laundrymen and dyers who worked alongside the Bièvre. The pattern of disease had changed so little

---

[67] Vieillard-Troiekouroff *et al.*, 'Anciennes églises'; M. Vieillard-Troiekouroff, *Les Monuments religieux de la Gaule d'après les œuvres de Grégoire de Tours* (Paris, 1976), pp. 210–11; Lombard-Jourdan, 'Du nouveau sur les origines chrétiennes de Paris'; P. Périn, 'Les Cimetières mérovingiens de Paris', *Paris et Ile-de-France*, 32 (1981), pp. 91–6.

[68] *Libri Historiarum*, VI, 25 (pp. 264–5). The classic work on such matters is M. Champion, *Les Inondations en France depuis le VIe siècle jusqu'à nos jours*, I (Paris, 1858). Flood of 1196: G. Brice, *Description de la ville de Paris* (1752 edn), ed. P. Codet, II (Paris and Geneva, 1971), p. 117. A. Vernet, 'L'Inondation de 1296–1297 à Paris', *Paris et Ile-de-France*, 1 (1949), pp. 49–50. 'Bourgeois de Paris', *A Parisian Journal*, trans. J. Shirley (Oxford, 1968), pp. 165, 275, 323, 347.

that medical topographies could be copied from eighteenth-century classics of the genre without fear of contradiction. Saint-Marcel was deservedly known as 'the sick faubourg'.[69]

It would be rash, of course, to assume that it had always been as insalubrious. And we have no direct evidence from the Middle Ages of the epidemics that might have followed in the wake of the flooding. Of the numerous water-borne diseases that could have been prevalent in such an ecology, malaria is the only one that I shall single out. This is partly for the reason stated at the outset: it is a disease that deserves greater prominence in our historical epidemiologies. But it is also because its presence in the area during the sixth century seems to be attested in the sources. Gregory of Tours records in one of his miracle books that Marcellus once expelled a huge serpent from Paris. Gregory had perhaps learned of the expulsion from Fortunatus's *Life*, which he cites as an authority. He then adds: 'the priest Ragnimodus, who is now bishop of Paris, went to Marcellus's tomb with a quartan fever. He knelt and for an entire day was occupied in fasting and praying; when evening came, he slept. A short while later he awoke from his sleep and rose from the tomb a healthy man.'[70]

References to the miraculous remission of periodic fever – usually of the tertian or quartan variety – provide the best evidence of malaria that we can hope for from this period. Marcellus was hardly the only Merovingian saint to cure malaria. Sufferers from fever are quite common in the miracle books of Gregory of Tours, to look no further afield.[71] Indeed, the account of Marcellus in Gregory's *Glory of the Confessors* is matched by notices of two other holy Parisians. The first of them, the virgin Criscentia, was buried in a suburb not far from what Gregory perplexingly refers to as the senior church (*ecclesia senior*) – which some have identified with the church of Saint Marcellus. 'A man whom the burning of a tertian fever was distressing with severe tremors scratched a bit of dust from the tomb and drank it; soon his tremors were calmed and all was well. The news was published and was of great benefit to many

[69] R. Cobb, *Paris and its Provinces 1792–1802* (Oxford, 1975), pp. 40, 63, 81. Cf. A. Sutcliffe, *The Autumn of Central Paris* (London, 1970), pp. 3ff. L. Chevalier, *Labouring Classes and Dangerous Classes* (London, 1973), pp. 86, 340ff.

[70] *Liber in Gloria Confessorum*, 87 (p. 804), trans. Van Dam, pp. 92–3.

[71] M. Weidemann, *Kulturgeschichte der Merowingerzeit nach den Werken Gregors von Tours*, 2 vols. (Mainz, 1982), II, p. 378.

people afflicted with this illness.'[72] The second holy Parisian is the nun Genovefa. She was buried, Gregory tells us, in the church of the Holy Apostles (actually, the construction of the church was undertaken, by Clovis, in order to house her tomb). 'The fevers of people suffering from chills very often are extinguished by her power.'[73]

A few reports of this kind will not, of course, establish the prevalence of malaria in Merovingian Paris. Nor are they evidence of an epidemic. But the direction in which they point is, nonetheless, suggestive. And whatever the diseases involved, the sufferers will probably have attributed them to miasma, the bad air that arose from standing water, such as that left behind after a flood.

VI

I have now proposed that we envisage Marcellus's dragon not only as a dragon of disease but as an animal to be conceived as intimately related to its local environment: a beast with an ecology. Much more than a symbol of epidemic disease, it *is* the epidemic (as the hagiographer of Mac Reiche insisted), or at least the cause of it. By whatever means, in the saint's flood-ridden eponymous faubourg, it spreads pestilence. In confronting the dragon and taming or killing it, the saint is restoring salubrity to the area. Such is the implication that the *Life* of Marcellus could have had for those to whom it was read in the sixth century.

It is tempting to proceed from that conclusion to an obvious question: what did Marcellus (if he existed) and his kind actually do? Just as I have not attempted to translate hagiographical dragon narratives into the terms of modern epidemiology, so I resist the notion that Marcellus's feat can be demythologised. The dragon is an animal that embodies or causes the disease. The corollary is that the saint has genuinely to subdue the monster. Reports of his doing so are not allegories of some other achievement.

It is, of course, conceivable that a historical Marcellus somehow dealt with a historical dragon – a snake perhaps, magnified in the telling to monstrous proportions. Le Goff entertains the possibility,

[72] *Liber in Gloria Confessorum*, 103 (pp. 813–14), trans. Van Dam, p. 104. On the *ecclesia senior* see Vieilliard-Troiekouroff, *Monuments religieux*, pp. 215–16.
[73] *Liber in Gloria Confessorum*, 89 (p. 805), trans. Van Dam, p. 94. On the accuracy and authenticity of the *Life* of Genovefa, see the references in Van Dam, p. 94 n. 100, and Wood, 'Forgery', pp. 376–8.

only to dismiss it. We may, however, recall the observation of a distinguished anthropologist that 'myths are not the creation of unbridled fancy, but in many cases, at least, are sober historical records'. It is also worth remarking that legends of monsters have sometimes been observed to develop from comparatively mundane beginnings. In June 1764, for instance, a large wolf appeared near the little French town of Langogne in Lozère. It had claimed about fifty lives before hunters could despatch it. Since wolves usually attacked humans only surreptitiously and in winter, the local people were unsure of the terrifying beast's identity. Rumours about its form and ancestry multiplied. And its renown was increased by the imaginative depictions sold on broadsheets. It became, within a relatively brief time, the monstrous *Bête de Gévaudan*.[74] A comparable explanation of the origin of Marcellus's dragon would not invalidate my theory of that beast as a monster of epidemics, given the pestilential attributes of snakes in the early Middle Ages. And it would be a kind of explanation that deserves greater intellectual respect than it has customarily been accorded since the demise of positivism. Even so, it could hardly be a satisfactory solution to the problem. A knowledge of the particular origin of the legend of Marcellus – were it attainable – would still leave us with no understanding of why the legend developed as it did, of why one feat of snake-killing should have been elevated to supreme importance in Marcellus's presumed career. The answer to the question of what Marcellus actually did must be something far less specific.

Once again, a sense of context is needed – an awareness of the environment in which representations of dragon-taming might prove 'contagious'. About the historical relationship between the context and the representation we can have no notion. The cast of mind, the interaction of metaphor and metonymy, that linked one to the other are of course irrecoverable. We do not even have an agreed theory to show how we may conceptualise the link. We must be content to describe.

What merits description in this context arose from the progressive weakening of local political leadership in the barbarian West of the

---

[74] Le Goff, 'Marcellus', pp. 163–4; quotation from *Imagination and Proof: Selected Essays of A. M. Hocart*, ed. R. Needham (Tucson, Arizona, 1987), p. 51; J. Devlin, *The Superstitious Mind: French Peasants and the Supernatural in the Nineteenth Century* (New Haven and London, 1987), pp. 75–6, and see also pp. 77–80.

fifth and sixth centuries, the time of Marcellus and Fortunatus. Bishop-saints gradually became far more than spiritual leaders, miraculous healers and fathers of the poor. Partly in default of alternative executants, partly (it may be) in order to enhance their often precarious position in the community, they took on an increasing variety of what had been thought of as secular public functions.[75] One bishop, Nicetius of Trier, of whom Fortunatus has left a verse eulogy, erected fortifications; more than one minted coins.[76] Others busied themselves responding to environmental threat or disaster. Examples are again forthcoming from Fortunatus's poetry. Sidonius of Mainz had dams constructed to contain the flooding of the Rhine. Felix of Nantes deployed earthworks for a similar purpose. Meanwhile, in the letters of Desiderius of Cahors we find a request to a fellow bishop for aid in laying water pipes.[77] Among such practical projects, it is to be expected that measures were taken to combat disease. The most striking example again comes from the correspondence of Bishop Desiderius. He received a letter from Gallus (II) of Clermont about instituting road blocks to prevent the spread of bubonic plague.[78]

Evidence such as this suggests that it is by no means wholly fanciful to envisage some bishops of the period as generally concerned with organising the community to withstand the progress of an epidemic, and more particularly with establishing the sort of drainage schemes necessary for reducing the risk of water-borne infections such as malaria. We have very little idea of the fate of Roman systems of drainage in the early medieval West. But if they

---

[75] R. Doehaerd, *Le Haut Moyen Age occidental: économies et sociétés* (Paris, 1971), pp. 122ff; F. Prinz, 'Die bischöfliche Stadtherrschaft im Frankenreich vom 5. bis zum 7. Jahrhundert', *Historische Zeitschrift*, 217 (1974), pp. 1–35; Heinzelmann, *Bischofsherrschaft in Gallien*, pp. 98–183; Brown, *Society and the Holy*, pp. 246–7; Geary, *Before France and Germany*, pp. 131–8. Cf. Le Goff, 'Marcellus', p. 173.

[76] Fortunatus, *Carmina*, III, 12, lines 21–2, ed. F. Leo, *MGH, AA*, IV, 1 (1881), p. 64; M. Prou, *Les Monnaies mérovingiennes* (Paris, 1892), pp. 355, 380, cited from I. Wood, 'The Ecclesiastical Politics of Merovingian Clermont', in P. Wormald *et al.* (eds.), *Ideal and Reality in Frankish and Anglo-Saxon Society* (Oxford, 1983), p. 51.

[77] *Carmina*, IX, 9, lines 27–30; III, 10 (pp. 216, 62–3). Desiderius, *Epistulae*, I, 13, ed. W. Arndt, Corpus Christianorum, Latin series CXVII (1957), p. 322. See further J. Durliat, 'Les Attributions civiles des évêques mérovingiens: l'exemple de Didier, évêque de Cahors (630–655)', *Annales du Midi*, 91 (1979), pp. 237–54.

[78] *Epistulae*, II, 20 (p. 341).

74

were maintained, restored or imitated, bishops would surely have been responsible.[79]

Their (on our estimation) purely practical undertakings could find spiritual counterparts. Thus Bonitus of Clermont achieved the ending of drought through ordering public fasts; indeed, a flood ensued – to end which more fasting was necessary. Gallus (I) instituted Rogations and a pilgrimage to protect Clermont from bubonic plague. The sheer saintly presence of Nicetius, along with that of the relics of two of his predecessors, was apparently enough to avert the same disease from Trier. In less dire circumstances, the relics of the martyr Clement restored to its original point of emergence a spring that (through a system of canals) had been irrigating fields near Limoges until it was mysteriously diverted into a swamp.[80] The slaying or taming of dragons may belong in this context – as another miraculous means of coping with a large ecological problem.

Between the practical and the miraculous approaches to the management of epidemics, then, no discontinuity seems to have been perceived. It is not inappropriate to discuss dragons and drainage in virtually the same breath. It could even be hazarded that traces of the practical approach are discernible in some of the hagiography earlier summarised. Why else do we find saints drawing circles around dragons or confining them under stones, and inscribing boundaries on beaches and islands? These, it was argued over a century ago, are to be interpreted as aspects of construction work on dams and drainage. The bishop marks out the ground before the workmen move in.[81] As before, I would not expect such precise congruences between the legends and their historical origins. It is the broad context that we should rather try to imagine. If these minor touches in the hagiography can be referred to some aspect of that

[79] For the classical background see Traina, *Paludi e Bonifiche*. For the early Middle Ages, see Doehaerd, *Haut Moyen Age*, p. 107; G. Bertrand *et al.* (eds.), *Histoire de la France rurale*, 4 vols. (Paris, 1975–6), I, pp. 78ff. A late antique legendary parallel: R. Lane Fox, *Pagans and Christians* (Harmondsworth, 1986), pp. 531–2. Cf. the dykes of St Illtud: Henken, *Welsh Saints*, p. 110.

[80] Wood, 'Merovingian Clermont', p. 52; Gregory of Tours, *Liber Vitae Patrum*, XVII, 4 (p. 731); *Liber in Gloria Martyrum*, 36 (p. 511). On Rogation processions to protect from pestilence, see I. Wood, 'Early Merovingian Devotion in Town and Country', in D. Baker (ed.), *The Church in Town and Countryside*, Studies in Church History XVI (Oxford, 1979), pp. 61–76.

[81] J.-F. Cerquand, 'Taranis et Thor', *Revue Celtique*, 6 (1883–5), pp. 417–56.

context, then I suggest that they reflect what I earlier called the practical but non-technological management of epidemics.

This concept obviously requires elaboration. I derive it, not from the evidence or historiography of Merovingian Gaul, but from the findings of some students of disease and colonialism in sub-Saharan Africa. It has come to be realised that first-world epidemic control may have been as unsuitable in a third-world ecology as first-world economics in a 'developing' economy. Indeed, the insensitive application of first-world techniques may have been positively damaging. Pre-colonial Africa was hardly free of epidemics; one should not attribute all of the continent's disasters to colonial expansion. But in certain areas a delicate ecological equilibrium had been arrived at between diseased waste and healthy settled land. That equilibrium was maintained by local leadership and custom. It required no extraordinary technology. This, for example, is how one leader managed trypanosomiasis:

> Shoshangane of the Gaza ordered his people to congregate around him in the tsetse bush of the Mzilizwe valley. The bush was cleared, the new land cultivated (and thus kept clear), but several large areas were deliberately left uncleared. Wild game was confined to them and outside them the game was hunted. Game guards controlled their movement. The tsetse vanished.[82]

Shoshangane was succeeded by his son in 1885. The latter was driven south by the Portuguese and forced to abandon Gazaland in 1889. The tsetse returned. For the 'ancient ecological equilibrium' had been destroyed.[83] (At about the same time, comparable disruption was being wrought by the arrival of immigrant workers in Manchuria: the third pandemic of bubonic plague ensued.[84]) It is not inordinately hard to visualise Marcellus as a Dark-Age Shoshangane managing epidemics by all the means at his disposal. In the case of my principal example, malaria, these perhaps included initiating drainage schemes or maintaining a corporate sense of purpose in the 'cleaning up' after a flood. But not the least of his skills, I would tentatively propose, was the oversight of the subtle adjustments that had always to be made between settlement on one

---

[82] G. Prins, 'But What Was the Disease? The Present State of Health and Healing in African Studies', *Past and Present*, no. 124 (1989), pp. 170–1.

[83] J. Ford, *The Role of the Trypanosomiases in African Ecology. A Study of the Tsetse Fly Problem* (Oxford, 1971), p. 145.

[84] W. H. McNeill, *Plagues and Peoples* (Harmondsworth, 1977), pp. 146–7.

76

hand (the settlement of those who observe his taming of the dragon) and water or wasteland (to which he confines the monster) on the other.

'Should a traveller, returning from a far country, bring us an account of men . . . who knew no pleasure but friendship, generosity, and public spirit; we should immediately, from these circumstances detect the falsehood . . . with the same certainty as if he had stuffed his narration with stories of centaurs and dragons, miracles and prodigies.' So thought David Hume.[85] In a narration that has lacked only centaurs among the implausibilities mentioned, I hope to have shown that – in the management of epidemics – dragons, miracles and public spiritedness may have been intimately linked.

[85] *Enquiry Concerning Human Understanding*, VIII, 1, ed. L. A. Selby-Bigge, rev. edn, ed. P. H. Nidditch (Oxford, 1975), p. 84.

XIV

MEDITERRANEAN PLAGUE IN
THE AGE OF JUSTINIAN

> During these times there was a pestilence, by which the whole
> human race came near to being annihilated.
> – Procopius, *Wars*, 2.22.1, trans. Dewing

Very occasionally the emperor Justinian deserves our sympathy. Epidemics are usually named after their victims: the biblical plague of the Philistines, for example, or the plague of
Athens famously described by Thucydides. Yet the pandemic (world-
wide epidemic) that struck the empire on an unprecedented scale during
Justinian's reign, spreading to northern and western Europe, many parts
of the Middle East, and possibly China, has always been treated differently. In the *Secret History* Procopius blamed the emperor's demonic
machinations for all the natural disasters of his reign.[1] Even though
Justinian himself contracted the disease and its ravages long outlasted
him, historians of the sixth century, following Procopius's lead, have
written of "the plague of Justinian."[2] This is unfair. In what follows
attention will be confined for the most part to plague in sixth-century
Byzantium. But the phenomenon is far larger, and to convey its "global"
impact, extensive chronology, and questionable biological identity, I
shall refer to it more neutrally as the early medieval pandemic (EMP).

ITINERARIES

There had doubtless been localized epidemics aplenty in the later
Roman and the early Byzantine empires. Yet, when the EMP arrived in
541, there had apparently not been a major one since the 520s. Looking

XIV

back to approximately a century before his own time, the author of the *Paschal (Easter) Chronicle* recorded a Great Death under the year 529, which may well be a mistaken reference to the EMP.[3] Much later on, though more plausibly, the tenth-century universal chronicler Agapius of Hierapolis mentions a "terrible epidemic" that broke out in 525–526 and lasted for six years.[4] Even these epidemics apparently paled beside that of 541. In the first place it was probably a novel disease. Well before Justinian's time, there may, in the eastern Mediterranean, have been highly restricted outbreaks of a disease with similar symptoms.[5] But those symptoms had not been noticed since the first century AD. To its sixth-century victims this disease seemed wholly without parallel – and not only in symptoms, but in mortality and terrifying speed.

Before worrying further about diagnosis, let us look in more detail at the pandemic's initial phases to establish the geography and character of its movement.[6] (Map 7) The disease arrived on the Mediterranean scene at Pelusium (modern Tell el Farama), a small entrepôt at the extreme eastern edge of the Nile Delta, around the middle of July 541. It had perhaps been transmitted from central Africa via Zanzibar and the Christian Ethiopian kingdom of Axum. Once it had erupted in Pelusium it spread swiftly, presumably by boat, in two directions simultaneously, westward along the north African coast, eastward to coastal Palestine.

In the eastward direction, it has been plotted as first reaching Gaza, on the coast. It then turned inland as well as continuing along the Palestinian littoral, following shipping lanes and caravan routes. Constantinople remained untouched until March or April of 542. But once arrived, the plague raged in the capital until August. By the summer it had also reached Syria. Of major settlements, Antioch was struck first in the early summer of 542, followed by neighboring towns, and the small inland city of Zora in southern Syria. At about the same time, Myra on the Lycian coast and Sykeon in Galatia also succumbed. The disease was spreading rapidly across Asia Minor. By the autumn of 542 it had extended itself to Adarbigana (Media Atropatene) in modern Azerbaijan and reached the army of Persia, which had retreated there from its war with Byzantium.

In its western onslaught, the EMP crossed overland to devastate Alexandria in September 541. It may have been carried to Sicily in late 542. In early 543, it had probably reached Tunisia and was advancing across the Mediterranean reaches of Roman North Africa. It was present in Italy and Illyricum throughout 543, reaching Rome at the end of that year or very soon after. In 543 it is also attested in southern Gaul and parts of Spain, although it seems to have subsided quite quickly in both areas.[7] On March 23, 543 Justinian issued a law in which he declared God's "education" (the epidemic) over; wages, which had soared, were to be restored to their preplague levels.[8] The plague had traversed the Mediterranean world and much of the Middle East in just under two years. It then mysteriously retreated, at least from Justinian's empire. But it may have reached Ireland in 544 or 545 and, just possibly, Wales in 547. There may also at this time have been "satellite" outbreaks as far apart as Finland and the Yemen.[9]

Doubtless the survivors of the 540s profoundly hoped that the pandemic really was over. In fact, so far as the Age of Justinian is concerned, this was only the first wave of many. Constantinople was struck again from February to July, 558, and Cilicia, Syria, and Mesopotamia in 560–561. A third wave reached Gaul in 571 and Constantinople in 573–574. A fourth wave broke in 590–591, with Rome and Antioch its leading casualties. A fifth wave was first evident in Thessaloniki in the summer of 597. It spread to Avar territory in 598, then moved to Constantinople, Asia Minor and Syria in 599, and North Africa in 599–600, finally attaining Ravenna and Verona in 600–601.

Thus battered, Justinian's century came to an end, but the pandemic did not. Eleven more visitations can be documented in the course of the seventh and early eighth centuries. They primarily affected the newly conquered "land of Islam," but there are some attested outbreaks in Byzantium and western Europe (including England in the 660s and perhaps Scandinavia), and others can be inferred because the pandemic had already shown itself to be no respecter of frontiers. The last epidemic in the Mediterranean was probably that which struck Naples in 747.[10] By 750 or quite soon after, the EMP had also disappeared from Islamic territories. It ceased almost as suddenly as it had begun.

I have surveyed the pandemic in these stark geographical and chronological terms first of all to give some idea of its scale. It affected all three continents of the then known world, although most of the Arabian peninsula, and perhaps the central Asian steppes, were free of it, their nomadic populations fortunately lacking the density necessary for its spread.[11]

Some of the geography and chronology given above is secure, based on reliable texts; other parts of it are more conjectural. The waves into which the chronology is divided are constructions of the most authoritative recent historians. They are a best attempt to make sense of the advance and retreat of the pandemic, its periodic disappearances – on average just over every eleven years[12] – until, for reasons that remain

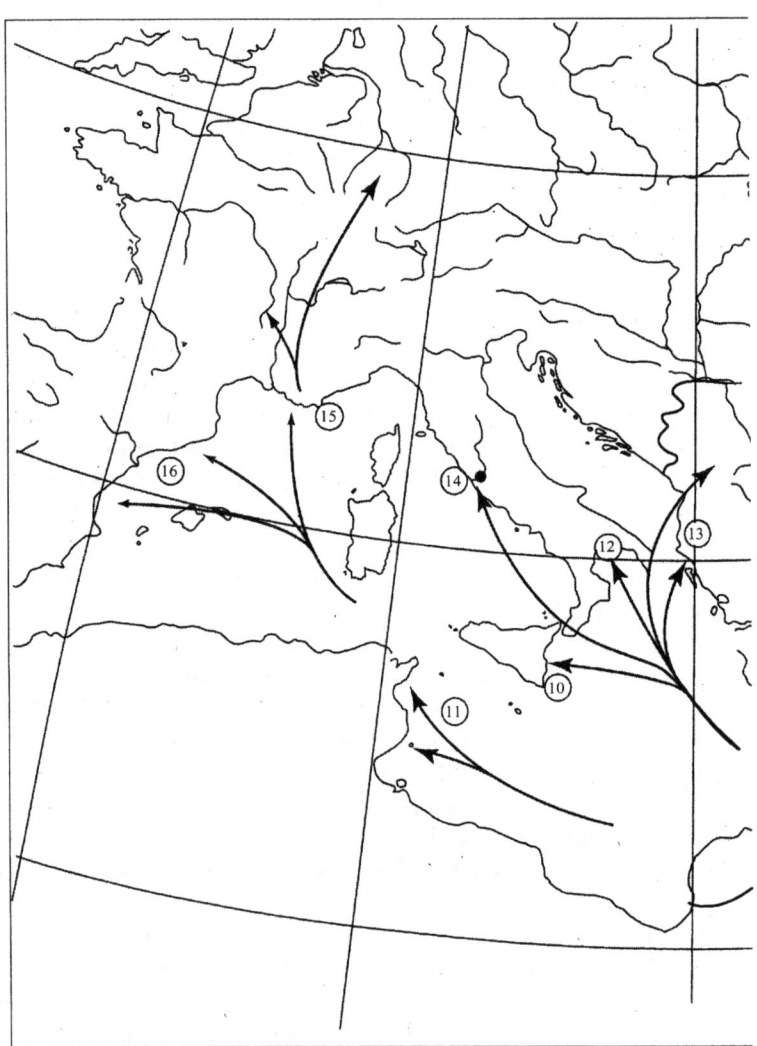

1. Pelusium, July 541
2. Gaza, Aug. 541
3. Jerusalem, 542
4. Antioch, summer 542

5. Myra, summer 542
6. Constantinople, Mar./Apr. 542
7. Sykeon, summer 542
8. Media Atropatene, fall 542

MAP 7. The first wave of the early medieval pandemic, (after Dionysios Stathakopoulos, *Famine and Pestilence in the Late Roman and Early Byzantine Empire: A Systematic Survey of Subsistence Crises and Epidemics* [Aldershot, 2004], chap. 6).

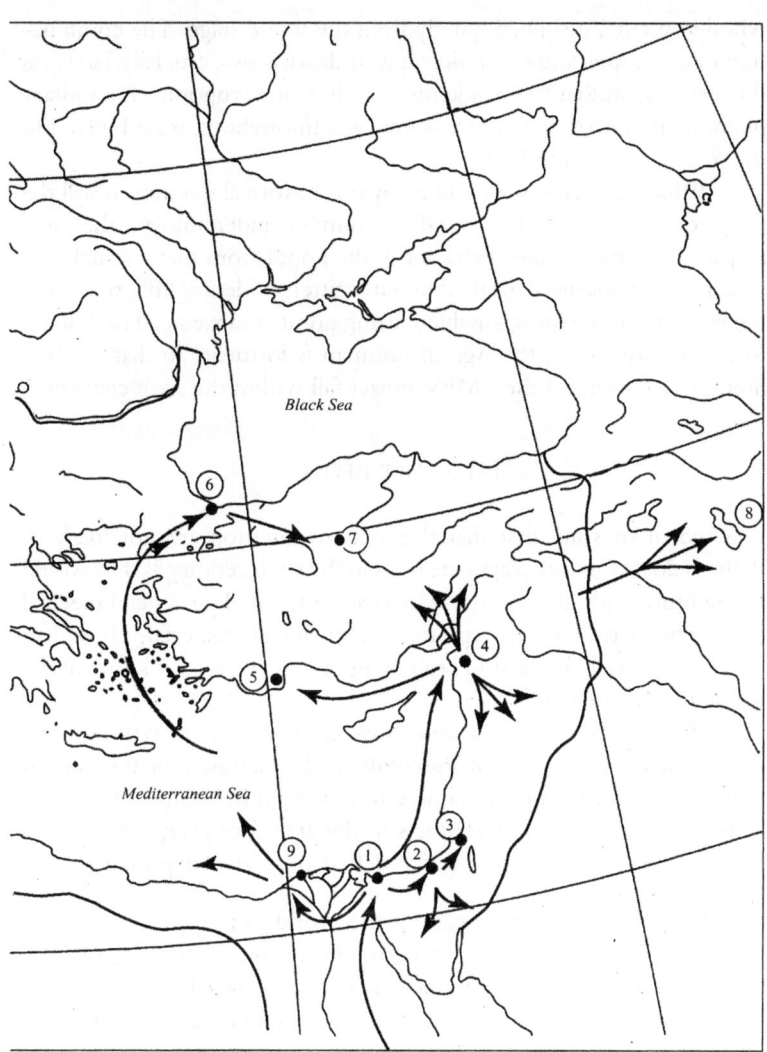

9. Alexandria, Sept. 541
10. Sicily, Dec. 542
11. Tunisia, Jan./Feb. 543
12. Italy, 543–544

13. Illyricum, 543
14. Rome, 543
15. Gaul, 543
16. Spain, 543

XIV

wholly obscure, it slipped quietly from the world stage. The combination of geography and chronology given above is also, crucially, based on the assumption that the pandemic, for all its interruptions, is a unitary phenomenon: that one disease is involved throughout, from Finland to the Yemen, Ireland to Iran.

What was that disease? The obvious historical question is still the most controversial. We have to take account of epidemiology – the overall pattern of the disease's behavior in the populations that it struck – as well as the symptoms described in our written evidence. Still, that written evidence is the indispensable starting point, and we need to "listen" to it. The student of the Age of Justinian is fortunate in that the best literary evocations of the EMP's impact fall within the sixth century.

DESCRIPTIONS

It is worth stressing first that the texts in question are not medical. Perhaps doctors wrote plague treatises in the sixth century as they would in the fourteenth; if so, nothing survives of them. The general medical texts of the period merely reproduce centuries-old material.[13] If we had only the medical "profession" to rely upon, we would not know of the pandemic's existence.

What we do have are vivid passages of historical writing. The most well known is that of Procopius in his narrative of the Persian Wars.[14] He had returned to Constantinople with Belisarius after the fall of Ravenna and was an eyewitness to the arrival of plague in the city. He describes its universality, which defied all rational explanation:

> It did not come in a part of the world nor upon certain men, nor did it confine itself to any season of the year, so that from such circumstances it might be possible to find subtle explanations of a cause, but it embraced the entire world, and blighted the lives of all men. . . . And it attacked some in the summer season, others in the winter, and still others at the other times of the year.

After mentioning its progress from coastland to interior, he sets out its "folk etiology," the way some people perceived its arrival.

> Apparitions of supernatural beings in human guise of every description were seen by many persons, and those who encountered them thought that they were struck by the man

they had met in this or that part of the body, as it happened, and immediately upon seeing this apparition they were seized also by the disease.

Then he elaborates on the symptoms, which baffled even the greatest physicians:

They had a sudden fever. . . . And the body shewed no change from its previous colour, nor was it hot as might be expected when attacked by a fever, nor indeed did any inflammation set in, but the fever was of such a languid sort from its commencement and up till evening that neither to the sick themselves nor to a physician who touched them would it afford any suspicion of danger. . . . But on the same day in some cases, in others on the following day, and in the rest not many days later, a bubonic swelling developed; and this took place not only in the particular part of the body which is called "boubon," that is, below the abdomen, but also inside the armpit, and in some cases also besides the ears, and at different points on the thighs.

Up to this point, then, everything went in about the same way with all who had taken the disease. But from then on very marked differences developed. . . . For there ensued with some a deep coma, with others a violent delirium. . . . And in those cases where neither coma nor delirium came on, the bubonic swelling became mortified and the sufferer, no longer able to endure the pain, died. . . .

Death came in some cases immediately, in others after many days; and with some the body broke out with black pustules about as large as a lentil and these did not survive even one day, but all succumbed immediately. With many also a vomiting of blood ensued without visible cause and straightaway brought death. . . .

Now in those cases where the swelling rose to an unusual size and a discharge of pus had set in, it came about that they escaped from the disease and survived, for clearly the acute condition of carbuncle had found relief in this direction, and this proved to be in general an indication of returning health; but in cases where the swelling preserved its former appearance there ensued those troubles which I have just mentioned.

XIV

Then Procopius records the mortality – so great that the dead could not be buried in the customary fashion:

> Now the disease in Byzantium ran a course of four months, and its greatest virulence lasted about three. And at first the deaths were a little more than the normal, then the mortality rose still higher, and afterwards the tale of dead reached five thousand each day, and again it even came to ten thousand and still more than that. . . .
>
> At that time all the customary rites of burial were overlooked. For the dead were not carried out escorted by a procession in the customary manner, nor were the usual chants sung over them, but it was sufficient if one carried on his shoulders the body of one of the dead to the parts of the city which bordered on the sea and flung him down; and there the corpses would be thrown upon skiffs in a heap to be conveyed wherever it might chance.

To our second eyewitness. Traveling through regions recently devastated by the plague, John of Ephesus also includes the folk etiology of the plague's transmission from Egypt:[15]

> When this plague was passing from one land to another, many people saw shapes of bronze boats and figures sitting in them resembling people with their heads cut off. Holding staves, also of bronze, they moved along on the sea and could be seen going whithersoever they headed. These figures were seen everywhere in a frightening fashion, especially at night.

He is eloquent on the state of the countryside between Syria and Constantinople when the first "wave" was at its height:

> In these countries we saw desolate and groaning villages and corpses spread out on the earth, with no one to take up and bury them; other villages where some few people remained and went to and fro carrying and throwing the corpses like a man who rolls stones off his field, going off to cast it away and coming back to take another stone . . . [we saw] fields in all the countries through which we passed from Syria to Thrace, abundant in grain which was becoming white and stood erect, but there was none to reap or gather in.

Mortality in the capital exceeds even Procopius's estimates:

> Thus the people of Constantinople reached the point of disappearing, only few remaining, whereas of those only who had died on the streets – if anybody wants us to name their number, for in fact they were counted – over 300,000 were taken off the streets.

The symptoms are, however, reminiscent of Procopius's description:

> From now on the common people ... could be seen to be smitten by a single great and harsh blow, and suddenly to fall, apart from a few. Not only those who died, but also those who escaped sudden death were struck with this plague of swellings in their groins, with this disease which they call *boubones*, and which in our Syriac language is translated as "tumours."

And not only people are afflicted:

> Also we saw that this great plague showed its effect on the animals as well, not only on the domesticated but also on the wild, and even on the reptiles of the earth. One could see cattle, dogs, and other animals, *even rats*, with swollen tumours, struck down and dying. (Emphasis added)

To these vivid evocations could be added the later testimony of the historian Evagrius, who saw plague not as divisible into waves but as lasting continuously from 542 until the time of his writing, the 590s.[16] For him too, the epidemic was universal, though utterly capricious in its geography and seasonality, sparing some cities but not others, seizing some quarters of cities but bypassing others, wiping out entire families while not touching any of those around them. Evagrius knew whereof he wrote. He contracted the disease as a schoolboy but survived; several members of his family and household perished, however. He describes symptoms different from those recorded by Procopius and John. In some, he writes, the plague was first evident in bloody and swollen eyes and moved down the body; others had severe diarrhea; others still buboes and fever. Some died suddenly after two or three days; others

XIV

went mad. Some contracted the disease from the company of the sick; others who had lost members of their family tried to infect themselves and could not, as if the disease were thwarting them. Because Evagrius had firsthand experience of the pandemic, his account has sometimes been read rather straightforwardly; it is in fact a highly artful exploration of every conceivable contradiction in the disease's behavior.

DIAGNOSES

For all students of the period, these texts and a few others like them are the materials for diagnosis. To the question of what the EMP was, three main answers have been given, one of them endemic (as it were) to historians of the sixth century, two others imported.

It is one of these imports that we might consider first. It provides in some ways the simplest response to any request for diagnosis. The plague was what its sufferers and observers said it was – no more, no less.[17] They – at least those who thought and wrote in Latin or Greek – characterized it as a *plaga* or *loimos* (or *thanatikon*).[18] They did not have a name for the disease (although writers in Arabic did, distinguishing this "plague" from other kinds of epidemic).[19] It was, simply, a great pestilence or mortality. But its particular etiology was conceived in culturally specific ways, such as headless supernatural seafarers, or an imbalance of humors caused by corrupt air, or divine chastisement. People experienced its symptoms as, variously, a severe fever, delirium, insomnia, acute pain in the *bubones*, and vomiting of blood.

And that is all there is to be said. Any given disease is at once a biological, a psychological, and a social phenomenon; and the biological must not be privileged in defining it. Today, diseases are isolated, named, and understood in the laboratory. Before the laboratory, however, different approaches prevailed: the diagnosis was more a judgment about the patient, and his or her environment, as a whole. The way the disease was conceptualized determined the way it was experienced, and that determined what it was. This approach to the problem of diagnosis is, in philosophical terms, a version of epistemological relativism. The nature of something is entirely relative to the way in which knowledge of it is acquired. Each age has its own culture and thus its own diseases. We cannot ask whether plague in the sixth century is the same as plague in the twenty-first – not because the answer is difficult, but because there are no criteria of sameness. There can therefore be no retrospective diagnosis, no imposition of our disease categories onto the very different ones of the past. Indeed, we might say that there are no *diseases*, there are only culturally specific *illnesses* – and our early medieval pandemic is one of them. Since the emperor contracted it and had his own experience of it, it really is, in that special sense, the plague of Justinian.

I have described this philosophically rigid approach in some detail because, though influential with respect to other periods, it has, so far, been alien to the historiography of the sixth century. When it arrives in late antique studies, it will encounter fierce resistance. Not surprisingly, historians of medicine and disease, reluctant to remain on the "surface" of the texts, and confident in the applicability to the remote past of the nosology of modern biomedicine, have long espoused retrospective diagnosis; and they have long known what the EMP really was. Theirs is the "endemic" approach to the question of diagnosis, to which we turn next before registering another import from outside the field.

The EMP was bubonic plague, *Yersinia pestis*, and its pulmonary and septicemic variants. It is a disease of rats (as John of Ephesus seemingly noted) and of their fleas, with human fleas and direct person-to-person transmission as occasional adjuncts. The details are familiar, are repeated in virtually any book with "plague" or "Black Death" in the title published before 2000, and need not be rehearsed at length here. I quote from the unexceptionable summary of a medically experienced historian:[20]

> Bubonic plague epidemics occurred as *Yersinia pestis*, a rodent disease that was communicated to humans through the bite of infected fleas. Humans have exceedingly poor immune defenses to this organism, and within 6 days of infection most victims develop a grossly swollen lymph node, a bubo, signifying the body's attempt to contain and arrest multiplication of *Y. pestis*. On the average, around 60 percent of those infected died within a week after the appearance of the bubo. . . .
>
> With the historically ironic exception of western Europe, *Y. pestis* today occurs naturally throughout the world among the wide variety of rodents and lagomorphs (i.e., rabbits and related species). . . . the "disease," then, is not always a disease, and it is ecologically very complex. Indeed, it is occasional ecological change or disturbance that brings

XIV

susceptible rodents into contact with *Y. pestis*. Historically the most important of these rodents is considered to be *Rattus rattus*, the common, commensal black . . . house rat, that literally "shares man's table." When infected by *Y. pestis* these susceptible animals die quickly of an overwhelming infection, with blood levels of the microbe so high that their rat fleas imbibe large numbers of organisms. . . .

Human plague usually arises after an epizootic plague has produced high mortality among susceptible rodents, when infected fleas, deprived of rodent hosts, begin to feed on humans. Although some historians speak of "endemic plague," no such phenomenon can exist. Humans do not normally carry the *Y. pestis* organism, and thus cannot infect fleas or otherwise pass the disease to new hosts. For human communities, plague is an acute infection ultimately derived from infected rodents. . . . Once a human is infected with *Y. pestis*, the organism rapidly replicates at the site of the flea bite. This area can subsequently become necrotic, where dead tissue blackens to produce a carbuncle or necrotic pustule often called "carbone" in many historical accounts. But in many cases the progress of infection is too rapid for this to happen. The lymphatic system attempts to drain the infection to the regional lymph node, where organisms and infected cells can be phagocytized (ingested by macrophages and white blood cells). That node becomes engorged with blood and cellular debris, creating the grossly swollen bubo. Because infected fleas usually bite an exposed area of the body, often a limb or the face, the location of the subsequent bubo is often visible. Frequent sites are the groin, the axilla, or the cervical lymph nodes. . . . the acute formation of a bubo, visible in 60 percent of bubonic plague victims, is pathognomonic of plague, meaning that no other disease commonly causes this reaction.

That seems to settle the matter. Those for whom retrospective diagnosis is philosophically permissible have mostly had no difficulty with the EMP. The telltale buboes are not only referred to in Byzantine histories such as those reviewed above; they appear in descriptions of plague sufferers that were written in Italy, Spain, Gaul, and Britain. To take only two further examples, for Gregory of Tours, writing in the 580s, this was *lues inguinaria*, "the groin plague"; for Paul the Deacon, recording around 790 an epidemic that struck northwest Italy in the sixth century, "there began to appear in the groins [*inguinibus*] of men . . . a swelling of the glands [*glandulae*], after the manner of a nut or date, presently followed by an unbearable fever."[21]

In such material there also seem to be represented the fever, delirium, diarrhea, and vomiting characteristic of modern cases of infection by *Yersinia pestis*; the black pustules that can form where the fleas bite; the rapid death that marks out the septicemic form of plague; the person-to-person transmission that is a sign of the pneumonic type (although the role of this in the EMP has been extensively and inconclusively debated);[22] and the patchy incidence combined with long-distance transmission (usually by shipborne infected rats or fleas) that has so often been a feature of later epidemics.

Ancient and modern pathology apparently match quite well. Moreover, discrepancies are easily explained by the nature of the ancient evidence. Some of the texts in question were written by eyewitnesses, but none of them can count as clinical descriptions. Complete accord with modern symptomatology would almost be suspicious. Even in modern times, not many people have wholly observed bubonic plague run its full course in a patient without either running away or intervening.

Today, then, virtually all students of the EMP reckon its diagnosis settled. The doubts come from outside, from those studying the Black Death of the fourteenth to seventeenth century. This is the last of the three possible approaches to diagnosis. The doubts will not easily be dispelled and those new to the plague of Justinian should be aware of them, even if ultimately they prefer one of the other two approaches just outlined: that of relativism (the disease was precisely what its sufferers said it was), or that of the conventional diagnosis (bubonic plague).

INFERENCES

First, though, it needs to be shown why the Black Death may be relevant. The EMP is commonly held to be the earliest of three pandemics of plague that have so far affected the globe. The second was the Black Death, which struck Europe in the 1340s and continued to return in waves for almost twice as long as did the EMP, finally receding from western Europe only in the eighteenth century and maintaining its grip on the Ottoman Empire for a good deal longer. The third pandemic began more slowly in China in the second half of the nineteenth century, reaching Canton and Hong Kong in 1894, whence it spread around the world.[23]

Understanding of these pandemics is to some extent inferential and even based on circular reasoning. Since, on the conventional diagnosis, all three were pandemics of the same disease, the early authoritative accounts of the third pandemic not only include historical backgrounds but at times draw on the historical record of the second pandemic, the Black Death, to supplement the data available for the third.[24] These accounts are then treated by historians of the Black Death simply as scientific views of the third pandemic, independent of historical interpretation. So the history of the Black Death is to some extent explained using evidence of the modern pandemic that was originally based in part on narratives of the Black Death – circularity. The summary account of bubonic plague quoted above is an attempt by a historian with medical experience to generalize across the first two pandemics to make a biological history of the disease. While perfectly serviceable as a clinical description and epidemiology, it blends historical evidence and modern reports. I chose it precisely because it illustrates how such summaries can then become the starting point for further retrospective diagnosis, however explicit the author may be about the use made of history.

Since evidence for the first pandemic is so much sparser and more reticent than that for the Black Death, the latter is called upon to help interpret the former. In particular, estimates of the mortality caused by the EMP are inevitably colored by those for the Black Death. And in a less vicious circle than the one connecting the second and third pandemics, the plague of Justinian also becomes part of the historical background for the fourteenth-century plague, since few books on the Black Death fail to allow it a vignette in an early chapter.

The axiom that there have been three pandemics of the same disease also affects modern laboratory work. The pathogen is named *Yersinia pestis* after the man who first isolated the bacillus and after the "great pestilence" that was the Black Death in early modern England. The assumption that the second and third pandemics were biologically identical is thus built into its very name.[25] Three biovars (strains) of *Yersinia pestis* have been differentiated according to the degree to which they ferment glycerol, and their official names each correspond to one of the three presumed pandemics – *antiqua, mediaevalis,* orientalis.[26] Although there is certainly some historical evidence to support the attribution, nothing is settled, and the issue might have been less prejudiced by historically neutral terminology.

It is because of these multiple scholarly and scientific connections between pandemics that the scholarship of the plague of Justinian cannot be detached from recent work on the Black Death.

DENIALS

The recent work can be summed up under the heading of "bubonic plague denial." The deniers have gathered momentum and garnered wide publicity in the years around the turn of the millennium. Yet aspects of their case have been aired for some time. In 1970, J. F. D. Shrewsbury argued on the basis of his (somewhat selective) "reading" of the third pandemic that the second one could not have killed one-half to one-third of Europe's population – as was, and is still, commonly thought – and that other diseases must have been involved.[27] He was taken to task for not giving sufficient "credit" to lethal pneumonic plague. His stance was not exactly one of denial, but it did bring to light some possible differences between second and third pandemics. In 1984, Graham Twigg published a book-length discussion of those differences and was either derided or ignored by medical historians. So powerful was their attachment to the bubonic paradigm that they felt no need even to engage with most of his arguments, let alone to refute them.[28] So, on the whole, and despite minor academic skirmishing, the matter rested for some time. Then, in the years around the turn of the millennium, two contradictory developments could be discerned.

On one hand, a few molecular biologists were able to extract DNA from the teeth of skeletons excavated from burial grounds very likely to contain plague victims of the later medieval and early modern periods. Comparison of the DNA with that of *Yersinia pestis* showed enough similarity for the biologists to proclaim (on the "one swallow *does* make a summer" principle) that the Black Death was an epidemic of bubonic plague and that all doubt about its identity had been removed.[29]

On the other hand, there was a return to, and amplified restatement of, Twigg's analysis of disquieting differences between the second and third pandemics – by two historical demographers, Susan Scott and Christopher J. Duncan, and by a historian of later medieval Europe, Samuel K. Cohn.[30] Both deny that *Yersinia pestis* could have been the primary agent of the Black Death and its subsequent waves. The symptoms and epidemiology were just too different.

There is space here neither to reflect adequately the detail of the deniers' hypotheses nor to convey the vigorous and knowledgeable

XIV

counterattack that has been launched on behalf of the plague of Justinian by Robert Sallares.[31] It must suffice to report that, in effect, the jury is still out – and likely to remain so for some years, because the literature of plague in all its aspects and periods is now so large and variegated that almost any plausible position can find some empirical support, and because of continuing disagreements among biologists, epidemiologists, and historians alike about crucial data and their interpretation.

What the jury still has to deliberate on seems to me to be the following, mainly epidemiological, aspects of the modern pandemic. These aspects contrast it strongly with both of the first two pandemics and hence continue to unsettle the traditional diagnosis of the EMP as bubonic plague.[32]

First, despite its potentially global impact, the third pandemic inflicted nothing like the mortality now generally attributed to the EMP or the Black Death. We shall come back to the effects of the EMP below; but if, on a cautious estimate, the mortality of the first two pandemics was of the order of 20–30 percent, that of the early-twentieth-century pandemic, before vaccines were available, was of the order of 1 percent or less (as, e.g., in India, 1896–1917).

Second, both the earlier epidemics spread with astonishing rapidity compared to the plague's rate of advance in the later nineteenth and early twentieth centuries, even though it then had the advantage of diffusion by steamship or railway train. We saw the first waves of the EMP traversing the eastern Mediterranean in a matter of months. In South Africa in 1899, with steam trains to propel it, plague still moved inland at some 20 kilometers a year.

Third, the geography and seasonality of the modern pandemic are contrary to what historians expect. Bubonic plague is, first of all, a disease of rats and their fleas, and it cannot stray far from that zoological substructure. It should peak in spring or summer; yet, as we saw, Procopius states that the initial wave of the early medieval pandemic was felt throughout the year, and there are many other such anomalies in reports of both the first two pandemics. Following on from that, since the rat's flea, *Xenopsylla cheopis*, is the crucial vector in the transmission of bubonic plague from rodents to humankind, and since that flea requires a *sustained* summer temperature of 20–25°C to reproduce, the extension of plague pandemics to Scandinavia and Iceland, even to Britain, verges on the biologically impossible. Not just the occasional warm spell, but clusters of long, warm summers are required for the biology of fleas to accord with the chronology of recurrent epidemics.

Fourth, neither of the stopgaps proposed by defenders of bubonic plague to explain some of these anomalies really serves its purpose. The human flea is a very inefficient vector of plague and is now rarely espoused as a way of "detaching" the disease from its rodent base and explaining its rapid spread. The pneumonic form of plague, precisely because it is so lethal, will not sustain an epidemic beyond the geography of rats and their fleas. It burns itself out too quickly. In Manchuria in the early 1900s, living conditions among the migrant workers who became victims of pneumonic plague were so apt to produce an epidemic that an evil scientist might have designed them as a laboratory experiment.[33] Yet even in such ideal conditions (ideal for the bacillus, that is) the mortality was far lower than is postulated by historians of the first two pandemics.

Fifth, the DNA results referred to earlier are liable to the charges that they have, so far, proved unrepeatable, and that they may have arisen from contamination of the sample being analysed by DNA of *Yersinia pestis* already present in the laboratory. More importantly, these results, even if accepted, prove simply that bubonic plague was present at around the right time, not that it was the sole or even primary agent of the pandemic.[34]

That introduces a sixth point. Even the staunchest defenders of *Yersinia pestis* concede that diseases such as typhus could also have been involved in the first two pandemics. There is nothing biologically dubious about postulating mixed or overlapping epidemics of a number of different diseases. Perhaps bubonic plague was prevalent in the Mediterranean and other diseases predominated in the colder north, in epidemics whose chronological continuity with Mediterranean or Middle Eastern plagues was the result either of chance or of some interaction between the ecologies of plague and the other diseases that is currently obscure to us. Such a hypothesis of mixed or overlapping epidemics of course has obvious disadvantages. It invites the application of Ockham's razor in that it perhaps multiplies diseases beyond necessity. In this frustratingly difficult sphere of investigation, however, the conclusions that we adopt may have to be the least implausible, not the most convincing.

A final point under this heading of "denial": All the biological evidence suggests that plague evolved recently, perhaps as recently as 2,500 years ago, and has remained stable since.[35] The three biovars ("ancient," "medieval," and "oriental") are genetically very similar and seem to be equally infective and virulent. New strains have appeared through random mutation, some of them extremely recently. But the range of variation within which the bacillus has any chance of success is

XIV

severely limited by the ecology of its hosts, the rat and the flea. More-over, there is no evolutionary pressure for the bacillus to accommodate itself to humankind, because it is only relatively occasionally a disease of humanity. It has no "incentive" to become milder with each pan-demic. That seems to rule out one possible explanation of why the first and second pandemics appear to have been vastly more serious than the third.

There are other questions that could be put to the first two pandemics – such as why hardly anyone in Europe, Byzantium, or Islam seems to have noticed the high and very visible mortality of rodents (and rodents only) that should have preceded an outbreak of plague, when the folk wisdom of the lands in which the modern pandemic origi-nated is replete with warnings to evacuate the area of a rodent epizootic (animal epidemic).[36] (John of Ephesus, it will be recalled, referred to dead rats, but only in a lengthy catalog of smitten fauna.) But these are "softer" questions about cultural matters, almost impossible to answer with any confidence. The seven preceding questions are, however, mat-ters of historical biology, epidemiology, and ecology on which progress ought to be possible. To these questions posed or implied by the deniers, upholders of the conventional diagnosis of the EMP must provide more substantial answers than they have so far managed.

As the debate continues, one other fundamental question deserves an airing: "So what?" That is, what turns on achieving the correct ret-rospective diagnosis of the EMP? The answer may be: "nothing." If correct, this is uncomfortable for both affirmers and deniers of *Yersinia pestis*. The reason nothing turns on the outcome of the debate is that both sides are trying to explain the evidence and the historical phe-nomena to which the evidence points. Neither side is trying to use its preferred diagnosis – bubonic or not-bubonic – as a way of either playing down the significance of the pandemic (as Shrewsbury did in his history of bubonic plague in Britain) or of showing that it has somehow been underestimated. Those who claim that the pandemic was not bubonic plague are simply trying, in the most economical way, to account for its speed of diffusion and the mortality it inflicted. They do not want to change our picture of the disease's impact. Those reaffirming the role of *Yersinia pestis* are claiming no more than that the traditional explanation is enough to account for its observable effects.

Arguments about diagnosis provide entertainment, and they are currently the focus of the most lively scholarship concerning any of the pandemics. That is why they have been conveyed here at length. But they do not necessarily advance historical understanding.

CAUSES

If we cannot be certain of the EMP's biological identity, we are, a fortiori, unlikely to be able to give a causal explanation of its arrival. The first and most obvious subject against which to measure our scepticism is demography. In the eastern Roman Empire, it is now widely held, the two centuries preceding the pandemic of the 540s had been ones of economic expansion, a quickening of the monetary economy, and sustained demographic growth.[37] There were numerous periods of food stress and occasional famines – their frequency perhaps increasing in the 520s and 530s.[38] A new imperial elite acquired large estates and sucked a demographically expanding peasantry into its orbit. It was, perhaps, able to do this because, in many parts of the Byzantine world, the peasantry was too numerous to survive independently on ever smaller subdivisions of available land. Yet, despite the food shortages, there is no sign from the eastern Mediterranean of the sixth century, as there is from the Europe of the late thirteenth and early fourteenth century, that the population had generally grown substantially beyond its means. The EMP did not prick the Malthusian bubble in Byzantium. In general, explanations for its arrival of a demographic kind seem unpromising. At best they offer a context in which the disease could have spread rapidly and devastatingly. Something more obviously causal and more catastrophic is needed.

An earthquake is one type of candidate for that catastrophe. An earthquake preceded the outbreak of plague in India in 1993. Constantinople was shaken by earthquakes in 525, 533, 548, 554, 557, and 740. Only that of 557 is closely tied to the EMP, preceding a new wave of it by eight months.[39] But perhaps we should not expect the correlation to be too close. If rodents were involved in plague, then several years may have had to elapse between environmental disaster, changes in rat population, and epizootic. If the disease was not bubonic plague, then the biological or ecological preconditions of the EMP remain to be determined. And in any case, earthquakes are far from unusual in and around the Mediterranean. The German geographer Alfred Philippson wrote, for example, that no day passes without an earthquake somewhere in Greece.[40]

More promising than an earthquake as a cause of the EMP is climate. The climatological history of the sixth century is in its infancy, and from the scanty evidence so far available it would be rash to infer a general trend, for example toward greater precipitation, which might have encouraged a growth in rat population.[41] There were dry years in

530 (Constantinople) and 536 (Iran), but heavy snowfall in 540 (Syria). Yet what has quickened the pulse of scientists, historians, and even television audiences has been the "years without summer" or the "dust-veil event" of 536–537. The cause was low solar emissions or some dust-producing terrestrial disaster – perhaps the impact of an asteroid or comet, perhaps a major volcanic eruption (although none of these is so far clearly evidenced from the years in question).[42] The effect, widely noticed across the globe from Italy to China, and suitably registered in the very slow growth of tree rings, was twelve to eighteen months of faded sunlight, and a resulting period of poorer climate across the northern hemisphere.

Here, if anywhere, is a big ecological upset. In the eyes of believers, it heralded plague by causing a migration of plague-bearing rodents from their normal central African habitats.[43] More plausibly, though again only if *Yersinia pestis* was involved, the reduced temperatures of the 530s expanded the area within which plague survived enzootically among those African rodents. It pushed the perimeter of its reservoir almost to the coast opposite Zanzibar Island. Here, Byzantine Red Sea trade, especially an expanding trade in ivory, brought both seafarers and susceptible Mediterranean rats. On the return journey the rats took the disease north to Pelusium.[44] It may have been so, and it may have been that this "event" ushered in not only plague, but also the Avars, the weakening of the late Roman state, and the rise of Islam.[45] But the ecological connections between meteorology and history on this scale remain indistinct.

EFFECTS

What, then, was the impact of the early medieval pandemic on the Age of Justinian? To attempt even a partial answer to that question is virtually to rewrite the demographic, economic, social, cultural, and political history of the Mediterranean world in the later sixth and early seventh centuries. In that respect providing the answer falls to all contributors to this volume; it can hardly be restricted to a chapter on the pandemic itself. Perhaps significantly, only one other contribution (Chap. 2, by John Haldon) includes the EMP as an ingredient in major change.

There is no great surprise here. First of all, those who study the EMP directly tend to attribute a far greater effect to it than do those for whom it is, in disciplinary terms, peripheral. In recent decades only one influential plague denier has emerged among those who write on the pandemic: Jean Durliat.[46] He denies, not the diagnosis of bubonic plague, but the mortality and hence the wider effects. The descriptions of Procopius, John of Ephesus, Evagrius, and their kind may be rhetorical exaggerations, elite responses to localized panic. Beyond these few "supercharged" evocations, the written evidence worryingly fails us, either because it is imprecise about the nature of epidemics or because it does not mention the EMP where we should expect it. Without the major literary texts, Durliat asks in effect, what indices would we have of the plague's impact? There are no traces of it in the Egyptian papyri, and very few in the hagiography, our two most abundant documentary sources for "everyday life." The inscriptions of the period do not register it either. And there are, so far, no genuine plague pits known to archaeologists, no direct proof of the hastily improvised mass burials described by Procopius and widely known from the period of the Black Death.[47] Perhaps then the disease was confined to major cities and routes linking them. Even here, moreover, its impact remains uncertain because (as we see confirmed elsewhere in this volume) city life continued: "business as usual," in the words of another, similar, denier.[48]

Other scholars of plague are more or less united in rejecting this minimalist view. Although they must concede that the immediate impact of the EMP remains invisible in the urban archaeology and the field surveys of the sixth and earlier seventh centuries, Durliat's reassessment remains vulnerable on several counts. The record of inscriptions offers the clearest example. Improvised multiple burials would not have been recorded in inscriptions. And the majority of the dead would inevitably have been the poor, for whom epigraphic immortality was never in prospect. Again, if the epidemic was not a far more widespread and serious phenomenon than Durliat suggests, why did Justinian legislate at the end of the first wave to counteract major wage and price increases, and why was there famine in Constantinople one year later? *Contra* Durliat, mortality estimates similar to those given for the Black Death are widely and confidently repeated in the literature: figures ranging between 20 and 30 percent.[49] They are based not only on the texts quoted above but on the repeated impression of widespread panic, chaos, and disruption conveyed by a substantial corpus of written evidence, not only Latin and Greek but, still more, Syriac and Arabic.[50] Lawrence Conrad argues convincingly that, "as the witnesses responsible for these accounts spoke different languages (and often did not know others), represented different social, cultural, and religious viewpoints, and frequently lived at considerable chronological and geographical removes from one

XIV

another, it is impossible to put these congruences down to the literary and emotional factors adduced by Durliat."[51]

There, however, clarity and consensus end – which may be one reason why the plague is mentioned, if at all, only in passing in many modern accounts of the period.[52] This, too, is unsurprising. A similar degree of ambivalence or caution prevails in the historiography of the Black Death. There was massive depopulation, not just from the initial pandemic but from recurrent waves of it – on average, one year in four between 1380 and 1480. The mechanisms of demographic recovery thus never had the chance to develop. This basic fact about prolonged demographic depression ought to color all socioeconomic interpretation of the later Middle Ages.[53] The problem for historians is that, in many cases, survivors of the pandemic prospered, in a land-rich, wage-inflationary environment. Demographic catastrophe was not, in the long term, matched by economic collapse. And if we cast the interpretative net more widely, there is no subject, from church sculpture to farming techniques, on which the Black Death can be said to have had a distinct and unequivocal impact: "Repeatedly we find that the Black Death was not an autonomous agent of change but worked in tandem with other processes."[54]

So it is with the early medieval pandemic: a major ingredient in the changes that we detect in the Age of Justinian and the seventh to eighth centuries, but only one such ingredient among several.[55] The EMP struck the Byzantine and Islamic Middle East less frequently than the Black Death did but was hardly a "light touch." Perhaps western Europe was more fortunate in the early Middle Ages; it is impossible to tell. In what follows, therefore, discussion is confined to the eastern Mediterranean, where the problems of interpretation seem slightly more tractable.

On one hand, the short-term impact (the "hammer-blow," as Peter Sarris puts it)[56] can, pace Durliat, be detected outside the usual literary evidence. Papyrology, for instance, records a quite rapid and marked improvement in the security of tenure enjoyed by Egyptian lessees of land from the mid-sixth century onward; presumably landlords suddenly found themselves in a buyers' market.[57] Nor is the history of coinage entirely unruffled by the EMP. The Byzantine state quickly responded to what must have been a drastic diminution of its tax revenues by reducing the size of its gold coinage, and perhaps also by tinkering with the weight of its copper issues.[58]

On the other hand, if we look to a broadly reliable index of manpower, recruitment to the army, it is far less clear that the state experienced insuperable difficulties.[59] In the later 540s and the 550s the armies of Byzantium fought successfully on three fronts: in Lazica, against the Moors in Africa, and, most decisively, in the Ostrogothic wars in Italy. Those who blame the pandemic for later defeats, inflicted first by the Persians, then by the armies of Islam, need to bear these successes of Justinian's reign in mind.

If there is so little certainty about the relations between the pandemic and such features of the political and military history of the period, still less can we pronounce on the role of plague in grander but vaguer phenomena like "the end of antiquity" or, à la Pirenne, the decline of the Mediterranean economy. A relatively sophisticated economy continued to function relatively unscathed well beyond the Age of Justinian in many parts of the empire – perhaps on much reduced populations, but not with that dramatic diminution of prosperity upon which several historians have insisted.[60] The "origins of the European economy," we are told by Michael McCormick, lie in the Carolingian world, not the tenth or eleventh century, where they had conventionally been placed.[61] That is, they lie in the period immediately following the EMP's recession from Europe. But there was too much else going on for the pandemic to be accorded a leading role in the economic *translatio imperii*.

USES

Michael McCormick treats plague as one way of tracking Mediterranean communications.[62] That prompts a final question: Is the EMP of any use? It was plainly not much use to its victims, other than in an eschatological sense; it was more obviously of use to those who survived into a world of greater economic opportunity. But has it anything to tell us today? If we could agree on a diagnosis, then we might enlarge our understanding of the ecology of the Age of Justinian. Until that unanimity is achieved, however, the way in which the disease spread by sea, by river, and from city to hinterland tells us, I submit, nothing that we did not already know. An unusual chronological cluster of inscriptions may, if interpreted as a sign of an epidemic, inform us that plague reached a locality where we had not previously suspected it. But this is progress at the microscopic level only. At the level of aerial photography, we use our already available evidence of Mediterranean communications and settlement to tell us about the likely behavior of the pandemic, not the other way around.

XIV

For all the immaculate scholarship that continues to be lavished upon it, the early medieval pandemic remains a black hole at the center of the Age of Justinian. It absorbs a great deal of our energy; it gives very little out.

NOTES

1   Procopius, *Secret History*, 18.36–44.
2   The pioneering work is Pauline Allen, "The 'Justinianic' Plague," *Byzantion* 49 (1979): 5–20. Dionysios Stathakopoulos, "The Justinianic Plague Revisited," *BMGS* 24 (2000): 256–276, surveys the literature.
3   Michael Whitby and Mary Whitby, ed. and trans., *Chronicon Paschale, 284–628 AD* (Liverpool, 1989), 111.
4   Alexander A. Vasiliev, ed., PO 8 (1912): 425. Here and throughout I am indebted to Dionysios Stathakopoulos for references and previews of works in press.
5   Robert Sallares, "Ecology, Evolution, and Epidemiology of Plague," in *The Justinianic Plague, 541–767 AD* (proceedings of conference held at the American Academy in Rome, December 2001), ed. Lester K. Little (Cambridge University Press, forthcoming), generously shown to me in typescript by its author, nn. 77, 212.
6   For full presentation of the evidence, see Dionysios Stathakopoulos, *Famine and Pestilence in the Late Roman and Early Byzantine Empire: A Systematic Survey of Subsistence Crises and Epidemics* (Aldershot, 2004), chap. 6, prefigured in Dionysios Stathakopoulos, "Crime and Punishment: The Plague in the Byzantine Empire, 541–749," in Little, *Justinianic Plague*. I cannot, however, always accept his speculative plotting of some of the disease's movements according to unusual chronological concentrations of funerary inscriptions.
7   See Alain Stoclet and Michael Kulikowski in Little, *Justinianic Plague*.
8   *Nov.*, 122.
9   J. R. Maddicott, "Plague in Seventh-Century England," *Past and Present* 156 (1997): 7–54; Stathakopoulos, *Famine and Pestilence*, 116.
10 Michael McCormick in Little, *Justinianic Plague*.
11 Lawrence I. Conrad, "Die Pest und ihr soziales Umfeld in Nahen Osten des früheren Mittelalters," *Der Islam* 73 (1996): 99–102; Peter Sarris, "The Justinianic Plague: Origins and Effects," *Continuity and Change* 17 (2002): 170 and n. 14.
12 Stathakopoulos, *Famine and Pestilence*, 123.
13 Marie-Hélène Congourdeau, "La Société byzantine face aux grandes pandémies," in *Maladie et Société à Byzance*, ed. Evelyne Patlagean (Spoleto, 1993), 25–26; Jean-Noël Biraben and Jacques Le Goff, "The Plague in the Early Middle Ages," in *Biology of Man in History: Selections from the "Annales: Économies, Sociétés, Civilisations"* ed. Robert Forster and Orest Ranum (Baltimore, 1975), 49 n. 3.
14 The following excerpts are from *Wars*, 2.22.1–10, trans. Dewing, 451–469.
15 The relevant (second) part of John's *Ecclesiastical History* survives in an eighth-century Syriac universal chronicle. Excerpts that follow are from Witold Witakowski, trans., *Pseudo-Dionysius of Tel-Mahre, Chronicle ... Part III* (Liverpool, 1996), 77, 80–81, 86–87 (modified).

16   *The Ecclesiastical History of Evagrius*, 4.29, ed. J. Bidez and L. Parmentier (London, 1898), 177–179, trans. Michael Whitby, *The Ecclesiastical History of Evagrius Scholasticus* (Liverpool, 2000), 229–232.

17   Andrew Cunningham, "Transforming Plague: The Laboratory and the Identity of Infectious Disease," in *The Laboratory Revolution in Medicine*, ed. Andrew Cunningham and Penry Williams (Cambridge, 1992), 209–244; Cunningham, "Identifying Disease in the Past: Cutting the Gordian Knot," *Asclepio* 54 (2002): 13–34.

18   Dionysios Stathakopoulos, "Die Terminologie der Pest in Byzantinischen Quellen," *JÖB* 48 (1998): 1–7; Liliane Bodson, "Le Vocabulaire des maladies pestilentielles et épizootiques," in *Le Latin médical: la constitution d'un language scientifique*, ed. Guy Sabbah (Saint-Étienne, 1991), 215–241.

19   Lawrence I. Conrad, "*Ṭāʿūn* and *Wabāʾ*: Conceptions of Plague and Pestilence in Early Islam," *Journal of the Economic and Social History of the Orient* 25 (1982): 268–307.

20   Ann G. Carmichael, "Bubonic Plague," in *The Cambridge World History of Human Disease*, ed. Kenneth F. Kiple (Cambridge, 1993), 628–630.

21   Gregory of Tours, *Libri Historiarum*, 10.1, trans. Lewis Thorpe, *Gregory of Tours, The History of the Franks* (Harmondsworth, 1974), 543; Paul the Deacon, *Historia Langobardorum*, 2.4, trans. W. D. Foulke, *History of the Langobards, by Paul the Deacon* (Philadelphia, 1907), 56.

22   The evidence is reviewed by Sallares, "Ecology," sec. 2.

23   Carol Benedict, *Bubonic Plague in Nineteenth-Century China* (Stanford, Calif., 1996).

24   Lien-Teh Wu, *Plague: A Manual for Medical and Public Health Workers* (Shanghai, 1936); L. Fabian Hirst, *The Conquest of Plague* (Oxford, 1953); R. Pollitzer, *Plague* (Geneva, 1954). See also Samuel K. Cohn, Jr., *The Black Death Transformed: Disease and Culture in Early Renaissance Europe* (London, 2002), 16.

25   For accounts of Yersin's achievement, see Cohn, *Black Death Transformed*, chaps. 1–2, and Cunningham, "Transforming Plague."

26   R. Devignat, "Variétés de l'espèce *Pasteurella pestis*: Nouvelle hypothèse," *Bulletin of the World Health Organisation* 4 (1951): 247–263, with Sallares, "Ecology," sec. 3.

27   J. F. D. Shrewsbury, *A History of Bubonic Plague in the British Isles* (Cambridge, 1970).

28   Graham Twigg, *The Black Death: A Biological Reappraisal* (London, 1984).

29   See, e.g., Didier Raoult et al., "Molecular Identification by 'Suicide PCR' of Yersinia Pestis as the Agent of Medieval Black Death," *Proceedings of the National Academy of Sciences of the U.S.A.* 97 (2000): 12880–12883. The literature is surveyed in Sallares, "Ecology," sec. 3.

30   Susan Scott and Christopher J. Duncan, *Biology of Plagues: Evidence from Historical Populations* (Cambridge, 2001); Cohn, *Black Death Transformed*.

31   Sallares, "Ecology."

32   I follow Graham Twigg, "Bubonic Plague: Doubts and Diagnoses," *Journal of Medical Microbiology* 42 (1995): 383–385.

33   Cohn, *Black Death*, 22–23.

34   James Wood and Sharon DeWitte-Aviña, "Was the Black Death Yersinial Plague?" *The Lancet, Infectious Diseases* 3 (2003): 327.

35   Sallares, "Ecology," fully reviews the genetic evidence. See also Scott and Duncan, *Biology of Plagues*, 63–65.

36   Cohn, *Black Death*, 17. Michael McCormick, "Rats, Communications, and Plague: Towards an Ecological History," *Journal of Interdisciplinary History* 34

(2003): 4, argues that early medieval texts do not distinguish rats from mice or other rodents. But that does not solve the problem: rodent mortality is very infrequently noticed in contemporary accounts of EMP.

37   Peter Sarris, "Rehabilitating the Great Estate: Aristocratic Property and Economic Growth in the Late Antique Eastern Empire," in *Recent Research on the Late Antique Countryside*, Late Antique Archaeology 2, ed. William Bowden, Luke Lavan, and Carlos Machado (Leiden, 2004), 55–71; Bryan Ward-Perkins, "Land, Labour, and Settlement," in *CAH* 14:319–321.

38   Stathakopoulos, *Famine and Pestilence*, 261–277.

39   McCormick, "Rats," 19; for wider context see *I terremoti prima del Mille in Italia e nell'area mediterranea*, ed. Emanuela Guidoboni (Bologna, 1989), 690ff.

40   *Das Mittelmeergebiet: Seine geographische und kulturelle Eigenart* (Leipzig, 1904), 28.

41   McCormick, "Rats," 20; Johannes Koder, "Climatic Change in the Fifth and Sixth Centuries?" in *The Sixth Century: End or Beginning?*, ed. Pauline Allen and Elizabeth Jeffreys (Brisbane, 1996), 270–285.

42   Joel D. Gunn, ed., *The Years without Summer: Tracing AD 536 and its Aftermath*, British Archaeological Reports Intermediate Series 872 (Oxford, 2000); David Keys, *Catastrophe: An Investigation into the Origins of the Modern World* (London, 1999), favors an eruption, perhaps of Krakatoa. M. G. L. Baillie prefers comets as his explanation for the EMP and much else; see his *Exodus to Arthur: Catastrophic Encounters with Comets*, 2nd ed. (London, 2000). Note also R. B. Stothers and M. R. Rampino, "Volcanic Eruptions in the Mediterranean before A.D. 630 from Written and Archaeological Sources," *Journal of Geophysical Research* 88 (1983): 6357–6371, a reference I owe to Morten Axboe.

43   Keys, *Catastrophe*, 18–19.

44   I follow unpublished work of Mark Horton of the University of Bristol, U.K.

45   As argued in Keys, *Catastrophe*.

46   Jean Durliat, "La Peste du VIe siècle: Pour un nouvel examen des sources byzantines," in *Hommes et richesses dans l'empire byzantin IVe–VIIe siècle* (Paris, 1989), 107–119, with the immediate response ("Rapport") by Jean-Noël Biraben, 121–125.

47   Michael McCormick's contribution to Little, *Justinianic Plague*, will contain a census of the archaeology of burials attributable to the EMP. For the meager trawl to date, see Stathakopoulos, *Famine and Pestilence*, 149–150.

48   Mark Whittow, *The Making of Orthodox Byzantium, 600–1025* (Houndmills, Eng., 1996), 66.

49   Stathakopoulos, *Famine and Pestilence*, 140; Allen, "The 'Justinianic' Plague," 11.

50   On social and religious responses to the EMP in Byzantium, see Stathakopoulos, *Famine and Pestilence*, 146–154.

51   Lawrence I. Conrad, "Epidemic Disease in Central Syria in the Late Sixth Century: Some New Insights from the Verse of Ḥassān ibn Thābit," *BMGS* 18 (1994): 56.

52   For a recent exception, in which plague, along with other environmental disasters of the 530s and 540s, becomes key to the whole subsequent, hyper-religious, tenor of Justinian's reign, see Mischa Meier, *Das andere Zeitalter Justinians* (Göttingen, 2003), esp. 340–341.

53   Colin Platt, *King Death: The Black Death and Its Aftermath in Late-Medieval England* (London, 1996), 177.

54 P. J. P. Goldberg, "Introduction," in *The Black Death in England*, ed. W. M. Ormrod and P. G. Lindley (Stamford, Eng., 1996), 13.

55 Conrad, "Die Pest und ihr soziales Umfeld," 102–112.

56 Sarris, "Justinianic Plague," 173.

57 Sarris, "Justinianic Plague," 178, cites Jairus Banaji, "Rural Communities in the Late Empire: Economic and Monetary Aspects" (PhD diss., University of Oxford, 1992), tab. 20.

58 Sarris, "Justinianic Plague," 175–177.

59 Michael Whitby, "Recruitment in Roman Armies from Justinian to Heraclius (*ca.* 565–615)," in *The Byzantine and Early Islamic Near East*, vol. 3, *States, Resources and Armies*, ed. Averil Cameron (Princeton, N.J., 1995), 61–124.

60 Ward-Perkins, "Land, Labour and Settlement," 327; Ward-Perkins, "Specialized Production and Exchange," in *CAH* 14:354, 388.

61 Michael McCormick, *Origins of the European Economy: Communications and Commerce, AD 300–900* (New York, 2001). For plague and economic change, see esp. 538–539. For plague and the overall "disease burden," 38–40.

62 McCormick, "Rats," esp. 25.

XV

The Millennium Bug: Health and Medicine around
the Year 1000

All calendrical systems involve arbitrary choices. They are also remarkably various,
and divide people as often as they unite. At 'Band Aid' for Ethiopia in 1984 Bob
Geldof asked emotively, 'do they know it's Christmas?' For the event's intended
beneficiaries, however, it was not Christmas at all. Indeed, in the calendar of the
Ethiopian church it was not even 1984.[1] As we embark on the third millennium of
the 'Common Era' we should approach all commemorations of the end of the first
millennium with a certain wariness. Did they know it was the year 1000? If so, did
they care?

This opening paper in our celebratory collection has two themes: first, what can
be said about the diseases characteristic of the period; second, what generalizations
are possible about the medicine that could be deployed against them. I want to use
the topic of chronology as a way of opening up the first theme, that of disease. In
the process, I shall also be demonstrating the arbitrary element in our choice of
period.

I

For many of the people who inhabited the worlds with which we are here
concerned (western Christendom, Byzantium, and Islam in the tenth to eleventh

For assistance in the preparation of this piece I am much indebted to Bob Arnott, Faith Wallis,
my co-editor, and my three referees, one of them anonymous. Surviving errors are naturally my own.

[1] A. Bryer, 'What Time is It?' (conference paper abstract), *Bulletin of British Byzantine Studies*, 25
(1999), 85.

XV

centuries) the year 1000 fell in either an immemorial past or a scarcely imaginable future.[2] Muslims, of course, inaugurated their (lunar) calendar with the Hijrah, the Prophet's departure from Mecca, although more commonly they dated events by referring to the ruler's regnal year. For them, in AD 1000, the thousandth year of the Hijrah lay centuries ahead. Many others—including most Jews, many Byzantine Greek scholars, some western chroniclers—reckoned in terms of the years elapsed since the creation of the world. This was the *anno mundi* (AM) system. For its adherents, the 'year of the world' 1000 had come and gone in earliest Biblical times. The AM system did, though, yield its own special date. This was 6000, at which (millenarians thought) history would end as the world entered its seventh 'day',[3] and there would follow, according to Revelation ch. 20, the thousand-year reign of Christ and the saints preceding the general judgement.

In western Christendom, the system of dating from Christ's incarnation, invented in the early sixth century but generalized only centuries later by the influence of Bede,[4] did not render *anno mundi* chronology obsolete. Nor did it eliminate alternative techniques, such as dating by regnal years, or by the fifteen-year cycle of tax Indictions of the later Roman Empire. A scribe-annalist embellishing Easter tables in a monastery in Berry wrote coolly beside the year 1000: 'a severe famine. There are 6,201 years from the beginning of the world'. Another monk in Lotharingia took care to note that the year 1000 was also Indiction 13.[5]

We are thus choosing to examine medical practice around a thousand years ago in cultures that would not all, at that time, have acknowledged that they were living in the tenth or eleventh century. Our focus is to that extent arbitrary: it reflects current obsession with anniversaries. As I hope to show later, there is some justification for looking back a thousand years or more into European history: western medicine before *c.* 1000 is in many ways very different from western medicine *c.* 1200. By contrast the *anni Domini* around 1000 correlate with no particular turning-point in the Byzantine or the Islamic medical past.

Those who did know it was 1000 were conceivably the minority within the worlds we are studying. Even so, about that minority, as also incidentally about others who had earlier awaited the fraught AM 6000, one question is worth raising. It pertains—at least potentially—to medical history. Hardly a novel question, it is prompted anew by recent fears of the real 'millennium bug': fears which sometimes verged on the pathological and were no less profound for having, like all apocalypticism thus far, been proved groundless. How deeply were people troubled by the approach of AD 1000? Was there millennial 'fever': a 'hystory' comparable to those controversially ascribed to the late twentieth century?[6] Is

---

[2] B. Blackburn and L. Holford-Strevens, *The Oxford Companion to the Year* (Oxford, 1999), pt II, is a learned conspectus of calendars and chronology.

[3] II Peter 3.8; Psalm 90.4.

[4] *Bede: The Reckoning of Time*, trans. F. Wallis (Liverpool, 1999), esp. p. lxx and commentary on Bede's ch. 66. R. McKitterick, 'Constructing the Past in the Early Middle Ages: The Case of the Royal Frankish Annals', *Transactions of the Royal Historical Society*, 6th series, 7 (1997), pp. 103–10, makes important qualifications about the extent of Bede's influence in this respect.

[5] R. Landes, 'Giants with Feet of Clay: On the Historiography of the Year 1000' [http://www.mille.org/1000-pg.html], at nn. 121, 169.

[6] E. Showalter, *Hystories: Hysterical Epidemics and Modern Culture* (London, 1997).

there any remaining validity in the charged depictions of *les terreurs de l'an mil* bequeathed to popular historiography by romantics such as Michelet?[7]

Our three chosen cultures naturally present a hugely variegated picture. The term 'apocalypse' had no exact equivalent in Arabic, and the Qur'ān stated that only God knew when the Last Hour would come.[8] Each generation of Muslims had thus to be on its guard, constantly re-evaluating possible signs of the end (which included the return of Jesus).[9] From Byzantium, some writers do create the impression that the tenth century was a time of heightened expectation. The historian Leo the Deacon expressed his fear that the ship of life was on the point of being halted. Niketas David had already looked at the cosmic 'week' and calculated that only six hours and eight minutes remained; he predicted the end of the world in 1028.[10] Or rather, in the equivalent of 1028, for he was reckoning in terms of the *era mundi*, the age of the world. Like Leo's, his own eschatological unease falls within a tradition going back to before the earliest year thought to mark the beginning of the seventh millennium AM—that is, AD 500. The belief that the last days were approaching had a long history by the 'tenth century' in Byzantium. It was a belief fuelled by the advance of Islam, and it demonstrably added to the pious zeal of a number of emperors, especially in the sixth and the ninth to tenth centuries.[11]

And Europe? Here the availability of critical years in both AD and AM systems suggests that apocalyptic expectation might be more emphatic. Yet it now seems clear that both the romantic historians who claimed to detect *terreurs* as 1000 approached, and also their critics who argued that everyone was 'millennium compliant'; were alike wrong. There *were* widespread movements in the later tenth century that may have had eschatological overtones: the Peace of God, large-scale pilgrimages, anti-Semitic agitation, popular heresies.[12] Scholarly interest in *computus*, the medieval 'science' of the calendar, increased.[13] Some major figures writing in the years around 1000—Ralph Glaber, Ademar of Chabannes, Ælfric, for example—had, especially in Ademar's case, voiced increasingly strident concerns about the impending *eschaton*.[14]

Two qualifications need to be entered, however. First, the years around 1000 were not the only ones to arouse anxiety. 'Y6K' in the *anno mundi* system, which had failed to arrive in AD 500, was postponed by various recalculations, the most

---

[7] J. Michelet, *L'histoire de France* (1835), bk. IV, ch. 1, in P. Viallaneix (ed.), *Oeuvres complètes*, IV (Paris, 1974), pp. 389–90.

[8] Qur'ān, VII.187, and elsewhere.

[9] I. K. Poonawala, 'Apocalyptic, ii: Muslim Iran', in *Encyclopaedia Iranica*, 7 vols. to date (London, 1985–), II, 157–60.

[10] C. Mango, *Byzantium: The Empire of New Rome* (London, 1980), p. 211.

[11] P. Magdalino, 'The History of the Future and Its Uses: Prophecy, Policy and Propaganda', in R. Beaton and C. Roueché (eds.), *The Making of Byzantine History: Studies Dedicated to Donald M. Nicol* (Aldershot, 1993), 3–34.

[12] Landes, 'Giants', at nn. 225 ff., offers, on a 'millennial' web site, the fullest review of the evidence and the historiographical controversies surrounding it.

[13] Ibid., at n. 110; Bede trans. Wallis, p. 363; though cf. Wallis, 'Medicine in Medieval Calendar Manuscripts', in M. R. Schleissner (ed.), *Manuscript Sources of Medieval Medicine* (New York and London, 1995), p. 108, for a different explanation of the increase.

[14] Landes, *Relics, Apocalypse and the Deceits of History: Ademar of Chabannes, 989-1034* (Harvard, 1995).

extreme being that of Bede who delayed it until 2048.[15] Bede had, in 708, complained of 'rustics' who irritated him daily with their enquiries about how many years remained in the final millennium of the world;[16] and AM 6000 was again expected in 801. Meanwhile, for advocates of dating from Christ's incarnation there were not only various estimates of when 1000 would fall, there was also the possibility of a turning-point in world history on the anniversary of the Passion, calculated to occur in 1033. Stranger candidates for the 'end time' also proposed themselves. A rumour supposedly swept Lotharingia in the 960s that the world would end when the anniversaries of the Passion, the Annunciation, and the creation of Adam coincided on Friday, 25 March, 970.[17] In 1096, the realization that the Feast of John the Baptist would fall on a Friday, and in a leap year with an extra lunar month, inspired apparently widespread eschatological dread in Ireland.[18]

There were, then, many possible occasions for anxiety, and they were spread out not over years or even decades but over several centuries. That is the first essential qualification; the second, inevitably, is that the seriousness of the 'fever' actually generated is now impossible to gauge. The standard—but far from triumphant—Augustinian response to such emotions was to forbid eschatological speculation. For Augustine the year 1000 was a symbolically perfect number (10^3), not a specific year.[19] Was agnosticism forced upon an excitable populace by clerics who insisted on postponing the significant date just enough for it to lose its threatening aspect—in what Richard Landes has called, somewhat paradoxically, a 'clearly documented case of a successful conspiracy of silence'?[20] Was computistic ingenuity, in other words, an effective therapy for millenarianism?

II

That is a question which historians—not only medical ones—must continue to discuss. Meanwhile, what other diseases might we associate with our period? It would be useful if, at this point, I could sketch a 'plagues and peoples around the year 1000', a pathological backdrop to the following articles which would show what the healers of the age were up against. This would be an imitation of W. H. McNeill's well-known feat of synthesis but on a much more limited time-scale.[21] It is instructive—if discouraging—to see what McNeill has to offer with respect to our period. The tenth century falls well after the 'confluence of the civilized disease pools of Eurasia.' And that is about the only way in which characterization seems possible. The analysis derives, unavoidably, from the generalities of conventional social history. As the millennium approaches so food production grows, and

[15] Idem, 'Giants', at n. 85.

[16] *Letter to Plegwin*, 15, trans. Wallis in *Bede: The Reckoning of Time*, p. 413.

[17] Landes, 'Giants', at nn. 130 ff.

[18] B. Hudson, 'Time is Short: The Eschatology of the Early Gaelic Church', in C. Walker Bynum and P. Freedman (eds.), *Last Things: Death and the Apocalypse in the Middle Ages* (Philadelphia, 2000), 101–23.

[19] *City of God*, XX.7.

[20] Landes, 'Giants', at n. 78, referring specifically to ecclesiastical historians, but with more general implication.

[21] W. H. McNeill, *Plagues and Peoples* (Oxford, 1997). See ch. 3 for what follows.

population too, first in the North (witness Viking colonization). European peoples have become part of a single disease pool, and once-lethal diseases have settled towards endemicity. Except in rural areas or on the fringes of Europe (such as Britain), where populations are not dense enough to sustain maladies at endemic level, virulent diseases have tended to subside into childhood afflictions (this is after all the period of Rāzī's celebrated description of measles and smallpox).[22] With that, the period is abandoned so far as European history is concerned: we jump forward to the Mongol irruption and its role in spreading the Black Death.

McNeill's picture, though somewhat a priori, is fuller and more vivid than the one given by the *Cambridge World History of Human Disease*.[23] Apart from sweeping reference to the multiplicity of epidemics and asides on the pathogenic role of the crusades, the pertinent sections on disease ecology have little to say that even verges on our period; indeed, the section on the Middle East and North Africa scarcely ventures earlier than the nineteenth century. With respect to our period, the section on diseases of the Middle Ages discusses only population growth, meat consumption, and female iron deficiency: its one specific reference is a mistaken one, contradicted elsewhere in the volume, to bubonic plague in twelfth-century Rome.

In 1993, the same year that the *Cambridge World History* was published, the doyen of plague historians, Jean-Noel Biraben, essayed an outline of diseases in medieval Europe.[24] He rightly points to ergotism as a disease whose worst outbreaks seem to have begun in the early tenth century,[25] and to serious epidemics (especially in 927 and 1105) of what, on the basis of work done a century ago, he asserts to have been influenza.[26] He then attempts a 'pathocoenosis' of the high Middle Ages, which at least includes the centuries around 1000. The term 'pathocoenosis' was coined by M. D. Grmek in an article of 1969 by analogy with Möbius's 'bio-coenosis.'[27] It is taken to designate 'the ensemble of pathological states present in a specific population at a given moment in time',[28] the interrelationships between diseases as well as between each disease and its ecology.[29] Inspired doubtless by Grmek's detailed and complex panorama of diseases in the ancient Greek world,[30] Biraben offers a chart of the medieval European pathocoenosis, derived from Wickersheimer's catalogue of Latin medical manuscripts in French libraries.[31]

[22] Trans. W. A. Greenhill, *A Treatise on the Small-Pox and Measles* (London, 1848). Emilie Savage-Smith informs me that the earliest preserved monograph on the subject (represented by an unpublished manuscript now in Aleppo) was not by Rāzī but by Thābit ibn Qurrah (d. 901).

[23] K. F. Kiple (ed.) (Cambridge, 1993), sections V.3, VII.2, 7.

[24] Now translated as 'Diseases in Europe: Equilibrium and Breakdown of the Pathocenosis', in M. D. Grmek (ed.), *Western Medical Thought from Antiquity to the Middle Ages* (Cambridge, MA, and London, 1998), 319–53.

[25] See also Kiple, *Cambridge World History*, section VIII.49. J. Sumption, *Pilgrimage* (London, 1975), p. 75, with references.

[26] For this and what follows, Biraben, 'Diseases', pp. 345–8.

[27] M. D. Grmek, 'Préliminaires d'une étude historique des maladies', *Annales*, 24 (1969), 1473–83, at p. 1476; R. Sallares, *The Ecology of the Ancient Greek World* (London, 1991), p. 225.

[28] M. D. Grmek, *Diseases in the Ancient Greek World* (Baltimore and London, 1989), p. 3.

[29] Compare J. Landers, *Death and the Metropolis: Studies in the Demographic History of London 1670–1830* (Cambridge, 1993), ch. 1, for the cognate term 'pathogenic load'.

[30] Grmek, *Diseases in the Ancient Greek World*.

[31] E. Wickersheimer, *Les manuscrits latins de médecine du Moyen Age dans les bibliothèques de France* (Paris, 1966).

Counting references to diseases in 118 texts dating from between the seventh and eleventh centuries yields precise statistics, the details of which are, Biraben writes, 'certain to be of interest': 60 mentions of fever (5.5 per cent of the total), broken down into intermittent fevers (13 mentions), various febrifuges (42), other fevers (5), and so on. Overall, the table shows a preponderance of non-infectious conditions, particularly of the digestive tract and the nervous system (above all migraine or paralysis). There are 58 references to gynaecological problems, 57 to gout, and 80 to ocular ailments. Under the 'infectious' heading, meanwhile, smallpox, leprosy, and rabies are rarely encountered; and most of the infections tabulated are too vaguely described to be represented by anything more than a single aggregate (113, or 38 per cent).

The way in which Biraben conceptualizes his evidence is revealing. At the start of the exercise, he takes the fact that the manuscripts seem to copy from one another as an indication that his results constitute, 'if not a *proper statistic of the diseases* of the era [which is how they were first introduced, and is what a pathocoenosis should ideally provide], at least a *reflection of the health concerns* of western European society'—which is not quite the same thing. By the time he concludes, the table has become '*in no way* a depiction of the distribution of diseases' (my italics throughout).[32]

The retreat from pathological reality to textual representation is symptomatic of the difficulties of the project. Pathocoenoses are exceedingly hard to establish. It is not just that the tenth to eleventh century in Europe is relatively so poorly documented, in many ways a more obscure period than the preceding centuries of what used to be called the Dark Ages.[33] The problem lies more in the nature of the evidence. Scholars attempting a panorama of the diseases of Greek antiquity, with the substantial Hippocratic corpus to draw upon, have just as much difficulty in seeing 'through' the texts to past biological reality: witness the continuing scholarly parlour game, 'What was the plague of Athens?', or, at the other end of the spectrum, the problem of interpreting 'fever.'[34] Historians of much later periods, too, are comparably afflicted by the difficulty of converting indigenous morbidity categories into those of biomedicine. Witness Ann Carmichael's work on Renaissance Florence and Milan,[35] with 'books of the dead' to help her, or Mary Dobson's on early modern England, its abundant bibliography of little help in cracking the code of febrile disorder in mid-eighteenth-century Sussex.[36]

This problem of diagnosis emerges forcefully in two of the following chapters where the evidence lends itself to a little nosography. In using the Old English compendium, the *Lacnunga*, in this way, Audrey Meaney has to make decisions

[32] Biraben, 'Diseases', pp. 345, 348.

[33] Although see now T. Reuter (ed.), *The New Cambridge Medieval History, Volume III c. 900–c. 1024* (Cambridge, 1999).

[34] Biraben, 'Diseases', pp. 324 ff.; Grmek, *Diseases in the Ancient Greek World*; Sallares, *Ecology of the Ancient Greek World*, ch. II.7, at pp. 225, 244 ff.

[35] A. G. Carmichael, *Plague and the Poor in Renaissance Florence* (Cambridge, 1986), ch. 2; eadem, 'Epidemics and State Medicine in Fifteenth-Century Milan', in R. French *et al.* (eds.), *Medicine from the Black Death to the French Disease* (Aldershot, 1998), 221–47.

[36] M. J. Dobson, *Contours of Death and Disease in Early Modern England* (Cambridge, 1997), ch. 5, esp. pp. 229 ff., 251, 256.

about such matters as the difference between 'tightness' and 'constriction' of the breast and about 'flying poison' which are inevitably somewhat arbitrary. To take another well-known example: is an Anglo-Saxon affliction such as 'elfshot' an evocative idiom for describing diseases that we might recognize if we saw them, or is it a 'culture-bound syndrome', an untranslatable folk illness?[37] Later in the collection, Cristina Álvarez-Millán faces a comparable challenge in translating the disease terminology of Rāzī's casebook, with its three different yet equally opaque terms for a gastric disorder and its species of melancholy that leads a woman to talk nonsense and laugh compulsively while blushing bright scarlet.

Diagnostic difficulties of this order are well-known. Less often acknowledged is the more intractable problem of deciding why the written evidence at our disposal was produced and thus of how directly—or how comprehensively—it relates to clinical reality. We obviously cannot assume that any text that seems to list ailments was intended to provide a *complete* list of important diseases, a pathocoenosis. Healers specialize: magicians, empirics, miracle-working saints, itinerant surgeons,[38] may each 'take on' only selected portions of the pathological panorama. Physicians may have been no less choosy—so that what can be elicited from the Hippocratic corpus or (to revert to Biraben) the texts of the early Middle Ages is not necessarily a full 'reflection of the health concerns of . . . society'.

A further assumption we should be chary of making is that evidence lending itself to tabulation of diseases was originally descriptive in purpose. Now the casebook drawn up by Rāzī's students seems designed to sustain clinical education—although even that work has to be assessed against the background of a literary tradition which may have constrained the varieties of disease included.[39] But what are we to make of a text such as *Lacnunga*, the provenance and purpose of which remain obscure?[40] Is it descriptive of ailments in anything like the same way: a manual for the complete practitioner? What can be deduced from the frequency with which it mentions particular complaints? To look to another article below (by Klaus-Dietrich Fischer): we would not necessarily infer from either the *Liber Passionalis* or one of its pseudo-Galenic sources that liver and gynaecological complaints predominated in the monastic scriptoria in which the text had its early medieval being. Like the womb, the liver may, for monks, have been more often a focus of learned discussion or a means of moral edification than a cause of pain.[41] The purpose of the *Liber* may have been more 'educational', in a very broad sense, than descriptive. In the *Politics* (1282a3) Aristotle drew a distinction between, in effect, the craftsman-physician, the learned 'professional', and the medically educated 'layman'. Many medical texts of late antiquity and the early Middle Ages which have been associated by historians with the first or second of those figures

[37] J. Neville, *Representations of the Natural World in Old English Poetry* (Cambridge, 1999), pp. 117–18; M. L. Cameron, *Anglo-Saxon Medicine* (Cambridge, 1993), pp. 10, 141–2. Compare B. J. Good, *Medicine, Rationality, and Experience* (Cambridge, 1994), pp. 53–5, 174–5.

[38] See further Savage-Smith below.

[39] C. Álvarez-Millán, 'Graeco-Roman Case Histories and their Influence on Medieval Islamic Clinical Accounts', *Social History of Medicine*, 12 (1999), 19–33.

[40] Cameron, *Anglo-Saxon Medicine*, p. 34.

[41] J. Cadden, *Meanings of Sex Difference in the Middle Ages* (Cambridge, 1993), pp. 48–9.

208

should perhaps be assigned to the third; and the third should be envisaged as capable of a great range of medical interests, philosophical as well as practical.[42]

We would like morbidity statistics of however rudimentary a kind. Yet the variety of the written evidence that we perhaps too trustingly classify as therapeutic can vitiate all attempts at aggregation. We are not told by Biraben which manuscripts from Wickersheimer's catalogue he used to compile his medieval pathocoenosis. Did it include the *Liber passionalis*? If so, how should that affect the weight we give to the 22 mentions of liver problems that Biraben includes?[43] How could such a tabulation accommodate a ninth-to-tenth-century compilation, the *Sapientia artis medicinae* (*Wisdom of the art of medicine*), which enumerates cures without describing them: 24 for the head, 12 for the eye, 25 for the thorax, etc.—so that, in one manuscript at least, the total is 365? Statistics of that particular kind tell us more about numerology than about clinical concerns.[44] We are back in the world of *computus*: a world hospitable to medicine, but not necessarily always of immediate practical value.

Such recalcitrant material might seem to invite the response that each text or piece of evidence can be interpreted only in relation to the cultural milieu in which it was produced and bears no clear imprint of pathological reality at all. On this view, nothing can be said about actual morbidity. All the historian can do is enumerate representations of disease, not the diseases themselves. Indeed it has become fashionable to accept without comment the epistemological relativism advocated, most notably, by Andrew Cunningham. Plague (his example) defined in the laboratory—caused by a bacillus—is simply not the same disease as plague experienced in the fourteenth century—in terms of the corruption of humours.[45] Hence, for the relativist, all illnesses are folk illnesses. There is as little transhistorical essence to plague as there is to neurasthenia or chlorosis.[46] The attempt to translate historical disease terms into modern ones is therefore not just difficult in practice: on conceptual grounds it is wholly impermissible. This is not the occasion to take detailed issue with such an increasingly influential approach[47]—except to point out that relativism is always (an elementary but still telling point) self-contradictory, because of its universalist claims. It is also in this particular instance self-defeating: the laboratory of today is so different from the laboratory

[42] See again Savage-Smith below; also Bennett for craft texts.

[43] Biraben, 'Diseases', p. 347.

[44] M. Wlaschky (ed.), 'Sapientia Artis Medicinae: ein frühmittelalterliches Kompendium der Medizin', *Kyklos: Jahrbuch des Instituts für Geschichte der Medizin an der Universität Leipzig*, 1 (1928), p. 108; F. Wallis, 'The Experience of the Book: Manuscripts, Texts, and the Role of Epistemology in Early Medieval Medicine', in D. Bates (ed.), *Knowledge and the Scholarly Medical Traditions* (Cambridge, 1995), 101–26, at pp. 121–2; eadem, 'Medicine in Medieval Calendar Manuscripts'.

[45] A. Cunningham, 'Transforming Plague: The Laboratory and the Identity of Infectious Disease', in idem and P. Williams (eds.), *The Laboratory Revolution in Medicine* (Cambridge, 1992), 209–44.

[46] On chlorosis see H. King, *Hippocrates' Woman: Reading the Female Body in Ancient Greece* (London, 1998), ch. 10.

[47] M. Hollis and S. Lukes (eds.), *Rationality and Relativism* (Oxford, 1982), remains a valuable introduction to the issues. See also the brief but trenchant attack on relativism in T. Nagel, *The Last Word* (New York, 1997). For an example of history of disease written in relativist spirit, see J. Arrizabalaga, J. Henderson, and R. French, *The Great Pox: The French Disease in Renaissance Europe* (New Haven and London, 1997).

of, say, Yersin (the eponymous discoverer of the plague bacillus) that, if the relativists are right, our own understanding of plague is incommensurable even with his, let alone that of the fourteenth century.

Philosophical issues apart, I contend that a cultural history of medicine, of the sort that historians have rightly favoured of late, needs pathological history just as it needs demographic history or the history of other aspects of the material world. And it can often (obviously not invariably) apply modern categories, suitably modified. If we are to make any progress with the history of pathology we obviously have to be fully sensitive to the nuances of past vocabularies of disease. Some terms will be more inscrutable than others. But we do not have to admit defeat totally in the effort to understand their possible biological referents.

III

Perhaps the first step is to concede that a single pathocoenosis for any one period may be unattainable, especially if our purview is both Europe and the Middle East. The second is to respect the different kinds of evidence and not to lump them together in the effort to produce unified tableaux. That evidence can broadly be divided into three types: first, archaeological; second, 'educational', an aspect of learned discourse, with no inevitable clinical application; third, therapeutic texts in all their multiplicity. Any one example of any of these types will give us no more than a keyhole view: all have their limitations, often severe ones. But the greater the number and variety of perspectives on the pathological past with which we can engage, the greater the chance that our analysis will not be completely disabled by problems of retrospective diagnosis.

Palaeopathology—essentially, in this context, the study of bones from burials—would seem to provide our (in several senses) hardest evidence for past afflictions. It enables the latest of laboratory techniques to be brought to bear on genuinely historical material, and it side-steps the problems set for us by the obscure terminology of the written record. To that extent, palaeopathology might furnish one minor element in the campaign against relativism. It demonstrates that diseases have a history, though it does not, of course, tell us how those diseases were experienced by the people who once animated the bones. In the particular case of plague, DNA analysis of dental pulp has already shown that people buried in two mass graves attached to quarantine hospitals in early modern France were indeed infected by the bacillus of *Yersinia pestis* rather than, for example, anthrax.[48] From the tenth century, however, the results so far available are less arresting. For many of the regions that come within our sphere in this collection, palaeopathology is virtually non-existent. To give us any idea of diseases characteristic of the period, scattered individual skeletons or bone assemblages are not enough. To my know-ledge, though, no tenth-century Islamic burial ground in the Middle East has been

[48] M. Drancourt *et al.*, 'Detection of 400-year-old *Yersinia pestis* DNA in Human Dental Pulp: An Approach to the Diagnosis of Ancient Septicaemia', *Proceedings of the National Academy of Sciences USA*, 95 (1998), 12637–40. The controversial diagnosis of the Black Death as anthrax was made by Graham Twigg in *The Black Death: A Biological Reappraisal* (London, 1984), a work that has been more often dismissed than properly evaluated.

comprehensively excavated. Of the Byzantine empire, the picture is hardly less bleak. The whole discipline of palaeopathology has been described as 'la lacune plus grave . . . une des priorités de notre discipline.'[49]

Western Europe does, in contrast, provide us with a handful of quite large excavations, from the right period, and thoroughly analysed by palaeopathologists. At the mid-tenth- to late-eleventh-century graveyard at Raunds in east Northamptonshire, for example, the total buried population was 363. Mortality peaked in infancy: 20 per cent of those excavated had not survived the first year of life. Like the overall age range, that is what can be expected of a pre-industrial population. As for the adults whose skeletons could be sexed, 100 were male and 82 female. Two lepers are reported, although the diagnosis of one of them is uncertain. Virtually all the adults over 17 years showed some degree of osteoarthritic degeneration, yet the prevalence of osteitis was surprisingly low (7.5 per cent). Osteoporosis of the orbits, probably associated with anaemia, could be detected in one-third of the sample.[50] A second, Italian, example: at Mola di Monte Gelato, about 35 km north of Rome, a farm belonging to an early medieval papal estate yielded remains of at least 243 people buried between c. 800 and 1100. Of adults whose sex could be determined, 25 were male, 23 female. Again, the age structure for the site was largely what could have been predicted, and signs of osteoarthritis were extremely common. Five cases of circulatory disorders were identified, as was one of a nasal polyp. And so on.[51] It is no discredit to the painstaking archaeologists responsible for these results that their samples are small and not necessarily representative, and that the results are far from distinctive.

Even when more excavations are available from the same period and different locales can be compared in greater detail, severe limits will remain to what excavation can reveal.[52] The history of a wide range of disorders is now susceptible to archaeological investigation.[53] Yet the selection of people for the original burial; subsequent disturbance of the site; incomplete excavation; misdiagnosis; and, above all, the fact that the investigation is confined to diseases that leave their osteological mark, whereas most ailments affect only soft tissue, which seldom survives—all these make even the largest and best excavated cemetery no more than another keyhole view of an enormous terrain. Techniques for the recovery of DNA from bones and their archaeological environments promise an exciting way in which that keyhole might be widened. Indeed, the palaeopathology of bubonic plague has already benefited. Future possibilities also include the identification of viral infections such as hepatitis and parasitic diseases such as malaria, of mutations that may lead to genetic disease, and even of susceptibility to mental illnesses such as schizophrenia. For the moment, however—certainly so far as the tenth century

[49] J.-P. Sodini, 'La contribution de l'archéologie à la connaissance du monde byzantin (IVe–VIIe siècles)', *Dumbarton Oaks Papers*, 47 (1993), p. 156, with references.

[50] A. Boddington *et al.*, *Raunds Furnells: The Anglo-Saxon Church and Churchyard*, English Heritage Archaeological Report 7 (London, 1996), ch. 13.

[51] T. W. Potter *et al.*, *Excavations at the Mola di Monte Gelato: A Roman and Medieval Settlement in South Etruria* (London, 1997), pp. 98–170. See also Pilsworth, below, pp. 255–6.

[52] J. W. Wood *et al.*, 'The Osteological Paradox: Problems of Inferring Prehistoric Health from Skeletal Samples', *Current Anthropology*, 33 (1992), 343–70.

[53] C. Roberts and K. Manchester, *The Archaeology of Disease*, 2nd edn. (Stroud, 1995).

is concerned—'biomolecular archaeology is still an immature research area.'[54] We must continue to seek evidence elsewhere.

That evidence will not necessarily fall into familiar categories. Take the example of Arabic magical–medicinal bowls, drinking from which was supposed to be rendered curative by the inscriptions engraved on them. These are both material and textual; they do not relate to the Aristotelian headings of either 'professional' or emprical medicine, though they were presumably considered to be of practical therapeutic value; and they survive in sufficient number for statistics to be compiled of the ailments for which they were designated. Emilie Savage-Smith's analysis of a collection of such bowls from Syria and Egypt shows the potential of this kind of evidence even though her datable objects are too late for our immediate purpose.[55] (After poisonous bites and stings, the most frequently mentioned problem was gastro-intestinal.)

The Middle East does seem, for our period, to have all the best evidence. Yet surprisingly little of it has been exploited in the pursuit of pathocoenosis. So, once more, I can merely register future possibilities. Under the non-medical heading must be listed the enormous dossier of private correspondence surviving, from as early as the tenth century, in the Cairo Geniza (the storeroom attached to the synagogue into which was deposited all writing that might include the name of God). The dossier may be eloquent about illness to an extent that its scholars have not fully revealed.[56] Still in the Middle East, and at the more obviously medical end of the spectrum, there are the major encyclopaedic texts of the period. Take the manual of 'medicine for the poor' or the medical handbook *Zād al-musāfir* (which circulated in Latin translation in Europe as the *Viaticum peregrinantis*) by the Tunisian physician Ibn al-Jazzār (d. 980).[57] Systematic comparison of the ailments enumerated in such texts with, for instance, those said by Qusṭā ibn Lūqā (d. 912) to be likely hazards of the pilgrimage to Mecca, might start to bring out both recurrent patterns and regional differences.[58] The results of the exercise could, in their turn, be compared with later medical works or travellers' accounts;[59] and that would elucidate chronological variation—provided, of course, that due attention were given to the provenance and presumed purpose of the texts under scrutiny. The western material, such as that scanned by Biraben, might also usefully be re-

[54] T. A. Brown and K. A. Brown, 'Ancient DNA and the Archaeologist', *Antiquity*, 66 (1992), 10–23, quotation at p. 16.
[55] F. Maddison and E. Savage-Smith, *Science, Tools and Magic: Part One. Body and Spirit, Mapping the Universe*, The Nasser D. Khalili Collection of Islamic Art vol. 12 (London, 1997), 72–100, at p. 24.
[56] To judge by D. Isaacs and C. F. Baker, *Medical and Para-Medical Manuscripts in the Cambridge Genizah Collections* (Cambridge, 1994). Cf. S. D. Goitein, *A Mediterranean Society*, V: *The Individual* (Berkeley, 1988), pp. 94–116.
[57] Compare M. G. Dugat, 'Études sur le traité de médecine d'Abou Djàfar Ah'mad', *Journal Asiatique*, 5th series, 1 (1853), 287–353; and G. Bos (ed.), *Ibn al-Jazzār on Sexual Diseases and their Treatment* (London, 1997).
[58] See J. Wilcox, 'Qusṭā ibn Lūqā and the Eastward Diaspora of Hellenic Medicine', in J. A. C. Greppin, E. Savage-Smith, and J. L. Gueriguian (eds.), *The Diffusion of Greco-Roman Medicine into the Middle East and the Caucasus* (Delmar, New York, 1999), 73–128.
[59] Compare J. Worth Estes and L. Kuhnke, 'French Observations of Disease and Drug Use in Late Eighteenth-Century Cairo', *Journal of the History of Medicine*, 39 (1984), 121–52; C. M. Doughty, *Travels in Arabia Deserta*, 2 vols., new edn. (London, 1921), well-indexed for illness.

worked in this way, and the Latin and vernacular (Old English) traditions compared.[60] Finally, we need further compilations of epidemics, however vaguely designated, to enable tentative plotting of the frequency and geography of crisis years.[61]

Easy to propose, hard to achieve. But we do not need to stay completely silent while awaiting further analysis. Low-level generalizations about the prevalence of ocular and intestinal disorders can be confirmed and even, occasionally, given a statistical fig leaf. We can also note surprising absences, such as reference to conditions resembling schistosomiasis. And we may, with greater confidence, make some negative statements about major infectious diseases. Our period is, for example, too late for bubonic plague. Indeed, that may be its least ambiguous feature. The pandemic that began as the Plague of Justinian had broadly ended in both Europe and the Middle East in the mid-eighth century, though there was some recrudescence in Islamic lands during the ninth, and perhaps later as well.[62]

'Absence', or at least 'lack of startling development', must be the key note in discussion of two other major infections of the years around 1000. First, leprosy. As the population increased from the tenth century onwards (partly, perhaps, because of the recession of plague), so the number of lepers in the societies that concern us presumably increased in proportion. There was, however, no great epidemic, contrary to what has often been supposed. Leprosy is not an epidemic disease and never has been, even in virgin populations—which those of our period certainly were not.[63]

Secondly, malaria. Looking at malaria in the Middle Ages is like stumbling upon an area of sudden calm in a chaotic battlefield. Elsewhere the debate is fast and furious: about why malaria in antiquity was apparently a less serious problem than it has been in modern times (or indeed since the 'fall of the Roman empire' to which, some still hold, it contributed); about how far we can chart the incidence of the disease from the osteological evidence of various hereditary anaemias which *may* confer immunity to it.[64] These debates primarily concern the ancient world. The Middle Ages have largely been omitted from discussion, and old conclusions have thus stood quietly unchallenged. The picture for instance presented by Angelo Celli (1857–1914) of a Roman Campagna in which the rise and fall of malaria could be charted quite neatly, and correlated with phases of depopulation and shifting settlement, would be of great interest in the present context. That is because Celli identified a phase of malarial advance beginning around the tenth century.[65] More recent study fails, unfortunately, to confirm the simplified demo-

[60] See Cameron, *Anglo-Saxon Medicine*, ch. 2, for a brief, insular, pathocoenosis.

[61] E.g. W. Bonser, *The Medical Background of Anglo-Saxon England* (London, 1963), pp. 59–94; P. Skinner, *Health and Medicine in Early Medieval Southern Italy* (Leiden, 1997), Appendix 3.

[62] L. I. Conrad, 'The Plague in the Early Medieval Near East' (unpublished Ph.D. dissertation, Princeton University, 1981); J. R. Maddicott, 'Plague in Seventh-Century England', *Past and Present*, 156 (1997), 7–54.

[63] M. Satchell, 'The Emergence of Leper Houses in Medieval England 1100–1250' (unpublished D.Phil. dissertation, University of Oxford, 1998). Compare R. I. Moore, *The Formation of a Persecuting Society* (Oxford, 1987), pp. 50 ff., 74.

[64] Grmek, *Diseases in the Ancient Greek World*, ch. 10; Sallares, *Ecology of the Ancient Greek World*, pp. 271–81. Compare Kiple, *Cambridge World History*, VIII.85, at p. 861.

[65] A. Celli, *The History of Malaria in the Roman Campagna from Ancient Times*, first published 1925 (London, 1933), ch. 5.

graphic, economic, and hydrological history of the region on which he based much of his account. The archaeology of the shift to nucleated hilltop settlement known as *incastellamento* now shows a rather more variegated picture; and the shifting along the spectrum between arable and pastoral proves to have been too complex for the ecology of malaria to be 'read off' from it. Nor can the intricate chronology of coastal sedimentation be translated into any straightforward narrative of the formation of malarial swamps.[66] Malaria was certainly present, and may well have been responsible for the epidemics chronicled by Celli that struck the biologically defenceless troops of invading Ottonian and Salian emperors. Yet, at its probable level of endemicity, the disease did not define the 'contours of death' around tenth-century Rome with the same rigour that it would manifest in early modern England.[67]

IV

So far I have been considering diseases and the ways in which we can try to recapture the pathology of the past. And I have treated the subject in some detail because the papers that follow have a different focus. In looking at pathology, however, I have, unavoidably, also introduced ways of conceptualizing the medical evidence of the age. And, in the last sections of this introductory paper, I want to turn to it more specifically. The scope of our collection was explained in the Preface; and each paper is preceded by a synopsis. So there is no need here either to repeat the rationale for our selection of topics or to give any specific foretaste of what is to follow. Instead, I want first to make some general points about the medical cultures under review, and then to emphasize what seem to me the major implications of the collection as a whole.

The first general point is that, even on an old-fashioned view of medical history that dwells too much on great men and technical advances, the centuries either side of the year 1000 are not without interest. This is, after all, the age of Bald's *Leechbook*, the most learned of the late Anglo-Saxon medical writings (Meaney); of Donnolo, the first Jewish physician to compose a medical work in Hebrew (Pilsworth); of Constantine the African, whose translations from Arabic into Latin mark the beginning of a whole new phase in European medical history (Pilsworth); of Rāzī, of course (d. 925) (Álvarez-Millán); and, towering above all, Ibn Sīnā (Avicenna; 980–1037). Pathological conditions are newly described, such as pannus (Savage-Smith) or, in the most *outré* example, the allergic reaction to roses.[68] Literary novelties are evident, as in the illustration of surgical instruments (Savage-Smith again). Finally, it is the age of Salerno, which would become the first prestigious and influential centre of medical education to emerge in medieval Europe, and which, like Constantine the African's work, has been held to mark a

---

[66] Compare P. Toubert, *Les structures du Latium médiéval: le Latium méridionale et la Sabine du IXe siècle à la fin du XIIe siècle* (Paris, 1973), though still much indebted to Celli; T. W. Potter, *The Changing Landscape of South Etruria* (London, 1979); P. Horden and N. Purcell, *The Corrupting Sea: A Study of Mediterranean History* (Oxford, 2000), ch. VIII.3–4.

[67] Celli, *Malaria*, pp. 64–72; Dobson, *Contours of Death and Disease*.

[68] M. Ullmann, *Islamic Medicine* (Edinburgh, 1978), p. 84.

turning point in western medical history—even though, in the period that concerns us, its fame was for practical medicine rather than the theory with which it was later associated.[69]

On the other hand (my next general point) our period is not, overall, a great one for hospitals. This is particularly so of western Europe. With one possible exception, there do not seem to have been any hospitals for the sick or poor in England before the Norman conquest other than monastic infirmaries, serving only monks (Meaney). It has been suggested that the pastoral organization of the Anglo-Saxon church around minsters removed the need for them: 'outdoor' charitable support could be informally provided by minster priests.[70] In Europe, more generally, the tenth to eleventh centuries present the hospital historian with an uninspiring picture. The wave of charitable foundations associated with the Carolingian reforms had been dissipated and the new fashion for establishing leper hospitals was yet to begin in earnest. Although the Byzantine empire could boast some spectacular multipurpose foundations in its capital, the broad run of Byzantine philanthropy emanated in this period from quite small and perhaps not very numerous hospitals and hospices (Bennett). Finally, the Islamic world presents an image which is both like and unlike that of Byzantium. Some highly impressive hospitals were established with charitable endowments, particularly in Baghdad, but few details of their structure or function survive from this period. Moreover, they were extremely scarce.[71]

What role, then, should be envisaged for medicine in the small number of hospitals that we do know about? It is conventional to say of almost all English hospitals and most European ones outside northern Italy that they became medicalized—that is, included doctors on their staff—only at the very end of the Middle Ages. I should prefer (though I have no space to defend the view here)[72] to see them rather as 'total therapeutic environments' in which nursing, iconography, and liturgy all played a greater quasi-medical part than many physicians could have done.[73] The sort of basic medicine dispensed by 'lay' attendants is perhaps exemplified for us in the manuscripts associated with Byzantine hospitals that David Bennett is able to draw upon below. Here are craft texts with no theoretical pretensions and requiring experience more than learning for their clinical application. They are only one stage up from nursing, and provide another means by which we might revise our over-estimation of the differences between Byzantine and western hospitals. As always, however, the most provocative evidence seems to come from furthest east. Rāzī was successively director of two hospitals, and his casebook seems to be a transcription of his clinical activity. Although there

---

[69] Skinner, *Health and Medicine*, ch. 7; L. García-Ballester *et al.* (eds.), *Practical Medicine from Salerno to the Black Death* (Cambridge, 1994).

[70] N. Orme and M. Webster, *The English Hospital 1070–1570* (New Haven, 1995), p. 23.

[71] E. Savage-Smith, 'Medicine', in R. Rashed (ed.), *Encyclopedia of the History of Arabic Science*, 3 vols. (London, 1996), III, pp. 933–6.

[72] See P. Horden, 'Religion as Medicine: Music in Medieval Hospitals', in P. Biller and J. Ziegler (eds.), *Religion and Medicine in the Middle Ages* (forthcoming).

[73] See also C. Rawcliffe, 'Medicine for the Soul: The Medieval English Hospital and the Quest for Spiritual Health', in J. R. Hinnells and R. Porter (eds.), *Religion, Health and Suffering* (London and New York, 1999), 316–38.

is no evidence of the circumstances of its composition, we might therefore be tempted to suppose that the casebook records his hospital practice. Whatever its provenance, we could legitimately infer that the type of medicine described in it bears some relationship to hospital therapeutics. Those therapeutics would then, like his casebook as Álvarez-Millán presents it, be somewhat un-theoretical. And that would again make two hospital cultures which we had thought quite differ-ent—the Byzantine craft-based one[74] and the Islamic one in which hospitals are supposedly beacons of learned Galenism[75]—seem surprisingly similar.

I shall come back to implications of the Islamic evidence shortly. But the subject of hospital nursing and empirical medicine turns our attention away from the 'big names' of medical history (such as Rāzī's) to the other end of the spectrum. My third general point is that, in any synopsis of medieval medical practice, we have to leave conceptual space for the scarcely documented, but surely numerous healers who had no direct contact with medical texts. They are hinted at in miracle collections[76] and charters (Pilsworth); in prohibitions of magical medicine which suggest the ubiquity of those whose services are outlawed;[77] in stray and miscel-laneous evidence such as an Old English riddle, the effectiveness of which seems to depend in part on the availability to its audience of leeches offering herbal remedies (Meaney).

For the healers of whom we do have some direct information, and who owned or read the surviving texts, it should be stressed once again how oblique the relationship may well have been between those texts and everyday therapy. The latter represented a practical wisdom in which medical theory was barely articulated background, or was even suppressed (Wallis). Such practical wisdom is hard for us to comprehend. We come to the medical history of the early Middle Ages, I suspect, with anachronistic presuppositions about how it should ideally have been. These derive from two related sources, both of which tend to make us characterize the centuries around 1000 in terms of what they were *not*, medically speaking, rather than in terms of their positive features. The presuppositions derive, first, from the medical world of the later Middle Ages (*c.* 1300–1500), the world of university medicine; and second, from the world of Arabic learned medicine. The university world accustoms us, I suggest, to a 'top-down' and perhaps also a 'trickle down' view of the role of theoretical learning. The texts that, thanks to Constantine the African and his successor translators, Latin Europe recovered from Islam are, for the most part, stable in form and systematic in structure. This is because they are grounded in Aristotelian philosophy and also because they are intended for the teaching of a syllabus. Widely yet carefully copied, methodically expounded, they have a clear shape and a well-defined purpose. They can readily be edited by philologists, which adds to their scholarly attractiveness. In them, philosophy is condensed into theory, from which are derived prescriptions for practice. That is the 'top-down' model. We have learnt from Michael McVaugh's study of medi-

---

[74] *Pace* T. S. Miller, *The Birth of the Hospital in the Byzantine Empire*, 2nd edn. (Baltimore, 1997).

[75] Compare M. W. Dols, *Majnūn: The Madman in Medieval Islamic Society* (Oxford, 1992), ch. 6a.

[76] *The Book of Sainte Foy*, trans. P. Sheingorn (Philadelphia, 1995), pp. 201, 206, 231 etc.; T. Head, *Hagiography and the Cult of Saints: The Diocese of Orléans 800-1200* (Cambridge, 1990), p. 183.

[77] V. I. J. Flint, *The Rise of Magic in Early Medieval Europe* (Oxford, 1991), pp. 59, 79, 314.

cine in the early fourteenth-century Crown of Aragon that the rudiments of such learned medicine can also 'trickle down' the social and professional hierarchy well beyond the confines of the university or those who aspired to its sophistication. A village wise woman may be so well versed in the rudiments of uroscopy that she can begin to sound like a medical student.[78]

Now a culture of this sort could develop in medieval Europe because it had already been created by medical scholars in medieval Islam. Here is the second source of our presuppositions about the medical world of the year 1000. The conventional wisdom is that, in ninth-century Baghdad as in, say, thirteenth-century Montpellier, theory and practice interlocked. Medicine, as distinct from the magical techniques of the unlettered, was philosophical. And philosophy translated into practice without losing too much in the process. So, at least, it is assumed, though chiefly on the basis of theoretical texts. And that assumption is likely to colour any overview of the Middle Ages: it will prejudice the comparison of Islamic and western medicine in the early Middle Ages in Islam's favour, just as the comparison of early and later medieval medicine is likely to be slanted in favour of the latter, with its university learning.

The relevance of the university model and the validity of the Islamic one, however, can both be called into question. That indeed is what, by implication, we do in the articles that follow. Let me, then, turn from general points about tenth-century medicine to setting out what seem to me the collection's most reverberant conclusions. I treat them in ascending order of geographical and chronological scope.

V

First, as Faith Wallis, Klaus-Dietrich Fischer, and Audrey Meaney demonstrate, the medical writings with which historians of early medieval Europe have to deal are indeed of a wholly different kind from those of the later university world. That is because they have a cultural and intellectual context of their own which renders the top-down model inapplicable, and thus transforms what, according to that model, are defects into positive characteristics, even virtues. European texts of the kind considered by Wallis, Fischer, and Meaney were not, it would seem, intended to provide a substitute for personal, *viva voce* apprenticeship: one might be reminded by these writings of certain aspects of the medicine of the day, but reading them would not enable one to learn medicine from scratch. They are somewhat like musical neumes: cues as to how a chant should be shaped by those who had already learnt it. (To continue the simile, university medicine is the equivalent of staff notation.) That might be why some texts which, to us, verge on unintelligibility[79] could still be worth copying.

Because these materials do not belong to the predictable, cosmopolitan world of university instruction—the world of syllabuses and lecture courses—they are also highly mutable and localized: a philologist's nightmare in which each community

---

[78] M. R. McVaugh, *Medicine before the Plague: Practitioners and their Patients in the Crown of Aragon 1285–1345* (Cambridge, 1993), p. 140, with n. 12.

[79] Compare Fischer and Wallis below.

of users is prone to create its own version of the text, combining and recombining a variety of materials. In this respect the medical writings of our age belong to the genre that has been labelled 'living literature'—a genre that also includes early Christian liturgical manuscripts, folk-tales, and medieval apocryphal visions and revelations.[80] Instead of practice that is aligned with text, and text which inhabits a clear theoretical framework, the theory (bequeathed by classical antiquity) has bled away and practical advice preponderates; but the relationship between the often disorderly prescriptions[81] and everyday clinical activity is likely to have been far from straightforward. As I suggested earlier, some of the texts with which we are dealing were perhaps never intended for sustained clinical use. Many of the major figures who deserve mention in any account of north-western European medicine in the tenth or eleventh century—figures such as Richer of Rheims, Fulbert of Chartres, and Gerbert of Aurillac—were not physicians; they were historians, bishops, scholars. They practised only occasionally and exemplify the Aristotelian medical category of the learned 'layman.'[82]

To appreciate this complexity on its own terms, we need a more sensitive and less anachronistic approach than that prompted by knowledge of the university world. David Harley's recent plea in the pages of this journal for a reconfiguring of medical history in terms of the rhetoric by which therapy is 'constructed' may offer one way forward.[83] Instead of seeing early medieval writings in terms of their lack of system, textual stability, and theoretical armature, we would locate them, more positively, within the very different rhetorical world that they did actually inhabit: a world of calendrical concerns, for instance, and of the monastic 'art of dying',[84] as well as the broad remit of scholar-churchmen. The difficulty with Harley's approach when applied to our period is that the medical rhetoric of the early Middle Ages is to a considerable extent beyond our recovery. Because the texts lie at often very oblique and changeable angles to the behaviour of those who read or heard them, we cannot assume that the verbal performance implied by them necessarily matched what physicians of the period said at the bedside. Even a text such as 'how to visit the patient', with which Faith Wallis begins, cannot automatically be treated as equivalent to a paragraph in a successful instruction manual.

Early medieval European texts were often tangential to practice, but can none the less be seen in a positive light and against an appropriate, if complex, cultural backdrop. This constitutes, I submit, the first overall conclusion of the papers that follow. It builds on work already done.[85] The second, more distinctive, outcome,

[80] See e.g. P. F. Bradshaw, 'Liturgy and "Living Literature"', in P. F. Bradshaw and B. Spinks (eds.), *Liturgy in Dialogue* (London, 1994), 138–53; J. Baun, *The Byzantine Apocryphal Imagination* (forthcoming).

[81] See especially Meaney, Fischer, and Bennett, below.

[82] See especially Fulbert of Chartres, *Letters and Poems*, ed. F. Behrends (Oxford, 1976), Letter 9, with D. Jacquart, 'La médecine au Xe siècle', in N. Charbonnel and J.-E. Iung (eds.), *Gerbert l'Européen* (Aurillac, 1997), 219–31.

[83] D. Harley, 'Rhetoric and the Social Construction of Sickness and Healing', *Social History of Medicine*, 12 (1999), 407–35.

[84] F. S. Paxton, '*Signa Mortifera*: Death and Prognostication in Early Medieval Monastic Medicine', *Bulletin of the History of Medicine*, 67 (1993), 639–43.

[85] See especially Wallis, 'The Experience of the Book'.

XV

to which I have already adverted in discussing hospitals, is that the emphasis on medicine as a craft rather than as a learned profession so evident in the western material is to be found further east as well. In the great sub-Galenic encyclopaedias of late antiquity, the seepage away of theory is already apparent. The particular contribution of David Bennett's paper, apart from focusing attention on the middle Byzantine period (much less studied than the early one),[86] is to display craft texts which are similar in many respects to the prescription lists of contemporary European medicine.

The third major conclusion of the collection is perhaps more radical, and emerges from its extension into the Islamic world. Here we meet the malign effect of the second source of misleading presuppositions to which I referred. Because Islamic medical culture from the ninth century onwards was so rich in theoretical texts, and because historians of Islamic medicine must largely depend on those texts, they have assumed that the top-down model must apply. That is, they have assumed that practice derived from theory in a quite straightforward way. The achievement of Cristina Álvarez-Millán and Emilie Savage-Smith is to show for the first time that even in medieval Islam, even in the learned circles of Rāzī and his pupils, or in tenth-century Spain, where Albucasis composed a detailed—and illustrated—discourse on surgery, practice simply did *not* match theory. Indeed, theory seems to exist in an independent literary realm with, conceivably, a separate audience: the same audience, I conjecture, as that which greeted accounts of technological marvels or geographical wonders but which had no direct concern with actual therapy (Aristotle's third category again, but in slightly different guise).[87] To this extent, then, it is not only the differences between Latin West and Byzantine East that may have been exaggerated; it is the differences between both those cultures and the Islamic Middle East. If we look away from the sphere of medical learning to where, in that vivid American phrase, 'the rubber meets the road', practical medicine seems to lack clear theoretical underpinning in *all three* cultures.

The final point to be made stems, by implication, from the foregoing. If theory and practice were so separate in medieval Islam, which provided the template for the university medical world of medieval Europe, then perhaps in that European world, too, practice was disjoined from theory once we move out of the university domain. I referred above to the 'trickle down', whereby a village cunning woman could pick up snatches of university terminology. But how significant was this phenomenon? How pervasive was the downward flow of learning? The fragmentary evidence of ordinary empiric practitioners, like the more abundant evidence of the vernacular medical receptaries, hints that, at this relatively humble level, the theoretical elaborations of the universities may have made less difference to cheap quotidian therapy than has been imagined.[88]

---

[86] A forthcoming issue of the journal *Medicina nei secoli* will be devoted to middle Byzantine medicine.

[87] R. Irwin, *The Arabian Nights: A Companion* (London, 1994), ch. 8: 'The Universe of Marvels'.

[88] Compare T. Hunt, *Popular Medicine in Thirteenth-Century England* (Cambridge, 1990), ch. 1; J. M. Riddle, 'Theory and Practice in Medieval Medicine', *Viator*, 5 (1974), pp. 178–81. For later medieval empirics see now P. Murray Jones, 'Thomas Fayreford: An English Fifteenth-Century Medical Practitioner', and K. Park, 'Stones, Bones and Hernias: Surgical Specialists in Fourteenth- and Fifteenth-Century Italy', both in French, *Medicine from the Black Death to the French Disease*, chs. 6, 8, respectively.

Our collection revolves around the year 1000. It deals with the admittedly obscure end of what were formerly known as the Dark Ages—always thought to be so different from what followed, and indeed, in their medicine, very different from the world of the universities. Yet perhaps the medicine of the end of the first millennium should not be merely the remote province of a few hardened specialists. Our subject may have far wider ramifications. The medical practice of the year 1000 can perhaps also tell us a great deal more than we had suspected about the medicine of the year 1500.

XVI

Continuity and Discontinuity in the History of Mediterranean Music Therapy

On a ridge above what is now Bosphorus University can be found a small cemetery.[1] It contains a plot of land where, according to tradition, some Janissaries were killed in a raid on Constantinople a year or two before it fell in 1453. In August 1959 the Municipality erected a plaque. It read: 'the grave of Nafi Baba, who fell at the Conquest' – that of 1453. This dating turned out to be a slight exaggeration. The local people knew of Nafi Baba. He had been the saintly head of a Bektashi *tekke* of Dervishes. But he had died, at the age of 81, in June 1912. His grandson had the mistake on the plaque rectified.

Another mistake was less easily corrected, however. After the saintly man's death in 1912, the villagers might well have been expected to make his tomb a place of pilgrimage, with candles, written prayers and votive offerings. But nothing of this could be found there. Instead, 150 feet away was a mausoleum covered with such things – with prayers not from illiterate villagers but from students at the nearby college. The grave was that of an army general, not a saint, who had died in 1916. Perhaps one student had been unable to read the Ottoman inscription and had fixed an offering to it. Perhaps he assumed that, since it was the most impressive tomb in the area, it must be the tomb of Nafi Baba. Just one candle would have been enough to establish the tomb as a holy place; other offerings would have followed. The likelihood of that is made clear by an example from a different cemetery on the Bosphorus. In a window set in a wall of the cemetery there are always lighted candles, clearly intended as offerings to some saint. This particular cult is said, on reliable testimony, to have been started in 1949 by a neighbourhood grocer. He wanted to encourage the sale of candles.

These examples are Turkish and concern saints. But I hope that they make a more general point about Mediterranean cults of all kinds (and cults elsewhere too). Cults can spring up quite suddenly. And they can spring up for very dubious reasons – reasons to do with fraud on the part of a cult's promoters or

---

[1]   All details in the first two paragraphs derive from Geoffrey Lewis, 'The Saint and the Major-General', *Anatolian Studies*, 22 (1972), pp. 249–53.

a simple mistake on the part of its devotees. Cults can evolve rapidly, bringing together previously quite distinct elements. They can change meaning. And we are easily tempted into thinking that they are much older than they really are – as with the cult of the saint who supposedly died around 1453, centuries before he was in fact born.

I am a medievalist studying medicine and the environment. If I have any claims at all to your attention, it is because I have been involved in two projects which both have a bearing on the subject matter of this conference.[2] I should like to treat this paper as an opportunity to see how they relate to each other. My hope is that they may provide a general framework for discussions of history and music in the Mediterranean – especially the history of the Mediterranean musical cult of the tarantula spider. Tarantism is, as you know, the musical healing cult with one of the longest documented histories in the Mediterranean area. It seems to me to raise in acute form the theme on which I want to focus: the theme of continuity and discontinuity.

Let me now try to characterize the two projects I referred to. The first is an enquiry into the unity, distinctiveness, and continuity of the Mediterranean area.[3] It runs from the Bronze Age to the beginnings of modernity, and is studied through the 'microregional' dynamics of Mediterranean ecologies. The first part of this project has been published under the title *The Corrupting Sea* and its co-author is Nicholas Purcell. In our vision, the constituents of the Mediterranean – the ingredients of its lasting unity – are microecologies that are defined, not by enumerating topographical features, but by understanding the systems of production that bring those features together into a whole. For that reason, microecologies are not easy to map. Their boundaries shift. They are highly unstable, as producers adjust their portfolios of strategies from year to year, anticipating the capriciousness of the Mediterranean environment. Their continuity over time has to be understood in terms of innumerable small *dis*continuities. We quoted Lévi-Strauss: 'it is not the resemblances, but the differences, which resemble each other'.[4] The ecology of religion, of cult in the widest sense, is part of this Mediterranean world as we described it. Each feature of the Mediterranean environment can, potentially, be 'sacralized' – can become an object of veneration.[5] Yet, as with microecologies in the economic sense, it is never enough simply to list topographical features that attained cult

---

2   'L'eredità di Diego Carpitella: Etnomusicologia, antropologia e ricerca storica nel Salento e nell'area mediterraneo', Galatina, 21–23 June 2002.

3   Peregrine Horden and Nicholas Purcell, *A Study of Mediterranean History*, vol. 1: *The Corrupting Sea* (Oxford, 2000) [vol. 2: *Liquid Continents*, forthcoming].

4   Claude Lévi-Strauss, *Totemism* (Boston, Mass., 1963), p. 77.

5   Horden and Purcell, *The Corrupting Sea*, ch. 10.

status. All such features must be understood in terms of the *systems* – religious, social, economic – that give them meaning. These systems, these contexts, change over time – often quite rapidly. Such changes offer another set of differences that resemble each other – complementary to those of the world of production, and, indeed, deeply connected to them.

To put it that way is to go against the grain of a venerable tradition of Mediterranean scholarship. This tradition takes its starting point from the apparent stability of the pre-modern Mediterranean, and especially from the way that certain features of the landscape seem always to have been foci of cult. Recall the pioneering but eccentric historical geographer of Anatolia, Sir William Ramsay, who wrote in 1892 on 'Permanent Attachment of Religious Veneration to Localities'.[6] Here is a more recent instance of this supposed permanent attachment:

> there is the example of the hot spring at Hammam Sayala near Béja in Tunisia, where miraculous cures are attributed to the intervention of a holy woman, Lella Sayala, to whom candles used to be burnt within living memory (perhaps they still are). Work on the spring... revealed Roman baths with a dedication by an imperial freedman to the *genius* or presiding spirit of the place, named Aquae Traianae. It is this spirit who is still invoked under the name of the Moslem holy woman Lella Sayala.[7]

But is it?[8] This is a nice example of a common enough phenomenon – the religious significance, at widely differing periods, of the sacred spring. The correspondence between ancient sites and the shrines of Islamic *marabouts* in the Maghreb is, moreover, very widespread. Yet on what grounds might one identify the modern cult as the direct descendent of the ancient one? Take another example: in the second century A.D. the satirist Lucian describes the importance of fish to the cults of North Syria. In Urfa, in the same region, are still to be seen great carp-ponds, now sacred to Abraham. What can be inferred from the similarities of cult object and place?

For Sir William Ramsay those similarities could only mean survival. But we must be cautious. It is easy to be mistaken in the interpretation of symbols. The carp of Urfa appear so bizarre that continuity is easy to credit. But this may rather be a case of the spontaneous regeneration of what is actually a rather common way of expressing sanctity. If a wider perspective is adopted, parallels multiply for even the strangest religious observances. In A.D. 563, for example,

---

[6]   *Transactions of the Oriental Congress in London* (London, 1892), cited from Horden and Purcell, *The Corrupting Sea*, p. 408.

[7]   Colin Wells, *The Roman Empire*, 2nd edn (London, 1992), pp. 243–4.

[8]   For what follows, with full bibliography, see Horden and Purcell, *The Corrupting Sea*, pp. 408–9.

the Emperor Justinian's last journey took him to the shrine of St Michael at Yürme, near Ankara. Here, it transpires, there was a miraculously healing fishpond not unlike those of Urfa. 'Les poissons sacrés sont la concrétisation vivante de la sainteté du lieu'; so says one authority on the cult of the *marabout*, who also discusses sacred tortoises, and a huge hairy eel with earrings that lives in a sacred pool. Bizarre zoological cults may not be so unusual.[9] I would endorse the sentiments of the late Julian Pitt-Rivers: nothing, he wrote, 'can be explained by being termed a "survival". On the contrary, the concept of survival is almost a confession of defeat before the challenge to find a contemporary sense in anything'.[10]

The seeming continuity or antiquity of a cult may conceal a number of different phenomena. First, there may be deliberate replacement (as when Christian shrines were deliberately intended to obliterate pagan veneration). Second, there may be deliberate revival in an antiquarian spirit; third, there may be unconscious recreation – given that there is perhaps a limited range of elements, both environmental and cultural, from which cults can be fashioned, and a recent cult may resemble an ancient one without being in any way its direct descendant.

Let me now turn from carp and hairy eels to the second of the two projects on which this paper depends. This project is represented in an edited collection with the title *Music as Medicine: The History of Music Therapy since Antiquity*.[11] Contemporary music therapists like to trace their ancestry a long way back. This is understandable. Theirs is a new profession that has only recently gained any status in the world of western biomedicine. They want the legitimation of history. They want what the therapist Juliette Alvin called 'the continuous thread'.[12] The history – in the sense of historical writing – to which they turn is, however, not always reliable. Great claims are made about continuity of practice since, even, *pre*-classical times. One of the aims of *Music as Medicine* was to provide a scholarly and sceptical history of musical therapeutics against which the historical claims of contemporary practitioners could be tested. *Music as Medicine* includes chapters on Chinese Ayurvedic medicine and some discussions of world ethnography: its scope is as nearly global as we could manage. But it does have a strong Mediterranean element. This is, first, because much of the book concerns music in the traditions of therapy that originated in

---

[9]   Émile Dermenghem, *Le culte des saints dans l'Islam maghrébin* (Paris, 1954), pp. 154–8.

[10]   Julian Pitt-Rivers, *The Fate of Shechem: Essays in the Anthropology of the Mediterranean* (Cambridge, 1977), pp. vii–viii.

[11]   Aldershot, 2000.

[12]   Juliette Alvin, *Music Therapy* (London, 1966), ch. 4.

classical (i.e. Mediterranean) antiquity; second, because we have three chapters (with an introduction by me) on the history of tarantism from its earliest recorded Italian cases, through its transplantation to eighteenth-century Spain, to modern revivals and reformulations (in a chapter by another speaker at this conference, Karen Lüdtke).[13]

I shall come back to tarantism. First, though, let me quickly note some of the larger discontinuities that seem to me to emerge from the collection.[14] They are, above all, cultural discontinuities. First, there is a discontinuity between (on one hand) the medical-philosophical tradition that descends from Graeco-Roman antiquity, and (on the other hand) the wider world of ethnomusicology and the societies that it principally discusses. Music therapists and ethnomusicologists know very little of one another – despite, I am sure, the efforts of many in this room. Also, they inhabit what seem to me to be different worlds. The world of the music therapist is one in which roles are clearly distinguished – the roles of patient and practitioner. In the wider world of ethnography, as I read it in the works of John Janzen, Marina Roseman, Steven Friedson, and others, sufferers become healers; words, drumming, and instrumental melody alike contribute to some all-encompassing ritual. Living human beings, dead ancestors, other spirits – all are involved. The sufferer may be a family or group as often as it is an individual. The music can be the disease, rather than (or as well as) the cure. It can be the diagnosis as well as the therapy.

Another discontinuity arises in the classical tradition and its descendents – a discontinuity between theory and practice, or, to put it differently, between philosophy and medicine. Music therapy in antiquity and the Renaissance, especially in Platonism in its various forms, is mainstream philosophy but marginal medicine. It is far more often talked about than practised. Much of its history is a mirage of activity constituted by ancient anecdotes, recycled throughout antiquity, bequeathed to the Middle Ages by Boethius in his *De musica*.

The last big discontinuity is between the pre-modern and the modern. I take the pre-modern to last from the time of Plato and Hippocrates to the dissolution of the classical tradition of medicine in the nineteenth century. In the pre-modern period, physicians sometimes recommend music to melancholic patients wealthy enough to hire musicians. A few sophisticates, such as Marsilio

---

[13] Horden (ed.), *Music as Medicine*, part IV. [To the historical bibliography add now Gino L. Di Mitri, *Storia biomedico del tarantismo nel XVIII secolo* (Florence, 2006).]

[14] For what follows, with full bibliography, see Horden, 'Musical Solutions: Past and Present in Music Therapy', in Horden (ed.), *Music as Medicine*, pp. 4–40.

Ficino, perform to themselves.[15] But, to generalise, in pre-modern times there is nothing like the intimate transactions that take place between modern therapist and patient, with the patient improvising the music. The music that today's patients make on drums or glockenspiel is a child of the age of Stockhausen. In any earlier age (say, before 1945) it would have been considered pointless cacophony, not music: a symptom of dysfunction, not its solution.

With those discontinuities in mind, I want to move to cults involving various creatures and the remedy for their bites. First, snakes and snake handlers. This is not from our book on music as medicine and is not strictly an example of music therapy, although the ancient medical writer Bolus of Mendes did list snakebite as one of many ailments that could be cured by the music of the *aulos*.[16] But, as with my opening examples, I want to use the material that follows to show how we should approach the history of cults that *are* musical.

There is a long and familiar history here.[17] It starts with the Marsi, Psilli, and other such ancient groups described by Pliny, Varro, and Solinus. It runs through the theatrical charlatanism of the *pauliani* of the sixteenth and seventeenth centuries – those who claimed to have inherited from their apostolic ancestor an immunity to snake bite, and who peddled an earth-based antidote. The story can also be taken into very recent times. And for this it is enough to mention the writings of Ernesto de Martino, Angelo Turchini, Brizio Montinaro, and others.

This centuries-long story is not, however, a simple or a continuous one. In the journal *Renaissance Studies*, Katharine Park has shown how the stereotypical image of the *pauliani* coalesces from a variety of elements quite quickly during the later Middle Ages. Their banners, their competitiveness, their theatrical routines with snakes, their selling of St Paul's earth – all these different aspects come together, from diverse sources, in a way which is relatively rapid. In the thirteenth and fourteenth centuries, remedies for snakebite associated with St Paul are magical or charismatic. The commercial element is not apparent until the late fifteenth century. And the *pauliani* do not appear as sellers of earth until the early 1500s. I quote Park's summary:

> We find the gradual convergence of the elements that will come to compose the figure of the *paulianus*: the man who, usually with one or more associates, put on

---

    [15]   Angela Voss, 'Marsilio Ficino, the Second Orpheus', in Horden (ed.), *Music as Medicine*, pp. 154–72.

    [16]   Martin West, 'Music Therapy in Antiquity', in Horden (ed.), *Music as Medicine*, p. 61.

    [17]   Katherine Park, 'Country Medicine in the City Marketplace: Snakehandlers as Itinerant Healers', *Renaissance Studies*, 15 (2001), pp. 104–20. [See further David Gentilcore, *Medical Charlatanism in Early Modern Italy* (Oxford, 2006), pp. 275–8.]

some kind of display with snakes in the city piazza, in order to sell a type of earth, called 'the grace of St Paul', which was in some way associated with his constitutional immunity to poison. The emergence of earth as the commodity in question seems to have come out of the interaction and convergence of two separate traditions: the medieval incantation involving the earth scraped from beneath the foot of snakebite victims or their proxies, and the renascent interest of fifteenth- and early sixteenth-century learned medical writers in ancient accounts of Lemnian earth. The latter attained new prominence with the appearance in northern Italian cities of an earth from Malta, which was revered by locals for its healing properties and which appears to have gained credibility among both lay people and medical men as analogous to – and cheaper than – Lemnian earth.[18]

We have, then, a revised and rather more fragmented account of *pauliani* than we are perhaps used to. Park writes of a 'gradual convergence'. By comparison with the millennia-long history sometimes attributed to *pauliani*, that convergence is, however, quick. I want to end this paper by using Park's work on the *pauliani* as a model for our interpretation of the early history of another cult focusing on a poisonous creature – that of the *tarantati*.

The cult of the tarantula spider in southern Italy, a cult that has involved music and dancing to cure the spider's bite, is the most superficially reassuring aspect of the history of music therapy precisely because it has been so long-lasting.[19] Few outline sketches of the topic fail to mention it. Not least because of De Martino's magisterial ethnography, it has a permanent place in the modern scholarship of the subject.[20] That is why we devoted to it no fewer than three chapters of the *Music as Medicine* collection. A young man who was bitten by a spider in 1996, and who was urged to dance by older family members, seems to bring back to life an otherwise obscure corner of the early modern world.[21] Such continuity, visible across the last few centuries, moreover fosters the temptation to extend the continuity much further back into the past.

Yet the continuity of recent times is not that of a 'permanent attachment', a 'survival'. It is more contingent in nature.[22] It depends on books, not ancient

---

[18]   Park, 'Country Medicine', pp. 112–13.

[19]   Horden, 'Commentary on Part IV, with a Note on the Origins of Tarantism', in Horden (ed.), *Music as Medicine*, pp. 249–54.

[20]   Ernesto De Martino, *La terra del rimorso: contributo a una storia religiosa del Sud* (Milan, 1961) [now translated and annotated by Dorothy Louise Zinn as *The Land of Remorse: A Study of Southern Italian Tarantism* (London, 2005)].

[21]   Karen Lüdtke, 'Tarantism in Contemporary Italy: The Tarantula's Dance Reviewed and Revived', in Horden (ed.), *Music as Medicine*, pp. 293–312. [See also her forthcoming monograph, *Dances with Spiders: Crisis and Celebrity in a South Italian Healing Cult* (Oxford, 2008).]

[22]   For what follows see Horden, 'Commentary on Part IV, with a Note on the Origins of Tarantism'.

customs. Why does tarantism spread from Italy to Spain and take root there with such rapidity? Because of the translation of a book, it seems – a book by Giorgio Baglivi. Why, for that matter, is it possible to recover a well-documented, protracted, and in many respects classic case of tarantism from Rhode Island, USA, in the early 1800s? Because of the English translation of the same book and an article in the *New York Magazine* of 1797. Why does modern neo-tarantism take the forms it does? Again, mainly, perhaps because of the indirect influence another book, that of De Martino.

Like the *pauliani*, the *tarantati* have a vivid and well-documented history in the early modern period (*c.*1500–1800), although much of the writing devoted to them at the time was stereotyped. (It is worth recalling that, apart from Epifanio Ferdinando's use of the case of Pietro Simone in his *Centum historiae* (Venice, 1621), the earliest first-hand account of tarantism that we have comes from an inquisitorial record of as late as 1723.[23])

Also like the *pauliani*, *tarantati* emerge in the evidence only in the later Middle Ages and their cult practice involves a fusion of several different elements. As is well known the first clear reference is fourteenth-century and is attributed to the Paduan physician William of Marra.[24] In a treatise on poisons probably addressed to Pope Urban V (who reigned from 1362 to 1370), the author asserts that the tarantula's venom engenders melancholy in the victim, and for this the best antidote is to rejoice. The vulgar and ignorant, he adds, say that the tarantula sings when it bites, so that music similar to that singing helps relieve the patient. William rejects this account. He prefers to think that the joy inspired by the music attracts the noxious humours within the body to its periphery, thus preventing the poison from entering the vitals. Of course there is no mention of dancing in his treatise, which is why students of tarantism have had to seek a precedent for that aspect elsewhere, for instance in the dancing epidemics associated with St Vitus that broke out sporadically in northern Europe of the thirteenth and fourteenth centuries.[25] Yet these are somewhat remote in time and place from fifteenth-century Apulia and hardly explain the specific character of the Italian tarantula cult.

Students of the *pauliani* have sometimes traced their history back to antiquity: Marsi and the like. The longevity of tarantism has encouraged similar attempts to discern its ancient roots. Marius Schneider apparently regarded

---

[23] David Gentilcore, 'Ritualized Illness and Music Therapy: Views of Tarantism in the Kingdom of Naples', in Horden (ed.), *Music as Medicine*, pp. 255–72.

[24] Gabriele Mina (ed.), *Il morso della differenza: Il dibattito sul tarantismo dal XIV al XVI secolo* (Nardò, 2000), pp. 30–38, 75–82.

[25] De Martino, *La terra del rimorso*, pp. 237–41.

tarantism as a survival of a ritual dating from the time of the megaliths.[26] Much more subtle and scholarly comparisons have been attempted between tarantism and various ecstatic cults of ancient Greece – Dionysiac, Corybantic, Orphic – as if some partial similarities, together with the fact that southern Italy was once part of Magna Graecia, were sufficient evidence of continuity. Here I am being rash enough politely to disagree not only with the great De Martino but also with my conference host, Gino Di Mitri.[27] I am simply not convinced that tarantism is so old.

Ancient cults do not, I believe, survive in this way undetected for many centuries. Even if they have been forced 'underground' they should, if they exist, still break surface occasionally in the medieval evidence (evidence significantly earlier than William of Marra in the 1360s). They do not break surface. Consider the two examples adduced by De Martino in his quest for the 'medieval origins' of tarantism. First, when Norman troops invading Sicily in the 1060s were beset with an epidemic of tarantula bites outside Palermo, the chief symptom, according to their chronicler Gioffredo Malaterra, was not dance-like agitation; it was excessive flatulence. The chief remedy, before the army simply decamped to a safer locale, was hot compresses, not musical exorcism. All this, note, took place in former Magna Graecia, and the details are given by a monk who had lived in Apulia since adolescence. Yet he seemingly knows nothing of the 'vulgar' beliefs reported by William of Marra.[28] The second of De Martino's two examples transports us to the First Crusade. In his massive *History of the Journey to Jerusalem* (*Historia Ierosolimitana*), Albert of Aachen (Aix) describes how the crusader's enfeebled camp followers, quartered near Sidon (modern Sayda, in Lebanon) were fatally bitten by *tarenta*. Yet, as De Martino acknowledges, Albert clearly refers to *snakes* called *tarenta* (perhaps the highly poisonous soft-scaled vipers still found in Lebanon). And the remedies suggested by locals were either the quasi-royal touch of one of the army's

---

[26] 'Tarantella', *Die Musik in Geschichte und Gegenwart: Allgemeine Enzyklopädie der Musik*, ed. F. Blume, vol. 13 (Kassel, 1966), cols 118–19; J. Godwin, *Harmonies of Heaven and Earth: The Spiritual Dimension of Music from Antiquity to the Avant-Garde* (London, 1987), p. 35.

[27] Gino Di Mitri, 'Le radiche orfiche e l'innesto paolino del tarantismo: ipotesi e indizi per un'archeologia del sapere', in Michele Paone (ed.), *Scritti di storia Pugliese in onore di Feliciano Argentina* (Galatina, 1996), pp. 11–28; idem, 'Mitografia, danza e drama sacramentale alle origini del tarantismo', in Gino Di Mitri (ed.), *Quarant'anni dopo de Martino. Atti del Convegno Internazionale di Studi (Galatina 24–25 ottobre 1998)* (Nardò, 1999), I, pp. 69–99.

[28] *Historia sicula (De rebus gestis Rogerii Calabriae et Siciliae comitis…)*, II.36, in L. A. Muratori (ed.), *Rerum Italicarum Scriptores*, vol. 5 (Milan, 1724), p. 570; De Martino, *La terra del rimorso*, p. 229.

leaders, or immediate sexual intercourse (presumably not with a leader). Again there is little here to remind us of 'classic' tarantism.[29]

It is for its failure to reckon with such counter-examples, as well as for its inherent implausibility, that the 'survivalist' argument has, on the whole, failed.[30] Not even its most careful exponent of recent decades, Carlo Ginzburg, could restore its credibility.[31] As you will know, his *benandanti* were members of an agrarian fertility cult, which had a modest musical component, and which was practised in the Friuli to the north-east of Venice. Not only has Ginzburg suggested that the cult members' out-of-body nocturnal battles against witches for the security of the harvest provided the actual popular counterpart of the fantasy of the Sabbath. He has also of course, in *Storia notturna: una decifrazione del sabba*, attempted to trace the history of such soul-journeys directly back to archaic Asian shamanism. It is a project that inspires admiration and scepticism in equal measure. The parallels drawn are too loose, the purported channels of transmission too elusive. And if Ginzburg cannot carry conviction on this millennial scale, then it is tempting to suppose that no one can. Rather than search the mists of time, we should reckon once more with the possibility that new healing cults, tarantism included, can develop quickly; unconnected elements can quite suddenly coalesce. Discontinuity is at least as likely as continuity.

That is the sceptical message that I bring to this conference in memory of a great Mediterranean ethnomusicologist from my two projects: one on the history of Mediterranean ecology, the other on the history of music therapy.[32]

---

[29]   Ibid., p. 230. I am most grateful to Susan Edgington for a preview of the relevant passage in her forthcoming edition of this text [now published as Albert of Aachen, *Historia Ierosolimitana, History of the Journey to Jerusalem*, ed. and trans. Susan B. Edgington (Oxford, 2007); see V.40, pp. 392–3].

[30]   See Walter Burkert, *Ancient Mystery Cults* (Cambridge, Mass., 1987), p. 53, for a very pessimistic view of the chances of ancient mystery cults' survival into the Middle Ages.

[31]   Carlo Ginzburg, *I benandanti: stregoneria e culti agrari tra Cinquecento e Seicento* (Turin, 1972), translated as *The Night Battles: Witchcraft and Agrarian Cults in the Sixteenth and Seventeenth Centuries* (London, 1983); idem, *Storia notturna: una decifrazione del sabba* (Turin, 1989), translated as *Ecstasies: Deciphering the Witches' Sabbath* (London, 1990).

[32]   My warmest thanks to Karen Lüdtke for advice on my text and to Gino Di Mitri for translating it into Italian for the original publication.

ADDENDA

I. How medicalised were Byzantine hospitals?

I have discussed the non-medical functions of hospitals in 'Memoria, Salvation, and Other Motives of Byzantine Philanthropists', in Michael Borgolte (ed.), *Stiftungen in Christentum, Judentum und Islam vor der Moderne* (Berlin, 2005), 137–46, of which a revised version appears as 'Alms and the Man: Hospital Founders in Byzantium', in John Henderson, Peregrine Horden and Alessandro Pastore (eds), *The Impact of Hospitals 300–2000* (Oxford: Peter Lang, 2007), 59–76.

II. The confraternities of Byzantium

See now the important additions to the dossier of Byzantine fraternities in Gilbert Dagron, '"Ainsi rien n'échappera à la réglementation." État, Église, corporations, confréries: à propos des inhumations à Constantinople (IVe–Xe siècle)', in V. Kravari, J. Lefort and C. Morrisson (eds), *Hommes et richesses dans l'Empire byzantin*, vol. 2: *VIIIe–XVe siècle* (Paris: P. Lethielleux, 1991), 155–82; also Jane Baun, *Tales from Another Byzantium: Celestial Journey and Local Community in the Medieval Greek Apocrypha* (Cambridge: Cambridge University Press, 2007), 371–85.

III. Ritual and public health in the early medieval city

On early medieval penitentials see the collection of articles in *Early Medieval Europe*, 14.1 (2006).

IV. Religion as medicine: music in medieval hospitals

p.144, end of n.50: Peter Brown's lectures have been published as *Poverty and Leadership in the Later Roman Empire* (Hanover, NH and London: University Press of New England, 2002).

VII. A discipline of relevance: the historiography of the later medieval hospital

For current directions in the historiography of the later medieval and early modern hospital see Carole Rawcliffe, *Medicine for the Soul: The Life, Death and Resurrection of an English Medieval Hospital. St Giles's, Norwich, c.1249–1550* (Thrupp: Sutton Publishing, 1999), and John Henderson, *The Renaissance Hospital: Healing the Body and Healing the Soul* (New Haven, CT and London: Yale University Press: 2006), the latter superseding the article by him cited in my n.9 and Davidsohn as in n.12, both on p.362. Also pertinent to the study of the 'mixed economy of care' is Marco H.D. van Leeuwen, *The Logic of Charity: Amsterdam, 1800–1850* (Basingstoke: Palgrave Macmillan, 2000). I have explored the role of the parish in this 'economy' in 'Small Beer? The Parish and the Poor and Sick in the Later Medieval England', in Clive Burgess and Eamon Duffy (eds), *The Parish in Late Medieval England*, Harlaxton Medieval Studies 14 (Donington: Shaun Tyas, 2006), 339–64.

VIII. Pain in Hippocratic medicine

p.312, n.42: the paper by Helen King with which I am in friendly debate can now be found in her *Hippocrates' Woman: Reading the Female Body in Ancient Greece* (London and New York: Routledge, 1998), chapter 6. The wider recent historiography of pain may be sampled in Esther Cohen, 'The Expression of Pain in the Later Middle Ages: Deliverance, Acceptance and Infamy', in Florike Egmond and Robert Zwijnenberg (eds), *Bodily Extremities: Preoccupations with the Human Body in Early Modern European Culture* (Aldershot: Ashgate, 2003), 195–220.

IX. Travel sickness: medicine and mobility in the Mediterranean from antiquity to the Renaissance

A preliminary version of this paper appeared as 'Regimen and Travel in the Mediterranean', in Renate Schlesier and Ulrike Zellmann (eds), *Mobility and Travel in the Mediterranean from Antiquity to the Middle Ages* (Münster: Lit Verlag, 2004), 117–31.

See now also Charles Burnett, 'Stephen, the Disciple of Philosophy, and the Exchange of Medical Learning in Antioch', *Crusades*, 5 (2006), 113–29, esp. the appendix, on the regimen for travellers that forms part of the *Royal Book* of al-Majusi and that could have been an extra example on my p.193.

p.183, n.18, line 2: my then forthcoming paper = 'The Earliest Hospitals in Byzantium, Western Europe, and Islam', in M. Cohen (ed.), *Journal of Interdisciplinary History*, special issue, 'Poverty and Charity: Judaism, Christianity, Islam', 35 (2005), 361–89.

pp.198–9: on Mercuriale see also Nancy G. Siraisi, 'History, Antiquarianism, and Medicine: The Case of Girolamo Mercuriale', *Journal of the History of Ideas*, 64 (2003), 231–51; and on Gratarolo see eadem, 'Medicine and the Renaissance World of Learning', *Bulletin of the History of Medicine*, 78 (2004), 1–36.

XI. Saints and doctors in the early Byzantine empire: the case of Theodore of Sykeon

I have discussed the interaction of saintly and secular healing a little further in 'Sickness and Healing', in Thomas F.X. Noble and Julia M.H. Smith (eds), *The Cambridge History of Christianity*, vol. 3: *Early Medieval Christianities, c.600–c.1100* (Cambridge: Cambridge University Press, 2008), 416–32.

XII. Responses to possession and insanity in the earlier Byzantine world

A version of this paper also appeared as 'Possession without Exorcism: the Response to Demons and Insanity in the Early Byzantine Middle East', in Evelyne Patlagean (ed.), *Maladie et société à Byzance*, Centro Italiano di Studi sull'Alto Medioevo Collectanea, 3 (Spoleto, 1993), 1–19.

XIII. Disease, dragons and saints: the management of epidemics in the Dark Ages

My hypothesis receives some further support from Robert Sallares, *Malaria and Rome: A History of Malaria in Ancient Italy* (Oxford: Oxford University Press, 2002), 231–4. On early medieval dragons, although not the one mainly discussed here, see now also Christine Rauer, *Beowulf and the Dragon: Parallels and Analogues* (Cambridge: D.S. Brewer, 2000).

XIV. Mediterranean plague in the age of Justinian

p.157, n.5: Little forthcoming = Lester K. Little (ed.), *Plague and the End of Antiquity: The Pandemic of 541–750* (Cambridge: Cambridge University Press, 2007).

Procopius references in nn.1 and 14 are to the old Loeb edition, trans. H.B. Dewing (Cambridge, MA: Harvard University Press, 1914–40); the reference in n.8 is to the standard edition of Justinian's *Novels* by R. Schöll and G. Kroll (Weidmann: Berlin, 1963).

XV. The millennium bug: health and medicine around the year 1000

Contributors to the special issue to which this paper is an introduction are cited by surname only. See further Peregrine Horden and Emilie Savage-Smith, 'Symposium on Medical Practice around the Year 1000', *Social History of Medicine*, 14 (2002), 387, with <http://www.sshm.org> [conference report].

p.218, n.86: *Medicina nei secoli* special issue = 11.2 (1999).

INDEX